Prostate Cancer: Advanced Researches

Prostate Cancer: Advanced Researches

Edited by **Karl Meloni**

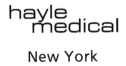

hayle
medical

New York

Published by Hayle Medical,
30 West, 37th Street, Suite 612,
New York, NY 10018, USA
www.haylemedical.com

Prostate Cancer: Advanced Researches
Edited by Karl Meloni

International Standard Book Number: 978-1-63241-329-1 (Hardback)

Printed in the United States of America.

Contents

Contents

Preface

Over the recent decade, advancements and applications have progressed exponentially. This has led to the increased interest in this field and projects are being conducted to enhance knowledge. The main objective of this book is to present some of the critical challenges and provide insights into possible solutions. This book will answer the varied questions that arise in the field and also provide an increased scope for furthering studies.

This book on prostate cancer brings forth a number of exciting discoveries made in the diagnosis and treatment of prostate cancer over the past decade. International experts have contributed to this book giving a descriptive and advanced review of drug therapeutics essential in prostate cancer. It is dedicated to the efforts and developments made by our scientific community, realizing we have a lot to learn in striving to cure this disease specifically among those with aggressive tumor biology. The book serves as a valuable resource for scientists and healthcare professionals related to this field.

I hope that this book, with its visionary approach, will be a valuable addition and will promote interest among readers. Each of the authors has provided their extraordinary competence in their specific fields by providing different perspectives as they come from diverse nations and regions. I thank them for their contributions.

Editor

Drug Therapeutics/Biological Agents

Prostate Cancer Progression to Androgen Independent Disease: The Role of the Wnt/β-Catenin Pathway

Jacqueline R. Ha, Yu Hao D. Huang and Sujata Persad
University of Alberta, Department of Pediatrics
Canada

1. Introduction

The development and progression of prostate cancer (CaP) is largely dependent on the dysregulation of the androgen/androgen receptor (AR) signaling pathway; though, the mechanism of CaP progression remains elusive. Initial treatments for CaP included prostatectomy or radiation to destroy cancerous cells (Feldman & Feldman, 2001). However, these treatments were not curative and more often than not there were recurrences and metastases of the cancer. Mainstay treatments that target the androgen/AR pathway through anti-androgen and androgen ablation therapies have been promising; yet again, these therapies seem to fail as the tumor progresses. This suggests that the androgen/AR dependence of CaP cells vary over time such that alterations in androgen availability, AR sensitivity and receptor promiscuity fuel a more aggressive CaP.

Approximately 80-90% of CaPs are originally androgen dependent (AD) at diagnosis (Niu et al, 2010). Androgens stimulate the proliferation and inhibit the apoptosis of cells, thus implicating that CaP cells require a certain level of androgens to maintain their proliferation and survival (Feldman & Feldman, 2001). This is primarily the reason why androgen ablation therapy is initially successful – it removes the stimulation these cells require for proliferation, ultimately causing the regression of the tumor. However, over time patients often fail androgen ablation therapy as the tumor becomes a more lethal androgen independent (AI) or castration resistant form. There is no effective therapy for AI-CaP.

The prostate requires androgenic steroids for its development and function. Testosterone is the main circulating androgen and is secreted from the testes as well as the adrenal glands (adrenal steroid conversion). Once in the blood stream, the majority of the testosterone binds to albumin and sex-hormone-binding globulin (SHBG) while a small fraction is freely dissolved within serum. Within the prostate, testosterone is converted to a derivative, dihydrotestosterone (DHT), by 5-alpha-reductase. DHT is a more potent and active form of testosterone and has a greater affinity for the AR relative to testosterone. Testosterone and DHT bind to the AR and causes its nuclear localization, transcriptional activation and its interaction with co-regulators/co-activators to mediate AR-directed gene transcription (Nui et al, 2010).

The AR is required for the development of prostate carcinogenesis from early prostate intraepithelial neoplasia (PIN) to organ-confined or locally invasive primary tumors

(Koochekpour, 2010). As a member of the steroid-thyroid-retinoid nuclear receptor superfamily of proteins, the AR is in its inactive form within the cytoplasm, bound to heat shock proteins (HSP) (He et al., 1999; He et al, 2000; Loy et al, 2003; Bennett et al., 2010) and components of the cytoskeleton (Veldscholte et al., 1992; Bennett et al., 2010), preventing AR nuclear localization and transcriptional activation. The binding of DHT or testosterone causes a conformational change leading to the dissociation of the AR from the HSPs and its subsequent phosphorylation (Nazarteh & Weigel, 1996; Feldman & Feldman, 2001). Once ligand bound, the AR is stabilized within the cytoplasm and translocates to the nucleus. The androgen-AR complex is in a conformational state to now homodimerize within the nucleus and bind to androgen response elements (AREs) in the promoter region of target genes (Feldman & Feldman, 2001) such as prostate specific antigen (PSA), a routine biomarker for prostate cancer diagnosis and progression (Bennett et al, 2010, Whitaker et al, 2008), and, probasin, a prostate-specific gene that has been exploited as a marker of prostate differentiation (Johnson et al., 2000). The AR has both a cytoplasmic and nuclear distribution, and shows a certain degree of trafficking either to or from the nucleus (Mulholland et al., 2002). There are varying reports on the subcellular distribution of the AR in different cell types; however, this two-step model for steroid hormone receptor activation is a clear representation of ligand activated translocation and the observed focal accumulations of the AR within the nucleus (Mulholland et al., 2002).

1.1 AR structure and function

The AR gene is located on the X chromosome (q11-12), and contains eight exons that produces a protein of approximately 920 amino acids (Bennett et al., 2010). Exon 1 codes for the N-terminal domain (NTD), exons 2 and 3 translate into the central DNA binding domain (DBD) which contains two zinc fingers for specific binding of DNA sequences (Feldman & Feldman, 2001), and exon 4 to 8 code for a hinge region and a conserved C-terminal ligand binding domain (LBD) .

The NTD (1-558) is a poorly conserved region that houses important sequence motifs for AR conformation and activity (Bennett et al, 2010). There are three regions of tri-nucleotide repeats, which include poly-glutamine (Q) and poly-glycine tracts (Choong & Wilson 1998; Bennet et al., 2010). The poly-Q tract is encoded by a polymorphic CAG repeat (Southwell, et al., 2008). The length of the repeats inversely affects the stability of the AR-NTD and C-terminal LBD interaction, and, AR expression and activity (Chamberlain et al., 1994; Ding et al., 2004; Bennett et al, 2010). CAG tri-nucleotide repeats can vary between 11 and 31 repeats; less than 18 repeats are thought be an indicator of CaP risk.

The NTD also contains the transcriptional activation function-1 (AF1) comprising two transcriptional activation units (TAU): TAU-1 and TAU-5. The AF1 subdomain of the AR is the predominant site for transactivation, where TAU-1 is required for ligand-dependent transcription of the AR; TAU-5 is responsible for the majority of the constitutive activity associated with the NTD, and the recruitment of the Steroid Receptor Co-activator (SRC)/p160 family of co-activators. For example, TIF2 (Transcriptional Intermediary Factor 2), SRC-1, and GRIP-1 are members of the SRC/p160 family which increase AR transcription through their interactions with the NTD and DBD (He et al., 1999; He et al., 2000; Hong et al., 1999; Xu & Li, 2003; Bennett et al, 2010). These co-activators also recruit other co-regulators such as histone acetyl transferase (HAT) activity containing enzymes such as cAMP response element binding protein (CREB)-binding protein (CBP)/p300 and p300/CBP-associated factor (p/CAF) to initiate chromatin remodeling (Lemon & Tijian,

2000; Bennett et al., 2010) in preparation for DNA transcription (Shen et al., 2005; Bennett et al., 2010).

The LBD folds into 12 helices. Interaction of ligands to the LBD promotes AR stability by the formation of the C-terminal transcriptional activation function -2 (AF2) domain and the subsequent interactions between the NTD/LBD (Bennett et al., 2010). The NTD interacts with the LBD through its sequence motifs [23]FQNLF[27] and [433]WHTLF[437] (He et al., 2000; Simental et al., 1991; Bennett et al., 2010), while co-activators/co-regulators (E.g. SRC/p160 family of co-activators) bind to the LBD by a highly conserved consensus sequence, the LXXLL (L is Leucine and X is any amino acid) motif (also known as the NR box) (Bennett et al., 2010). The LBD LXXLL binding region primarily serves to recruit LXXLL motif containing co-activators/co-regulators and structurally enables the NTD FXXLF containing region to interact with the LBD (Bennett et al., 2010). The LXXLL motifs of such co-regulators form a two-turn amphipathic α-helix which binds to the hydrophobic cleft of the LBD (specifically AF2) (Yang et al, 2002).

The LBD AF2 domain is comprised of helices 3, 4, 5 and 12 (Gelmann, 2002). The ligand binding pocket is formed by helices 3, 5, and 10. Helix 12 is thought to lie across the ligand binding pocket and stabilize the ligand-AR interaction and increase ligand-activated transcription. The AR NTD and C-terminal domain (CTD) interaction in conjunction with Helix 12 serve to stabilize agonist ligand binding and receptor transcriptional activity (Masiello et al., 2004). Furthermore, the interaction of AR-interacting proteins or co-regulators such as androgen receptor co-activator, ARA70, (which binds to both the AR-DBD and AR-LBD) can increase the receptivity of the AR-LBD to other activating ligands such as hydroxyflutamide (non-steroidal anti-androgen) and estrogens (Miyamoto et al., 1998; Miyamoto & Chang, 2000; Rahman et al., 2004; Bennett et al., 2010). However, it was shown that the AR NTD and CTD interaction was not required for transcriptional activity. For example, ligands used at high concentrations and peptides that blocked the NTD and CTD interaction did not absolutely inhibit transcriptional activity of the AR (Kemppainnen, et al., 1999; Chang & McDonnell, 2002; Masiello et al., 2004).

The AR is opposed by co-repressors which inhibit its transcriptional activation. Nuclear receptor co-repressor (NCor) and silencing mediator for retinoid and thyroid hormone receptors (SMRT) disrupts the NTD-LBD interaction and the binding of SRC/p160 co-activators (Bennett et al., 2010). NCor and SMRT are able to recruit histone deacetylases (HDAC) to promote the repackaging of DNA and prevent the binding of transcriptional machinery, activators, and receptors (Liao et al., 2003; Bennett et al., 2010). However, NCor requires the presence of a ligand (agonist or antagonist) whereas SMRT is able to mediate its effects in the presence or absence of ligands (Cheng et al., 2002; Heinlein & Chang, 2002; Liao et al., 2003; Bennett et al., 2010). The LBD also houses the nuclear export signal (NES) (amino acids 742-817) and the nuclear localization sequence (NLS), found at the junction between the hinge region and DBD (50 amino acids, 625-676) (Bennett et al, 2010). Upon ligand binding the NES becomes inactive and the NLS is bound by co-activators such as Filamin-A and importin-α. These interactions direct the nuclear localization of the AR (Cutress et al., 1998; He et al., 2002; Loy et al., 2003; Ozanne et al., 2000; Rahman et al., 2004; Schaufele et al., 2005; Heinlein & Chang, 2002; Bennett et al., 2010). Upon the loss of ligand interactions, the NES co-ordinates the shuttling of the AR to the cytoplasm where AR can tether to cytoskeletal proteins to again, prepare for ligand binding (He et al., 2000; Bennett et al., 2010).

The DBD (559-624) is comprised of two zinc fingers domains created by three α-helices and a 12 amino acid C-terminal extension (Feldman & Fledman, 2001). The first zinc finger contains a P-Box motif for specific nucleotide interactions and the second, a D-Box motif which functions as a DBD/DBD site for receptor homodimerization (Bennett et al, 2010). It is thought that Lysine (Lys;K) 580 and Arginine (Arg;R) 585 in the first zinc finger bind to the second and fifth nucleotide pairs in the first ARE repeat: GGTACA, respectively to the second and fifth nucleotide pairs in the first ARE repeat: GGTACA (Gewirth & Sigler, 1995; Luisi et al., 1991; Schwabe et al., 1993; Rastinejad et al., 1995; Gelmann, 2002). The second zinc finger stabilizes the binding complex by making hydrophobic interactions with the first zinc finger and contributes to the specificity of receptor DNA binding (Rastinejad et al., 1995; Gelmann et al, 2002). Due to the similarity of the hormone response elements (HREs) of the nuclear receptor family, there is an overlap of nucleic acid sequences in which these receptors can bind. Steroid receptors recognize a palindromic sequence spaced by three nucleotides (Haelens et al., 2003). The AR, glucocorticoid, mineralcorticoid and progesterone receptors recognize the 5'-TGTTCT-3' core sequence (Haelens et al., 2003). However, it has been found that ARs can also recognize specific AREs that consist of two hexameric half-sites separated by 3 base pairs (Claessens et al., 1996; Rennie et al., 1993; Verrijdt et al., 1999; Verrijdt et al., 2000; Shaffer et al., 2004). Although ligand specificity brings about hormone specific responses, the specificity of hormone receptors has been questioned, as each receptor can bind to similar or the same sequence (Shaffer et al, 2004). It is thought that protein-protein interactions play a role in discriminating AR and other steroid mediated effects (Adler et al., 1993; Pawlowski et al., 2002) to enable ARE dependent gene transcription rather than the activation of other HREs.

1.2 AR and post translational modifications

Despite the AR's role in genomic upregulation of androgen dependent gene transcription, its activation can signal through alternative means at the plasma membrane and cytoplasm (referred to as non-genomic signaling) (Feldman & Feldman, 2001). For example, the AR can trigger intracellular calcium release and the activation of protein kinases such as the Mitogen Activated Protein Kinases (MAPK), Protein Kinase A (PKA), AKT and PKC (Bennett et al., 2010). Phosphorylation of the AR by MAPK, JNK, AKT, ERK, and p38, increases AR response to low level of androgens, estrogens, and anti-androgens as well as enhances the recruitment of co-activators (Bennett et al., 2010). Furthermore, the AR itself is a downstream substrate for phosphorylation by receptor-tyrosine kinases and G-protein coupled receptor signaling. The phosphorylation of AR is mediated by the recruitment of kinases in the presence or absence of androgens. Phosphorylation at Serine (Ser) residues, Ser80, Ser93, and Ser641 is thought to protect the AR from proteolytic degradation (Blok et al., 1998; Bennett et al., 2010). Alternatively, AR degradation is regulated by the phosphorylation of specific residues recognized by E3 ubiquitin ligase. For example, MDM2 E3 ubiquitin ligase promotes polyubiquitylation of the AR by recognizing AKT dependent phosphorylated serine (Lin et al., 2002; Koochekpour, 2010). Moreover, transactivation of the AR largely relies upon the phosphorylation of Ser213, Ser506, and Ser650 (Bennett et al., 2010). Phosphorylation of the AR is required for its effects within the nucleus and the AR should remain hyperphosphorylated to mediate its transcriptional role (Koochekpour, 2010). Studies have also shown constitutive phosphorylation of the AR at Ser94 as well as on other serine residues such as Ser16, 81, 256, 309, and 424. The loss of phosphorylation results in the loss of transcriptional activity and nuclear localization (Grossmann et al., 2001; Gioeli et al., 2002; O-Mallet et al., 1991; Koochekpour, 2010). Specifically, Yang et al., (2005) demonstrated that dephosphorylation of AR at the NTD by protein phosphatase 2A (PP2A), resulted in the loss of AR activity.

The AR receptors can also be acetylated, and sumoylated. These types of post translational modifications have also been shown to affect receptor stability and activity. The KXKK motif of the hinge region is a site for acetylation. Mutations of lysine to alanine reduced the transcriptional activity of AR by favoring NCoR interactions (Fu et al., 2004; Koochekpour, 2010). Sumoylation of the AR is hormone dependent and competes with ubiquitination of lysine residues. Sumoylation is thought to repress AR activity. Disruption of sumoylation on Lys386 and Lys520 resulted in an increase in AR transactivation (Poukka et al., 2000; Koochekpour, 2010).

1.3 AR in CaP progression

The efficacy of many CaP treatments is often temporary, as CaP cells often become refractory to hormone ablation therapies. The current therapeutics are largely targeted towards the inhibition of AR activation, such as anti-androgens, chemical castration (treatment with gonadotropin releasing hormone (GnRH) super agonists to inhibit testosterone secretion from the testes), or surgery (orchidectomy) (Bennett et al, 2010). AI-CaP or castration resistant CaP is thought to occur due to the androgen deprivation therapies as they may induce altered protein activity and expression in the cancer cells. Despite androgen blockade in AI-CaP patients, expressions of AR target genes such as PSA remain high. Furthermore, hormone refractory CaP continues to rely on AR expression, suggesting that the AR is necessary to maintain proliferative and anti-apoptotic effects. Therefore, CaP acquires the phenotype of oncogenic addiction to the AR for its continued growth and resistance to therapy (Koochekpour, 2010). The progression of CaP from an hormone sensitive AD to a hormone resistant AI state is likely due to mechanisms involving alterations in AR expression, amplification, mutations, and/or AR activity.

AR mutations in primary CaP are relatively low when compared to metastatic CaP where frequencies are as high as 50% (Marcellie et al., 2000; Koivisto et al., 1997; Taplin et al., 1995; Tilley et al., 1996; Taplin et al., 1999; Feldman & Feldman, 2001). Germline or somatic mutations of the AR leads to AR overexpression and hypersensitivity due to point mutations and promiscuous mutant AR proteins. Germline mutations of the AR are rarely found. Familial inheritance of CaP with at least two first degree relatives account for 20% of cases and transmission compatible with Mendellian inheritance is described to be 50% of the cases observed (Koochekpour, 2010). Genetic susceptibility seems to be more significant in patients <55 years old (Koochekpour, 2010). Recently, a R726L mutation was reported in only Finnish patients with sporadic or familial CaP (Gruber et al., 2003; Mononen, et al., 2000; Koochekpour, 2010). Genomic alterations to the AR have been found in both non-coding and coding sequences such as polymorphisms of CAG and GGC repeats, single nucleotide polymorphisms, as well as silent and missense mutations (Ingles et al., 1997; Gruber et al., 2003; Crocitto et al., 1997; Koochekpour, 2010). Koochekpour, (2010) screened 60 CaP patients of African-American and Caucasian families with a history of familial CaP. Using exon-specific PCR, bi-directional sequencing and restriction enzyme genotyping, they found that one African-American family had a novel germline AR misssense mutation (exon 2 of DBD A1675T; T559S) in three siblings with early onset CaP. This mutation was transmitted in an X-linked pattern and located at the N-terminal region of the DBD. Koochekpour et al., (2010) reason that the location of this particular mutation likely affected AR ligand binding.

Somatic mutations are largely single base substitutions: 49% at the LBD, 37% at the NTD, and 7% at the DBD (Koochepour, 2010). For those CaP that harbor gain of function mutations the result is primarily an increase in ligand promiscuity. The AR is activated by testosterone and DHT; however, mutations in the LBD make the AR less stringent of its partners. For example, in LNCaP cells, a Threonine (Thr; T) to Alanine (Ala;A) mutation (T877A) caused the expansion of ligand binding activity (Veldscholte et al., 1992; Feldman & Feldman, 2001). This mutation permitted AR activation by androgens, estrogens, progesterones as well as the non-steroidal antagonist, flutamide. A study by Gaddipati et al., (1994) found that 25% of patient metastatic tumors had a T877A mutation. Patients that were treated with flutamide often experienced a worsening of symptoms over time. Once flutamide was withdrawn, patients tended to do better. Interestingly, some patients also experienced a rise in serum PSA levels upon flutamide treatment. Taplin et al., (1999) studied patients that were on flutamide treatment relative to those that were not given this particular treatment. Tumor cells that had the T877A mutation increased in proliferation while patients who were not treated with flutamide harboured different mutations of the AR that were not activated by flutamide. Therefore, there seems to be a strong selective pressure for AR mutants arising from flutamide treatment such that discontinuation of flutamide resulted in tumor regression before growth resumed again (Feldman & Feldman, 2001). Other mutations such as the H874Y (Histidine to Tyrosine) mutation in the CWR22 cell line have been found to affect co-activator interactions by altering the conformation of Helix 12 of the LBD. Helix 12 regulates co-activator binding and creates a specific groove with helices 3, 4, and 5 (Darimont et al., 1998; McInerney et al., 1998; Nolte et al., 1998; Shiau et al., 1998; Westin et al., 1998; Song et al., 2003). Helix 12 rotates over the ligand binding pocket and assumes favorable or unfavorable positions depending on agonist or antagonist binding, respectively. Helix 12 mutations have also been detected in CaP patients, such as Q902R (Glutamine to Arginine), and M894D (Methionine to Aspartic Acid) (an androgen insensitive mutation) (Taplin et al., 1995; Thrompson et al., 2001; Song et al., 2003). The importance of Helix 12 and the NTD-LBD interaction for AR activity is underscored by the fact that spontaneous mutations in Helix 12, NTD, and LBD caused either complete or partial androgen insensitivity (Thomspon et al., 2001; Song et al., 2003). Additionally, a L701H mutation was also identified in conjunction with the T877A mutation in MDA PCa 2a cell lines (Zhao et al., 1999; Feldman & Feldman, 2001). L701H mutation alone decreased the ability of AR to bind DHT, but increased binding of other non specific adrenal corticosteroids. The presence of the T877A mutation together with L701H potentiated this interaction by more than 300% as both mutations were located within the LBD (Zhao et al., 2000; Feldman & Feldman, 2001). Hence, the susceptibility of the AR to minimize its ligand specificity in AI-CaP makes AR dependent disease progression difficult to treat. On the other hand, other anti-androgens such as Casodex (bicalutamide) do not seem to have the same response to T877A AR (Feldman & Feldman, 2001). Novel truncated AR mutants, mRNA splice variants and mutant AR lacking exon 3 tandem duplication (coding for C-terminal portion of the DBD) have also been found in the CWR22R derived cell line 22RV1 (AI-CaP) (Marcias et al., 2009; Koochekpour, 2010). Furthermore, an important study by Han et al., (2001) demonstrated that prostate tumors from a genetically engineered mouse model upon androgen ablation resulted in AR gene mutations within AR NTD. Specifically, amino acid substitution A229T and E231G (Glutamic Acid to Glycine) within the AR NTD signature motif: ARNSM (Ala-Arg-Asn-Ser-Met), increased ligand independent basal activity, whereas, E231G increased responsiveness to androgen receptor co-activator

ARA160 and ARA70. The ARNSM motif is unique to the AR and the most highly conserved region of the AR NTD.

Another possible mechanism for the progression of AI disease is mediated by AR amplification. Overexpression of the AR causes hypersensitivity of the AR under low levels of androgens. Visakorpi et al., (1995) were the first to show that the AR was amplified in 305 hormone refractory tumors subsequent to androgen ablation therapy. Although these tumors were clinically presenting as AI-CaP, there was increased levels of the AR, and, continued proliferation of the tumor still required androgen. This suggested that some AR amplified tumors may require the presence of residual androgens that remain in the serum after monotherapy (Palmberg et al., 2000; Feldman & Feldman, 2001). Similarily, mouse models of CaP progression characterized by high expression of AR, increased AR stability, and AR nuclear localization, had hypersensitive tumor growth promoting effects upon DHT administration. DHT concentrations of 4 orders of magnitude lower were able to stimulate growth relative to DHT levels required for AD LnCaP cell proliferation (Gregory et al., 2001; Feldman & Feldman, 2001).

Although AR gene amplification and hypersensitivity serves to be a sound model for AI-CaP progression, the AR may be activated by alternative means including activation by co-regulators, increased androgen production, and/or intermediary downstream signaling pathways. Greater levels of co-activator expression such as SRC-1, ARA70, and TIF2 were demonstrated to be elevated in CaP and correlated with increased CaP grade, stage, and decreased disease free survival. For example, Cdk-activating phophatase B, an identified co-activator of the AR was overexpressed and also highly amplified in tumors with high Gleason scores (Koochekpour, 2010). Local production of androgens within the prostate can also increase AR transactivation by compensating for decreased serum testosterone resulting from androgen ablation therapy. Studies have shown that serum testosterone levels can decrease 95%, contrasting the DHT levels within prostate tissue which only reduce by 60% (Labrie et al., 1986; Feldman & Feldman, 2001). Locke et al., (2008) demonstrated that there was de novo and organ synthesis of androgens in LNCaP xenograft mouse models, suggesting that CaP cells had steroidogenic properties that enable them to survive in androgen depleted environments. Moreover, this was also indicative of greater levels of intratumoral 5-alpha-reductase activity. It is likely then, that during AI-CaP disease progression, there is a switch in androgen source whereby testicular androgens are replaced by prostatic androgen. Bennett et al., (2010) have deemed this as 'androgen self-sufficient'. There is also a hypothesis that conversion of adrenal steroids can sustain the androgen signal by supplying adrenal androgens such as DHEA and androstenedione (Trucia et al, 2000). After castration, adrenal androgens could account for as much as 40% of the total DHT in the prostate (Labrie et al., 1993; Trucia et al., 2000).

Hormone receptors that are activated by ligand independent mechanisms are known as 'outlaw' receptors (Feldman & Feldman, 2001). Certain growth factors such as Insulin Growth Factor (IGF)-1, Keratinocyte Growth Factor (KGF), and Epidermal Growth Factor (EGF) have been demonstrated to activate the AR and induce the expression of AR target genes. Culig et al., (1994) showed that there was a 5-fold increase in PSA levels in LNCaP cells upon IGF-1 stimulation. Moreover, the addition of Casodex abolished the activation of the AR by IGF-1, KGF and EGF, indicating that the LBD was necessary for this activation. Overexpression of these growth factors has been observed in CaP; however, it is unclear whether it is the AR pathway or indirect downstream effects that are mediating tumorigenesis. In fact, patients with AI-CaP can fail Casodex therapy suggesting that other mechanisms are in play for ligand independent activation of the AR. Furthermore, patients who received androgen ablation therapy have tumor cells that overexpress growth factor receptors, the receptor tyrosine kinases. Craft et al., (1999) demonstrated that an AI-CaP cell line, generated from xenografts implanted in castrated mice, consistently overexpressed Her-2/neu (from the EGF receptor family of receptor tyrosine kinases) (Feldman & Feldman, 2001). Interestingly, AD-CaP cell lines could also be converted to AI-CaP cells by overexpressing Her-2/neu. This pathway was not blocked by Casodex, which indicated that the LBD of the AR was not necessary to transduce the effects of Her-2/neu. Although Trastuzumab (Herceptin) is used primarily to treat breast cancer, Herceptin had anti-proliferative effects on AD- and AI-CaP xenografts when combined with the chemotherapeutic drug paclitaxel. Yeh et al., (1999) believe that Her-2/neu activated AR via the MAPK pathway, as inhibitors of MAPK decreased HER-2/neu mediated activation of the AR. In effect, a positive feedback loop is created where the AR can activate kinases and in turn, where kinases can activate the AR through its phosphorylation (in the presence or absence of ligand), regardless of the varying levels of androgens (Feldman & Feldman, 2001).

The AR pathway is thought to be in interplay with other signaling pathways. AR activation due to cross regulation by receptor tyrosine kinases and their downstream effectors provides alternative and sustained routes for AR activation despite androgen depletion. Currently, there has been accumulating evidence that the Wnt signaling pathway plays a significant role in CaP tumor progression. Although it is rare to find genetic mutations in components of the Wnt pathway such as APC or β-catenin in CaP, the deregulation of this pathway is thought to be an early event in tumorigenesis. Moreover, β-catenin, the key regulator of the Wnt pathway, is a direct co-activator of the AR.

2. Wnt signaling pathway: An overview

The Wnt signaling pathway, responsible for a vast array of biological functions, is activated by 19 Wnt isoforms (For a complete list of Wnt isoforms, refer to Chien et al., 2009). The Wnts are a family of secreted glycolipoproteins, which are conserved in all metazoan animals. Wnt ligands activate the Wnt pathway by binding to a seven-pass transmembrane frizzled (Fzd) receptor in conjunction with its co-receptors, LDL receptor related proteins 5 and 6 (LRP5/6). Other factors such as R-spondin, Norrin and Wise may also facilitate Fzd stimulation (Kharaishvili et al., 2011). Signaling by these powerful morphogens functions to direct cell proliferation, cell adhesion, tissue development, oncogenesis, tumor suppression, and cell-fate determination (MacDonald et al., 2009). As a result, defective Wnt signal transduction plays a critical role in a range of hereditary diseases and cancers such as polycystic kidney disease (Wuebken & Schmidt-Ott, 2011), Alzheimer's disease (De Ferrari et al., 2007), hepatocellular carcinoma (Ji et al., 2011), colorectal cancer (Fearon, 1995) and other malignancies. Here, we will focus on the role of Wnt signaling in the development of prostate carcinogenesis.

Wnt signaling can be divided into two categories: the canonical Wnt pathway and the non-canonical Wnt pathway. The former is activated by a certain subset of Wnt proteins that affects a potent oncoprotein, β-catenin, while the latter operates independently of β-catenin signaling. The canonical Wnt pathway is the most well understood and has been implicated in regulating cell-cell adhesion as well as cell cycle control. The planar cell polarity (PCP) pathway and the calcium (Ca^{2+})-dependent pathway have been identified as non-canonical, however evidence has yet to show whether these two pathways are truly distinct or simply part of a larger signaling network.

2.1 The non-canonical (β-catenin independent) Wnt pathway

In β-catenin independent signaling, Wnt pathways are activated via Fzd receptors and do not involve LRP5/LRP6. Binding of non-canonical Wnts, namely Wnt4, Wnt5a, and Wnt11, to Fzd can influence cell polarization, and embryonic processes such as convergent extension and cochlea development (Veeman et al., 2003; Shih et al., 2007). The asymmetrical distribution of transmembrane receptors and intracellular proteins such as Fzd and the scaffold phosphoprotein Dishevelled (Dvl) respectively, regulate the activation of Rho-family GTPases. The end-stop of the planar cell polarity (PCP) pathway is signaling via Rho-associate kinase (ROCK) and c-Jun NH-terminal kinase (JNK) (Macheda & Stacker, 2008). The second β-catenin independent signaling pathway is characterized by the release of intracellular calcium ions by the stimulation of G-proteins. Increased calcium levels are sufficient to elicit a response from two calcium-sensitive enzymes: 1) calcium/calmodulin-dependent kinase II, (CaMKII), 2) protein kinase C (PKC) (Kuhl, 2004; Kohn & Moon, 2005). The Wnt/Ca^{2+} pathway has been postulated to play a role in tumor progression as the upregulation of Wnt5a in melanoma cells furthered invasiveness by restructuring the actin cytoskeleton (Weerartna et al., 2002).

There is emerging evidence that the non-canonical pathway competes with canonical Wnt signaling. Certain non-canonical Wnts such as Wnt11 and Wnt5a have been shown to antagonize Wnt/β-catenin signaling, although the mode of action is still unclear (Railo et al., 2008). Proposed mechanisms include competitions for Dvl molecules and alternative degradation pathways involving Siah-APC instead of GSK3β-β-TrCP (Veeman et al., 2003; Topol et al., 2003; Kharaishvili et al., 2011).

2.2 The canonical Wnt (β-catenin dependent) pathway

In the absence of Wnt, β-catenin is targeted for degradation by the 'destruction complex' comprising adenomatous polyposis coli (APC), glycogen synthase kinase 3β (GSK3β) and casein kinase (CK1), all of which are anchored to a scaffold protein, Axin. Phosphorylation of β-catenin by CK1 at Ser45 primes the sequential phosphorylation at Thr41, Ser37, and Ser33 by GSK3β. Phosphorylation at Ser33 and Ser37 allows recognition of β-catenin by an E3 ubiquitin ligase subunit, β-TrCP (β-transducin repeat-containing protein), resulting in ubiquitination and subsequent proteasomal degradation (MacDonald et al., 2009). Strict regulation of cytosolic β-catenin levels via the destruction complex ensures to some extent the nuclear availability of β-catenin. However, in the presence of a Wnt signal, β-catenin is stablized to increase in cellular levels and subsequently translocate to the nucleus where it becomes transcriptionally active — the hallmark of the canonical Wnt pathway.

The canonical Wnts, primarily Wnt3, Wnt3a, and Wnt6, bind to Wnt-Fzd-LRP 5/6 complexes to activate Dvl, which then disables GSK3β activity and stimulates LRP5/6 phosphorylation. Phosphorylation of LRP5/6 on its cytoplasmic tail leads to Axin docking at the plasma membrane, thus preventing the constitutive destruction of β-catenin (Davidson et al., 2005; Shih et al., 2007). Consequently, β-catenin accumulates in the cytoplasm and ultimately translocates to the nucleus, where it acts as a co-activator of T-Cell Factor/Lymphoid Enhancer Cell (TCF/LEF) family of DNA-binding proteins to mediate Wnt target gene transcription. Interestingly, the mechanism underlying the nuclear localization of β-catenin remains unclear as β-catenin does not contain a Nuclear

Localization Sequence (NLS) nor does it utilize the conventional importin nuclear transport system (Clevers, 2006). It is likely that NLS containing chaperones such as APC, Axin and RanBP3 (Ran binding protein 3) shuttle β-catenin into the nucleus (Clevers et al., 2006). To date there has been no mandatory chaperone identified as an essential carrier for the nuclear transport of β-catenin. Furthermore, TCF-pygopus complexes have also been implicated in β-catenin's nuclear retention (Stadeli, et al., 2006).

In the absence of β-catenin, the TCF/Groucho complex represses gene expression. The interaction between β-catenin and TCF results in the physical displacement of repressor Groucho, leading to the transactivation of downstream target genes often overexpressed in cancer. (Clevers, 2006; Macdonald et al., 2009) For a comprehensive, updated overview of Wnt target genes, refer to http://www.stanford.edu/~rnusse/wntwindow.html.

2.3 Canonical Wnt pathway and CaP progression

CaP development has been linked to Wnt signaling abnormalities and the stabilization of β-catenin (Chesire et al., 2002; Yardy & Brewster, 2005). The canonical Wnts are secreted during early prostate development but are thought to rapidly diminish in the adult prostate (Yu et al., 2009). Expression of Wnts in mature prostate is therefore unfavorable. Studies have shown constitutive activation of the canonical Wnt pathway due to the deletion of exon 3 on β-catenin which caused hyperplasia, squamous cell transdifferentiation (Bierie et al., 2003), and high-grade prostatic intraepithelial neoplasia (HGPIN) in the adult prostate and sustained growth even after androgen ablation (Yu et al., 2009).

Although exon 3 mutations of β-catenin only occur in 5% of primary CaP, 20% of advanced CaP showed an overall increase in β-catenin levels (Chesire et al., 2000; Gerstein et al., 2002). This suggests that aberrant expression of β-catenin is likely responsible for late CaP tumorigenesis. For instance, in mouse prostate expressing SV40-large T-antigen (LPB-Tag), a powerful deactivator of p53 and retinoblastoma (Rb) family of tumor suppressors, the integration of a non-degradable β-catenin gene provided additional morphological changes by transforming areas of benign HGPIN into invasive adenocarcinoma, along with an elevated expression of matrix metalloproteinase (MMP)-7 (Yu et al., 2011). MMPs are proteases known to facilitate membrane invasion by catalyzing the breakdown of the extracellular matrix (Bonfil et al., 2007). In this sense, gain of cell transformation and cell aggression via β-catenin/Wnt signaling may be attributed to the upregulation of MMPs, which are known Wnt target genes. Further, cell motility is endowed by epithelial-mesenchymal transition (EMT), a process by which epithelial cells acquire mesenchymal cell phenotypes such as enhanced invasiveness and greater migratory capacity (Kalluri & Weinberg, 2009). Accumulation of free β-catenin due to a loss of its cytoplasmic binding partner, E-cadherin, contributed to EMT in colon epithelial cells (Novak et al., 1998) while nuclear localization of β-catenin promoted and maintained EMT induced by c-FosER fusion protein in mammary epithelial cells (Eger et al., 2000; Eger et al., 2004). Likewise, GSK3β, a negative regulator of β-catenin, was downregulated in LNCaP/HIF-1α and IA8 EMT positive CaP cell lines, suggesting that β-catenin stabilization correlated with EMT characteristics in prostate tumorigenesis (Jiang et al., 2007). Additionally, Zhao et al., (2011) showed that shRNA knockdown of β-catenin expression in LNCaP/HIF-1α cells caused a reversal of mesenchymal properties and metastatic potential. This repression of β-catenin also attenuated invasive potency, increased E-cadherin expression, retained cytoplasmic β-catenin, and downregulated mesenchymal markers such as vimentin, N-cadherin and

MMP-7 (Zhao et al., 2011). Last but not least, the activation of Wnt signals in LNCaP cells resulted in expression of neuroendocrine (NE) markers, NSE and Chr.A, signifying Wnt/β-catenin in the development of neuroendocrine differentiation (NED) (Yang et al., 2005). This is confirmed by *in vivo* studies, which have revealed areas of NED in mouse prostates expressing dominant active β-catenin and T-antigen (Yu et al., 2011).

While β-catenin is the point of interest in terms of Wnt signaling and cancer progression, dysfunction of other components within the Wnt pathway can be equally detrimental. A classic example is the APC truncation that occurs in over 80% of colorectal cancer (Quyn et al., 2008). APC is an integral part of the 'destruction complex' that prevents β-catenin from exhibiting its oncogenic properties. Accordingly, APC loss-of-function fosters cell proliferation and differentiation, specifically the growth of adenomatous polyps in the colon. Although there are relatively rare incidences of APC mutations in human CaP, the *APC gene* has been shown to be modified in primary and metastatic CaP, through processes such as promoter hypermethylation and somatic alterations (Jeronimo et al., 2004; Brewster et al., 1994; Bruxvoort et al., 2007). Moreover, deletion of the *APC gene* in mouse CaP models stimulated the rapid development of AI-CaP (Bruxvoort et al., 2007). Despite these data, the role of APC in CaP remains controversial as a recent study found APC variants in several clinical specimens of CaP to be non-functional (Yardy et al., 2009). In the same study, the scaffold protein, Axin, was modified in 6% of advanced CaP cell lines with four Axin polymorphisms identified (Yardy et al., 2009). Furthermore, a strong correlation was shown between Axin2 and CaP progression (Pinnarbasi et al., 2010). Finally, the knockdown of Wnt receptors, Fz2 and Ror2, and the removal of the co-receptor, LRP5, significantly reduced DU145 cells' invasive capacity and new bone formation in MDA CaP 2b – a bone-derived CaP cell line, respectively (Li et al., 2008, Yamamoto et al., 2010). Evidently, Fz2 and Ror2 function to facilitate CaP aggression while LRP5 mediates CaP induced bone metastases.

Wnt antagonists are a family of secreted proteins capable of obstructing Wnt signaling. Common antagonists include certain members of the Dickkopf (DKK) family, the secreted Frizzled-related protein (sFRP) family and the Wnt inhibitory factor (WIF) family, all of which are frequently downregulated in human cancers (Kharaishvili et al., 2011). These inhibitors are categorized based on their binding preference. Members of the sFRP and WIF-1 class bind directly to Wnt ligands, which may either block Wnt-Fzd interaction or form nonfunctional Fzd complexes. The DKK protein family binds to co-receptors of the Wnt receptor complex, LRP5/6, to inhibit canonical Wnt signaling (Kawano & Kypta, 2003). In PC-3 cell lines, approximately 88% exhibited hypermethylation of the WIF-1 promoter region, which corresponded to a decrease in WIF-1 expression (Yee et al., 2010). This was observed in 64% of primary CaP tumors (Wissmann et al., 2003). On the other hand, the restoration of WIF-1 expression in PC-3 reverted EMT and enhanced paclitaxel-induced apoptosis, and, in xenograft mouse models decreased tumor size by approximately 63%; this was accompanied by an increase in epithelial markers, E-cadherin and Keratin-18, and a decrease in the mesenchymal marker, vimentin (Yee et al., 2010, Ohigashi et al., 2005). Similar results in PC-3 were obtained by the reintroduction of Frzb/sFRP-3, a potential tumor suppressor that prevented EMT, and decreased MMP-2, MMP-9 and AKT activation (Xi et al., 2005). Additional studies of PC-3 cell lines demonstrated that sFRP-1 negatively regulated AR function, however, by neither Wnt/β-catenin signaling nor the non-canonical pathways (Kawano et al., 2009). Instead, the sFRP-1/Fzd complex may have been responsible for another pathway, closely resembling that of Wnt5a signaling. The therapeutic relevance of sFRP-1 remains elusive, as its attributes are largely dependent on certain cellular contexts. Examination of sFRP-1 treated prostate epithelial cells showed the downregulation of Wnt/β-catenin signaling, but unexpectedly, a reduction in apoptosis and stimulation of cell proliferation (Joesting et al., 2005). Unlike sFRP-1, sFRP-4 appeared to suppress anchorage independent growth, proliferation rate and mesenchymal expression in PC-3 cells, irrespective of AR functionality (Horvath et al., 2007).

The roles of DKK family of antagonists are becoming increasingly clear. Hall et al., (2008) reported that DKK-1 expression was elevated in early CaP development but became suppressed as CaP cells metastasized to the axial skeleton. Enforced DKK-1 expression in osteoblastic CaP cells was also shown to reduce bone formation and induce osteolytic activity (Hall et al., 2008). In this regard, DKK-1 was required at a high level initially to inhibit osteoprotegerin, a suppressor of osteoclastogenesis, downstream of the Wnt pathway, which led to osteolytic lesions that facilitated tumor growth (Glass et al., 2005, Hall et al., 2008). Once CaP cells had invaded the bone, DKK-1 levels subsequently minimized as new bone formation required Wnt activation to propagate osteoblastic activity. This was in line with more recent experimental data showing that intercardiac injection of stably expressing DKK-1 Ace-1 cells (a CaP cell line that produces mixed osteoblastic and osteolytic lesions) into mice, increased the appearance of a subcutaneous tumor mass and decreased Ace-1-induced osteoblast activity (Thudi et al., 2011). Taken together, these results support the association between DKK-1 overexpression in CaP metastases and a decreased overall patient lifespan (Hall et al., 2008).

3. β-catenin in CaP progression

3.1 β-catenin

Despite the clear regulatory role of upstream Wnt factors such as the Wnt ligands, inhibitors, and receptors in CaP progression, the major mediator of Wnt signal activation is β-catenin. β-catenin is a 781 amino acid protein composed of three distinct regions: the central armadillo domain containing 12 imperfect repeats of 42 amino acids, the amino (N) – terminal containing phosphorylation sites vital for ubiquitin mediated proteosomal degradation and the carboxyl (C) – terminal housing the transactivation domain required for gene activation (Huber et al., 1997). β-catenin serves two major functions. At the adherens junctions, β-catenin links E-cadherin to the actin cytoskeleton via α-catenin. The β-catenin-E-cadherin interactions maintain efficient cell-cell adhesion and structural integrity of tissue architecture. This adhesive property of β-catenin juxtaposes against its oncogenic functions exerted within the nucleus, where TCF/LEF transcriptional factors complex with β-catenin to activate gene transcription. β-catenin's remarkable capability to partake in both cell signaling and adhesion can be explained by the existence of differing molecular forms of the same protein. Gottardi & Gumbiner, (2004) discovered that a TCF-specific form of β-catenin was generated after Wnt activation. This selective type was incompatible with cadherin's binding domain. The majority of E-cadherin-β-catenin dimers were found only when β-catenin was bound to α-catenin. Other organisms such as *C. elegans* utilize several β-catenins to differentially control cell adhesion and signaling, vertebrates transform β-catenin into distinct structural configurations to maintain the same degree of coordination and regulation. The failure to do so, as frequently occurs in cancer, is a common mechanism by which carcinogenesis is facilitated. Therefore, it is key to fully unravel the complex machineries associated with this potent oncogene. This section of the review will discuss the structural basis of β-catenin's functionality, in terms of subcellular interactions, Wnt-mediated localization, and Wnt-independent signaling.

3.1.1 Armadillo repeat domain

The armadillo repeats (residues 141-664), each repeat consisting of 3 α-helices, helices 1 (H1), 2 (H2), and 3(H3), are densely packed, forming an overall cylindrical conformation. The armadillo tandem repeats form a superhelical molecule featuring a long, positively charged groove, which constitutes binding sites for the majority of β-catenin's interactors (Xing et al., 2008). The floor of this groove is made up of H3 helices. Although the groove shows high binding affinity for various molecular partners, the full-length protein interactions are rather weak, pointing to the significance of the terminal regions (Piedra et al., 2001; Castano et al., 2002). The proteolysis-resistant armadillo domain is also highly conserved and structurally rigid relative to the unstable terminal domains, which are sensitive to trypsin digestion (Xing et al., 2008; Huber, 1997). The inflexibility of the domain is caused by the extensive contacts between the 12 repeats, ensuring the stability of the continuous hydrophobic core (Huber et al., 1997). Deviations from the regular repetitions of residues create imperfect repeats, particularly on repeat 10, where an insertion of 20 amino acids between H1 and H2 surrounds the groove and affects ligand binding (Huber et al., 1997). The extra sequence hosts a binding surface for 14-3-3ζ, an important modulator of β-catenin transactivation by AKT (Fang et al., 2007; Xu et al., 2007). Other irregularities include a missing H1 in the seventh armadillo repeat and the kinked helices of the first repeat, but their functional roles are not clearly determined (Xu et al., 2007). Huber et al., (1997) hypothesized the seventh armadillo repeat as a site of potential hinge action since the lost helix would grant some local flexibility. Additional crystallographic analysis and mutational studies defined the importance of repeat 7 for TCF interaction and armadillo protein function (Graham et al., 2000; Tolwinski & Wieschaus, 2004).

3.1.2 Features of the armadillo groove

The long, positively charged groove is comprised of 12 armadillo repeats and forms β-catenin's ligand-recognition domain, which hosts mutually exclusive interactions with its numerous molecular partners. The positive charge of the groove and its negatively charged ligands assist β-catenin interaction. Superimposition of 3D crystal structures of a variety of β-catenin complexes, including TCF, the cadherins and APC, exposed a binding region (repeats 5-9) shared by the common ligands (Choi et al., 2006). Specifically, repeats 6-8 forms a special part of the groove containing a series of asparagine (Asn) residues that engage the polypeptide backbone of a diverse cohort of ligands (Gottardi & Gumbiner, 2001). Ligands recognizing β-catenin all contain a conserved consensus sequence, containing Aspartic Acid (Asp) and Glutamine (Glu) amino acids that form two disulfide bridges between Lys435 and Lys312 of β-catenin, respectively (Choi et al., 2006). Graham et al., (2000) dubbed these covalent bonds as "charged buttons" as they were required to affix the partners to β-catenin's armadillo domain. Despite the commonalities, each ligand interacts with the groove in a distinct manner: E-cadherin's cytoplasmic domain interacts with the entire span of the armadillo domain; TCF interacts with repeats 3-5 by its amphipathic helix C-terminal; ICAT, an inhibitor of TCF-β-catenin complex formation, is limited to only repeats 11 to 12 (Choi et al., 2006). In each case, the ligand appears to undergo conformational adjustments to properly accommodate the rigid groove (Gottardi & Gumbiner, 2001). This is supported by the fact that most of β-catenin's partners are poorly structured in the absence of β-catenin or other ligands. Measurements of cadherin, TCF, APC and Axin by techniques such as NMR, circular dichroism and fluorescence anisotropy have confirmed the native instability of these proteins. For example, as independent entities, the entire β-catenin binding domain of E-cadherin was found to be completely unstructured and TCF failed to adopt its secondary structure (Huber & Weiss, 2001; Knapp et al., 2001; Choi et al., 2006).

3.1.3 N- and C- terminal domains

The unstructured terminal tails flanking the armadillo repeat domain are highly flexible, and are proposed to regulate ligand binding. For instance, the interaction between the C-terminal (residues 696- 781) and the armadillo repeats limit the binding of E-cadherin and other co-factors such as the TATA-binding protein (Piedra et al., 2001). The N-terminal (residues 1 – 134) can also interact with the central domain, however, with low affinity when the C-terminus is absent, while the deletion of the N-terminus resulted in a tighter binding of the C-terminal to the armadillo domain (Castano et al., 2002). These results indicate that the two termini are interdependent and interact with the armadillo domain in a fold-back fashion. The possibility of this mechanism, nonetheless, is challenged by recent quantitative analyses of ligand interaction from isothermal titration calorimetry (ITC). Choi et al., (2006) reasoned that competitive inhibition by the terminal tails does not occur, instead, the tails may directly influence the binding of ligands or other allosteric sites on the arm domain to facilitate β-catenin interaction. The possibility of weak transient interactions was negated by data obtained from Nuclear Magnetic Resonance (NMR) spectroscopy – The NMR spectrum of ^{15}N-tagged C-terminus of β-catenin was negligibly affected by the armadillo repeats (Xing et al., 2008; Gottardi & Peifer, 2008). The proximal regions of the C-terminal have also been shown to form an α-helix, designated as Helix C, which modulates Wnt-mediated transcription (Xing et al., 2008). The significance of this particular helix is well documented: truncated *Drosophila* armadillo lacking the Helix C failed to initiate transactivation, whereas truncation of the C-terminus up to the Helix C preserved signaling capacity (Gottardi & Peifer, 2008). Equally, Helix C was found on transcriptionally active forms of β-catenin in C. *elegans* but not on an adhesive form which preferred the cadherins (Schneider et al., 2003; Gottardi & Peifer, 2008). Moreover, experiments delivering truncated armadillo void of the N-terminus into the nucleus revealed an absence of β-catenin- TCF complexes, suggesting that the N-terminus influences, if not to a greater extent than the C-terminus, the gene transcription and chromatin remodeling functions possessed by β-catenin (Chan & Struhl 2002; Tolwinski & Wieschaus, 2004). Further crystallographic and NMR investigations suggested the dynamism of the unstructured tails distal to the Helix C: the negatively charged N- and C-tails respond to the positively charged groove in a highly variable manner and do not interact in a static conformation (Xing et al., 2008). Hence, the tails may "shield" the armadillo repeat domain from any non-specific interaction, or act as "intramolecular chaperones" of the armadillo repeat domain to facilitate ligand binding and to prevent self-aggregation of the repeats (Xing et al., 2008).

3.1.4 β-catenin and the destruction complex

The 'destruction complex' responsible for β-catenin turnover was described to encompass four major entities – the scaffold protein, Axin, the nuclear chaperone, APC and the phosphorylation kinases, GSK3β and CK1. In the absence of Wnt stimulation, cytoplasmic β-catenin is phosphorylated at site Ser45 by CK1, priming the sequential phosphorylation at sites Ser33, Ser37, and Thr41 by GSK3β. In addition to the subsequent recognition by β-TrCP followed by proteosomal degradation, GSK3β and CK1 mediated phosphorylation has a major impact on the functionality of β-catenin. Unmodified β-catenin at GSKβ residues Ser33, Ser37 and Thr41 has been characterized as intrinsically more active than the pool of β-catenin that are phosphorylated (Staal et al., 2002; Maher et al., 2010). In other words, transactivation by β-catenin can be altered by phosphorylation. Using monoclonal antibodies detecting for β-catenin specifically unmodified at Ser37 and Thr41 (active β-catenin), Maher et al., (2010) indicated that active β-catenin exists in a monomeric form and was found in far fewer proportions relative to the total pool of β-catenin. That being said however, the low levels of active β-catenin were almost exclusively located in the nucleus. Furthermore, Maher et al., (2010) observed that β-catenin phosphorylated at Thr41/Ser45 was spatially uncoupled from β-catenin phosphorylated at Ser33/Ser37/Thr41. This suggested that phosphorylation at Ser45 by CK1 extended beyond a simple priming gesture (Maher et al., 2010). Since the majority of the Thr41/Ser45 phosphorylated β-catenin translocated to the nucleus, it is entirely possible that phosphorylation at Ser45 configures an active form of β-catenin (Maher et al., 2010). In contrast, β-catenin phosphorylated at Ser33/Ser37/Thr41 was generally cytoplasmic and was ultimately subjected to protein degradation. The F-box protein, β-TrCP, recognizes β-catenin at its doubly phosphorylated destruction motif, thereby causing ubiquitination at specific lysine residues by the larger SCFβ-TrCP complex (Wu et al., 2003) The helical region just prior to the destruction motif (residues 20-31) is also required for successful β-TrCP interaction (Megy et al., 2004).

The scaffold protein Axin facilitates the phosphorylation-dependent degradation of β-catenin by anchoring β-catenin, APC, CK1 and GSK3β to specific binding sites. The β-catenin binding domain of Axin includes a highly conserved helical region that interacts with armadillo repeats 3 and 4 of β-catenin's positively charged groove (Xing et al., 2003). The helical region on Axin is C-terminal to the GSK3β binding site and runs roughly parallel to the superhelix formed by β-catenin's armadillo repeats. This places GSK3β at the N-terminus of β-catenin to augment the phosphorylation efficiency of GSK3β by **20,000 fold (Dajani et al., 2003). Alternatively, the anchored CK1 and GSK3β can phosphorylate Axin to increase its affinity for β-catenin (Mo et al., 2009). External factors, such as WTX, a tumor suppressor encoded by a gene mutated in Wilms tumors, may aid the degradation of β-catenin by binding directly to β-TrCP (Major et al., 2007). WTX antagonized Wnt signaling in mammalian cells, and this effect was abrogated by the siRNA knockdown of WTX expression (Major et al., 2007). Co-immunoprecipitation assays indicated that WTX can also interact with Axin, APC and β-catenin. In effect, WTX is likely to be another component of the destruction complex, exerting its influence on β-catenin perhaps just prior to ubiquitination (Kennell & Cadigan, 2009).

APC is of particular interest, as it has been proposed to participate in a range of roles in the destruction complex. Firstly, as a nuclear exporter of β-catenin, it is able to restrict TCF interaction and thus gene transcription (Henderson, 2000; Rosin-arbesfeld et al., 2000; van de Wetering et al., 1997; Xing et al., 2004) This model can be partly supported by the nuclear accumulation of β-catenin in colorectal cancer cells (SW480) expressing mutated APC, as well as elevated β-catenin levels due a complete loss of the *APC gene* observed in *Drosophila* (Kennell & Cadigan, 2009). More directly, transient transfection of wild type APC into

SW480 diminished nuclear levels of β-catenin and increased the degradation of β-catenin (Henderson, 2000). Treatment with leptomycin B (LMB), a nuclear export inhibitor of APC, or the mutagenesis of the NES on APC, abolished the reduction in transcriptional activity and total β-catenin levels (Neufeld et al., 2000). As well, the loss of functional NES resulted in increased levels of β-catenin within the nucleus. Taken together, these data support the role of APC as a nuclear chaperone of β-catenin.

Structurally, APC binds to β-catenin by either its three 15-amino acid repeats (15 aa) or seven 20-amino acid repeats (20 aa) at its central domain (Rubinfeld et al., 1993; Su et al., 1993). The 15 aa repeats are not modified by phosphorylation and bind to armadillo repeat 5-8 of β-catenin, overlapping the regions of TCF binding site (Spink et al., 2001). In spite of this physical arrangement, the 15 aa repeats cannot hinder TCF-β-catenin interaction (Spink et al., 2001). Likewise, truncated APC maintaining the intact 15 aa repeats retains the ability to bind to β-catenin but fails to down-regulate β-catenin expression (Munemitsu et al., 1995). The 20 aa repeats are thought to be more functionally important; though, peptide competition studies showed unphosphorylated 20 aa repeats adopt the same binding surface on β-catenin as the 15 aa repeats (Spink et al., 2001; Xing et al., 2004). Despite their sequence similarities, the different β-catenin-binding repeats have crucial differences. The 20 aa repeats are highly conserved and can be phosphorylated on the SXXSSLSXLS consensus motif (Xu et al., 2007). Phosphorylation at this motif by GSK3β and CK1 drastically increases APC interactions with β-catenin by 300- to 500- fold (Xing et al., 2004). In fact, phosphorylation of the third 20 aa repeat has by far, the tightest binding affinity for β-catenin (Liu et al., 2006). Interestingly, the deletion of this site accounts for the majority of APC mutations in colorectal cancer (Bienz & Clevers, 2000; Nathke, 2004; Polakis et al., 1995, Xu et al., 2007). Crystal structures of the complex between the 20 aa repeats and the armadillo groove of β-catenin has led to greater insight. Xing et al., (2004), determined that the phosphorylated 20 aa repeats of APC binds to the armadillo repeats 1-5, and a single 20 aa repeat with its flanking residues covers the entire span of β-catenin's structural groove. Consequently, the large binding area, along with the high affinity between the phosphorylated 20 aa repeats and the armadillo groove, may play critical roles in regulating β-catenin function. Indeed, binding competition assays have confirmed phosphorylated APC disrupts β-catenin-TCF interaction, in part, due to APC residues N-terminal to the 20 aa repeat which adopt a conformation identical to that of TCF and E-cadherin (Xing et al., 2004)

Consistent with results showing reduced β-catenin levels upon expression of APC, Axin interacts with APC through its regulator of G-protein signaling (RGS) domain to promote the destruction of β-catenin (Hinoi et al., 2000). On the other hand, APC requires the Ser-Ala-Met-Pro (SAMP) repeats, in conjunction with the 15 aa and 20 aa repeats, in the central domain to effectively interact with Axin (Behren et al., 1998, Hart et al., 1998, Kennell & Cadigan, 2009). Although APC cannot independently induce GSK3β-dependent phosphorylation of β-catenin, the synergy between APC and Axin considerably increased levels of GSK3β modified β-catenin (Hinoi et al., 2000; Kennell & Cadigan, 2009). This suggests APC, along with the kinases, are essential in forming complexes with Axin to mediate the degradation of β-catenin. The current models hold that APC sustains the efficiency of the 'destruction complex' by controlling the release and the recruitment of β-catenin. The basis of these models is that the phosphorylated 20 aa repeats on APC, not the 15 aa repeats nor the unmodified 20 aa repeats, competitively inhibits β-catenin-Axin interaction (Xing et al., 2003). In one system, Axin recruits β-catenin bound to the 15 aa repeats, which then allows the efficient phosphorylation of the N-terminal serine and threonine residues by

GSK3β and CK1 (Xing et al., 2003). The latter kinases then phosphorylate the third 20 aa repeat on APC, dramatically increasing its affinity for β-catenin so that the Axin-β-catenin complex is derailed. Axin's β-catenin binding domain becomes free for the next available substrate while APC is dephosphorylated as it moves way from GSK3β's active site. Subsequently, β-catenin dissociates from APC and β-TrCP targets the released β-catenin for ubiquitination and degradation. An alternative model suggests phosphorylated APC first transports β-catenin to the 'destruction complex', where dephosphorylation of APC reduces its binding affinity, causing β-catenin to bind preferentially to Axin (Kennell & Cadigan, 2009). While β-catenin is recognized by β-TrCP, GSK3β and CK1 phosphorylate APC to renew the cycle once again. In both scenarios, a candidate dephosphorylation agent is protein phosphatase 2A (PP2A). This multimeric phosphatase promotes β-catenin turnover and causes β-catenin stabilization when inhibited (Xing et al., 2003). In *in vitro* studies, PP2A was shown to directly dephosphorylate APC (Xing et al., 2003).

3.2 β-catenin and cell adhesion

The progression of many cancers, including prostate metastasis, involves the loss of cell adhesion and contact inhibition. This can be attributed to the aberrant regulation of cell adhesion molecules (CAMs), which comprise the cadherins, integrins, selectins and immunoglobulin. E-cadherin is a calcium-dependent transmembrane glycoprotein responsible for mediating intercellular adhesion as well as structural integrity. The cytoplasmic domain of E-cadherin interacts with the entire span of β-catenin's armadillo repeat domain, and features multiple, quasi-independent binding regions (Huber & Weis, 2001). However, only the last 100 residues of the E-cadherin cytoplasmic domain make contact with the large binding interface on β-catenin – and this extensiveness may render the interaction resistant, in most cases, to single point mutations on β-catenin's E-cadherin binding sites (Huber & Weis, 2001; Gottardi & Gumbiner, 2001). The cytoplasmic domain can be subdivided into five regions, I-V, based on their distinct interaction with β-catenin's armadillo repeats. The most functionally relevant are region II and IV, where certain phosphorylation events occur to affect binding affinity. An α-helix in region II is packed against β-catenin Tyr654 on armadillo repeats 11-12. *pp60c-src* -induced phosphorylation of Tyr654 reduced the affinity of E-cadherin for β-catenin by 6-fold as the *in vitro* transfection of *pp60c-src* led to junctional instability and gain of invasive phenotype associated with metastasis (Roura et al., 1999; Behrens et al., 1993; Huber & Weis, 2001). In general, overexpression and constitutive activation of tyrosine kinases contributes to abnormal growth, in situ carcinogenesis and metastasis (Lilien & Balsamo, 2005). Region IV hosts consensus sequences for casein kinase II (CK-2) and GSK3β-mediated serine phosphorylation. The residues, Ser 684, 686 and 692, enhance E-cadherin binding to β-catenin by either salt bridges or hydrogen bonds, but only when they are phosphorylated. These sites are part of the extended PEST (Pro-Glu-Ser-Thr) sequence responsible for cadherin degradation; masking of the PEST domain when β-catenin binds consequently prevents degradation. Furthermore, site-directed mutagenesis of these key residues resulted in the loss of cell-cell adhesion and the attenuated β-catenin/E-cadherin interaction (Huber & Weiss, 2001).

Another key component of the adhesion complex is α-catenin, a protein linking the actin filaments to the E-cadherin bound β-catenin. The amphiphathic helix (residues 118-141) N-terminal to the first armadillo repeat of β-catenin forms the major binding surface for α-catenin (Huber &Weis, 2001). Residues 146-149 adopt a helix in a direction different from that of residues 118-141. The conserved residue Tyr142 is a critical regulator this region as it affects α-catenin-β-catenin interaction: phosphorylation of Tyr142 dissociated β-catenin from α-catenin with the simultaneous loss of cell adhesion (Piedra et al., 2003; Ozawa et al., 1998; Lilien & Balsamo, 2005). Crystal structure of chimeric protein, α-β-cat, a fusion complex between the binding domains of β-catenin and α-catenin, revealed that the amphiphathic helix structure collapses past residue 142, as the firm helix would introduce steric clash (Huber & Weis, 2001). Thus, the non-helical region between residues 142-144 creates a hinged region, which can accommodate both β-catenin and α-catenin simultaneously (Wu et al., 2007). While this supports the notion that α-catenin can directly interacts with the actin cytoskeleton while bound to the E-cadherin/β-catenin complex to facilitate structural integrity, recent evidence have led to an alternate mechanism that more accurately describe the mode of interaction. A prerequisite for actin interaction is for α-catenin to be in its homodimeric form; however, the homodimerization interface impedes β-catenin binding sites located on α-catenin (Drees et al., 2005). The monomeric form of α-catenin primarily binds to β-catenin but exhibits low affinity for actin. Thus, α-catenin cannot interact with both β-catenin and actin concomitantly. It seems, overall, α-catenin modulates actin dynamics in the presence of E-cadherin (Drees et al., 2005; Wu et al., 2007).

In CaP, both the deregulation of the E-cadherin/α-catenin complex and the down-regulation of E-cadherin/β-catenin complex were correlated with a high Gleason score and in some cases, low patient survival (Richmond et al., 1997). Furthermore, activated AR was found to repress E-cadherin gene expression and contribute to mesenchymal-like appearance and tumor metastasis (Liu et al., 2008). DHT was essential both *in vitro* and *in vivo* to induce the down-regulation of E-cadherin (Liu et al., 2008). Androgen-mediated EMT, characterized by a loss of E-cadherin, was inversely correlated with levels of AR expression in prostate tumor epithelial cells (Zhu et al., 2010). Thus, minimal AR activation was needed for maintenance of EMT (Zhu et al., 2010). The loss of α-catenin expression has also been observed in PC-3 cell line which was pivotal to the maintenance of cell-cell adhesion (Ewing et al, 1995; Verras & Sun, 2006). In addition, Sasaki et al., (2000) and Yang et al., (2002) demonstrated that the reintroduction of E-cadherin to E-cadherin negative cell line, TSU-Pr1, shifted the localization of β-catenin from the cytoplasm to the cell membrane. Furthermore, there was a reduction of nuclear levels of β-catenin and a corresponding decrease in AR mediated transcription by β-catenin (Yang et al, 2002). Conversely, the loss or reduction of E-cadherin expression from TSU-Pr1 cell lines enhanced AR mediated transcription due to the increased cytoplasmic and nuclear levels of β-catenin (Verras & Sun 2006). Hence, in CaP progression the integrity and presence of E-cadherin affects the redistribution of β-catenin and functionally affects AR induced cell growth and survival.

3.3 β-catenin and post translational modifications

A plethora of post-translational modifications occur on β-catenin to tightly regulate its cellular activity. This includes Ser/Thr phosphorylation, tyrosine phosphorylation, ubiquitylation, acetylation and O-glycosylation. The aforementioned modifications can occur on the N-terminus, the C- terminus, or the surface of the armadillo repeat domain, suggesting they do not alter β-catenin's 3-dimensional conformations on a large scale. Notably, tyrosine phosphorylation, in addition to its role of disassembling adherence junctions as discussed earlier (Section 3.2), has long been implicated to affect the transcriptional activity of β-catenin. For example, phosphorylation of Tyr654 can increase β-catenin's interaction with the basal transcriptional machinery TATA-binding protein by disassociating the C-terminal from the armadillo repeat domain. Mutation of Tyr654 to glutamate released β-catenin from cadherins and enhanced its activity as a co-activator of transcription, although there is no data suggesting that nuclear β-catenin is phosphorylated at this site (Piedra et al., 2001; Lilien & Balsamo, 2005) Interestingly, phosphorylation of Tyr142 by c-Met acts as a molecular switch that transforms the adhesive form of β-catenin into one that preferentially binds to BCL9-2, effectively increasing the transcription of Wnt target genes. β-catenin containing a mutated Tyr142 did not efficiently bind to BCL9-2, resulting in a dramatic decrease in Wnt target gene transcription (Brembeck et al., 2004). Similar outcomes were mimicked by the CK2-mediated phosphorylation of Thr393, which potentiated Wnt signaling by instilling β-catenin with resistance to proteosomal degradation and an elevated co-transcriptional function (Song et al., 2003).

β-catenin was recently reported to be post-translationally modified by O-linked N-acetylglucosamine (O-GlcNAc). While there was minimal O-GlcNAcylation of β-catenin in CaP, normal primary prostate cells exhibited significantly higher levels of O-GlcNAcylated β-catenin (Sayat et al., 2008). O-GlyNAcylation refers to a covalent modification of serine and threonine residues of mammalian glycoproteins (Brockhausen et al., 2009). This involves the attachment of a single monosaccharide of O-GlcNAc to the hydroxyl of serine or threonine amino acid residues by an O-glycosidic bond (Brockhausen et al., 2009). The addition and removal of O-GlcNAc groups is a reversible process that utilizes two *nucleocytoplasmic* enzymes, O-linked β-N-acetylglucosamine transferase (OGT) and β-D-N-acetylglucosaminidase (O-GlcNAcase), respectively (Guinez et al., 2004). The functional aspect of the O-GlcNAc modification of β-catenin was first reported by Sayat et al., (2008) and demonstrated that increasing cellular levels of O-GlcNAc-β-catenin resulted in diminished levels of nuclear β-catenin and a corresponding increase in cytoplasmic β-catenin. Moreover, TOPFlash-luciferase activity showed that the transcriptional function of β-catenin was inversely correlated to its O-GlcNAcylated levels (Sayat et al., 2008). Taken together, these data suggests that O-GlcNAcylation of endogenous β-catenin negatively regulated its nuclear localization and transcriptional activity in CaP and primary prostate cell lines. Such results have clear implications on the nuclear availability of β-catenin and to its transcriptional function including AR transactivation. However, the question of how O-GlcNAc modification may affect AR-β-catenin transcriptional activation, interaction and TCF-AR competition remains to be answered.

Levy et al., (2004) showed that lysine acetylation positively modulates β-catenin's transcriptional activity. Specifically, acetylation at residue Lys345 located in armadillo repeat 6, increased binding affinity of β-catenin for Tcf-4, and required the acetyltransferase activity of coactivator p300. Mutation on Lys345 severed the coopertivity between p300 and β-catenin, which served to reduce β-catenin's co-activation function. Interestingly, competition assays revealed that the acetylated form of β-catenin had lower affinity for the AR while the non-acetylated form better competed for the AR. This suggests a reciprocal relationship between the β-catenin-TCF interaction and the β-catenin-AR axis.

3.4 β-catenin and transactivation
The nuclear localization of β-catenin is the hallmark of the canonical Wnt pathway. Nuclear β-catenin activates gene transcription by forming a complex with TCF/LEF family of DNA-

binding proteins to mediate the transcription of Wnt target genes such as cyclin D1 and c-myc. Although the exact sequence of events that occur once β-catenin has translocated into the nucleus remains elusive, there are several models explaining the role of β-catenin in gene activation. The simplest explains β-catenin as a co-activator by providing a transcriptional activation domain to TCF/LEF (Sokol, 2011). Another model proposes that β-catenin heterodimerizes with TCF/LEF to supplant repressor proteins, Groucho/TLE, CtBP or HDACs, and thereby switching TCF/LEF from a quiescent state into one that is transcriptionally active (Stadeli et al., 2006; Sokol, 2011). Since TCF is DNA bound, changes in chromatin structure are also necessary to lift the transcriptional blockade imparted by the repressor proteins (Narlikar et al., 2002; Daniels &Weis 2005). β-catenin was found to interact with numerous other chromatin modifying proteins such as histone acetyltransferases (HATs), cyclic AMP response element-binding protein (CBP) or its close relative p300, TATA binding protein (TBP) and Brg-1 to assemble a multimeric complex in conjunction with TCF/LEF (Daniel & Weis, 2005).

The TCF/LEF family consists of Tcf-1, Tcf-3, Tcf-4 and Lef-1, and may function to either activate or repress the transcription of a plethora of genes depending on the availability of β-catenin in the nucleus (Ravindranath & Connell 2008). While Tcf-1 and Tcf-4 may play dual roles as both an activator and repressor, Lef-1 exists predominately as an activator whereas Tcf-3 is often a repressor (MacDonald et al., 2009). Upon Wnt activation, approximately 50 residues of Tcf-4 within the N-terminal interact with β-catenin in two distinct binding surfaces (Wu et al., 2007): an extended region (residues 13-25) that interacts with armadillo repeats 4-9 and an α-helix formed by residues 40-50 that binds to armadillo repeats 3-5. In the former interaction, Asp16 and Glu17 form salt bridges with armadillo residues Lys435 and Lys508, respectively, which fastens Tcf-4 to the positively charged groove (Poy et al., 2001). Asp16 is particularly important as it accounts for high affinity binding to β-catenin. In addition, hydrophobic interactions between the Tcf-4 side chains are critical for effective binding. Compared to wild type Tcf-4, the truncated proteins lacking these side chains showed almost a 60% reduction in transcriptional activity (Poy et al., 2001). The second binding interface involves the N-terminal to the DNA-binding high motility group (HMG) domain and overlaps the binding interface for transcriptional repressors Groucho/TLE (Wu et al., 2007). Thus, these proteins are displaced when β-catenin binds with a higher affinity.

Along with β-catenin, many other co-activators of TCF have been identified. BCL9 is an adaptor protein proposed to aid transactivation by providing docking sites for other transcriptional machinery such as pygopus (Sampietro et al., 2006). BCL9 has not only been found to interact with β-catenin/TCF complex to activate transcription, but also been found to sequester β-catenin in the nucleus (Kireghoff et al., 2006). The crystal structure of a β-catenin/BCL9/Tcf-4 complex revealed that BCL9 interacted with β-catenin at a region N-terminal to the structural groove of the armadillo repeat domain. The β-catenin binding domain on BCL9 forms an α-helix, but unlike other co-activators, the helix does not overlap the binding sites of other β-catenin partners and can be mutated to prevent proper β-catenin-BCL9 binding without compromising the integrity of other indispensible interactions (Sampietro et al., 2006). Sampietro et al., (2006) demonstrated that simultaneous mutations within hydrophobic pockets of the first armadillo repeat, especially on residues L156A and L159A, effectively abolished BCL9 binding but not that of E-cadherin and α-catenin, the only two known proteins that bind to the same region on β-catenin. This suggests that BCL9 interacts with β-catenin through unique, hydrophobic contacts and underscores the therapeutic potential of small molecule inhibitors to prevent the transcription of Wnt target genes via precise interferences of the BCL9-β-catenin complex.

A variety of antagonists and agonists functions to further regulate β-catenin/TCF-mediated transcription. A devoted nuclear antagonist, ICAT (inhibitor of β-catenin and TCF), inhibits binding of β-catenin to Tcf-4 *in vitro* and has been shown to decrease Tcf-4-induced reporter activity (Tago et al., 2000; Tutter et al., 2001; Daniel & Weis 2002). This inhibitory attribute is due to its high affinity for the armadillo repeats 5-10, which are shared between TCFs, APC, and cadherins. Moreover, the helical domain of ICAT can inhibit co-activators, namely p300; in fact, ICAT exhibits bipartite inhibition: its helical domain disrupts CBP/p300 binding, while its extended region prevents β-catenin-TCF interaction (Daniel & Weis, 2002). Positive modulators of β-catenin/TCF-mediated transcription include Galectin-3 (gal-3) and Daxx. Interestingly, the overexpression of gal-3 in the nucleus is associated with tumorigenesis and metastasis in colon, prostate, and tongue squamous carcinoma cells (Danguy et al., 2000; Honjo et al., 2000; Van de Brule et al., 2000). Shimura et al., (2004) demonstrated that gal-3 promotes transcription of Wnt target genes, cyclin D1 and c-myc, and colocalizes with β-catenin to induce transcriptional activity of Tcf-4 up to 13 fold. The binding region of gal-3 (residues 1-131) overlaps with that of α-catenin and may cause displacement of β-catenin from the plasma membrane (Shimura et al., 2004). Another positive co-regulator is Daxx, which potentiates β-catenin/Tcf-4-mediated transcription possibly by removing binding of repressors Groucho/TLE (Huang et al., 2009). Surprisingly, Daxx can also down-regulate DNA binding capacity of nuclear hormone receptors including the AR (Shih et al., 2007).

4. Wnt/β-catenin-AR mediated cross-talk

Alterations in β-catenin distribution and expression have been reported in patient CaP samples with a general trend of increased β-catenin levels in AI-CaP and a greater nuclear presence of β-catenin with increased Gleason grade (Whitaker et al., 2008). As mentioned previously, recent evidence has demonstrated that the Wnt signaling pathway partakes in mediating CaP progression. Activating mutations of β-catenin, the major regulator of this pathway, are found in 5% of prostate cancers (Song et al., 2003). Such mutations directly contribute to altered growth of the CaP, but also increase AR activity (Cronauer et al., 2004). However, since mutations of β-catenin occur focally, it is still a subject of debate whether such alterations to β-catenin represent a late event in prostate cancer progression (Verras & Sun, 2006). It is unlikely that mutational activation of β-catenin is the primary cause. Evidence is clear that increased AR expression results in sensitivity to androgen and that increased AR expression alone is sufficient to transform primary CaP into a more aggressive AI phenotype. The recent identification of a physical interaction between AR and β-catenin and AR and TCF was an exciting new development for understanding the mechanism underlying CaP progression. In effect, the observed accumulation of β-catenin and increase in AR activation are likely in interplay to arbitrate selective gene expression programs that potentiate prostate carcinogenesis.

4.1 The AR-β-catenin Interaction: Structure

β-catenin contains five LXXLL motifs situated within the armadillo region. The LXXLL motifs are found on the second alpha-helix of armadillo repeats 1, 3 7, 10, and 12 (Pai et al., 1996; Huber et al., 1997; Mulholland et al., 2005; Song et al., 2003). However, deletion mutants of repeats 7, 10 and 12 indicated that these regions were not necessary for AR/β-catenin binding (Yang et al., 2002; Song et al., 2003; Mulholland et al., 2005). A possible explanation for this observation was that the leucine residues of the armadillo repeats may be buried within hydrophobic cores, thus inaccessible to binding the AR LBD (Mulholland et al., 2005). On the other hand, Yang et al., 2002 showed that the central armadillo repeats 1-6 of β-catenin were responsible for the LBD interaction. Using a yeast two hybrid system, Yang et al., 2002 showed that deletion of the AR N-terminal activation domain alone (134-671) or deletions that combined the central armadillo domain (671-781; repeat 1-7) of β-catenin and the N-terminal of the AR resulted in no interaction. This indicated that the primary binding region of the AR encompassed the N-terminus and the first seven armadillo repeats of β-catenin (Yang et al., 2002). However, when deleting repeat 6, the interaction was essentially abolished. These results were confirmed using site directed mutagenesis protocols to generate internal deletions mutants of β-catenin that either lacked repeats 7, 10, 12, 6, or 5. Again, deletions of repeat 7, 10 or 12 had no effect in LBD-β-catenin interaction; deletion of repeat 6 or 5 abolished this interaction. In addition, analysis of AR transcriptional activity (measured by luciferase reporter construct, MMTVpA3-Luc), using β-catenin mutants lacking repeat 6 together with an AR expression vector, showed no enhancement of AR transcriptional activity in CV-1 (AR null) cells. The study by Yang et al., (2002) clearly described that armadillo repeats 1-6 were required for β-catenin AR interaction and AR directed transcriptional activity. However, the LXXLL motifs within β-catenin may not directly contribute to AR binding (Yang et al., 2002).

The LBD is thought to be sufficient for AR-β-catenin interactions. As mentioned previously, β-catenin alone can increase androgen dependent transcription. Using an androgen responsive MMTV LTR luciferase promoter assay, Song et al., (2003) demonstrated that when cells were co-transfected with a GAL4-AR LBD fusion protein and herpes simplex virus VP16-β-catenin fusion protein, there was a rescue of agonist dependent AF2 activity in the AR LBD. Moreover, co-transfection of the NTD and VP16-β-catenin had a synergistic effect on reporter expression (Song et al., 2003). This indicated that the LBD can change its conformation to form a binding area that accommodates co-activator binding. Accordingly, Song et al., (2003) reported that binding of β-catenin to the AR modulated the NTD through its interaction with the AF2 region and this interaction was adjacent but not identical to the AF2 binding site for TIF2. Residues K720 and Valine (V) 716 located on Helix 3 were necessary for AR- β-catenin and AR-TIF2 interaction, respectively (He et al., 1999; Song et al., 2003). Mutation to the AR LBD specifically at K720A reduced AR NTD interactions by 50% and completely abolished β-catenin binding. AR LBDs with either V716R or K720A were both able to maintain DHT ligand binding. Thus, the synergistic effects of β-catenin and NTD were mediated by the independent binding of each to the AR LBD (Song et al., 2003). In addition, two-hybrid interactions with GAL4-AR LBD and AR mutants that lost either the NTD [23]FQNLF[27] or the [433]WHTLF[437] motifs were able to reduce binding to the GAL4-AR LBD (Song et al., 2003). However, in the presence of VP16-β-catenin, there was still a mild interaction of the AR mutants with β-catenin. This suggested that the NTD/CTD interaction of the AR was required for the efficient interaction of the AR and β-catenin. Although, Song et al., (2003) reported that the effects of β-catenin on AR dependent transcription in the presence of TIF2 and/or NTD were small, β-catenin could modulate TIF2 activation of AR mediated MMTV-Luc reporter activity and enhanced the effects of AR NTD. In this case, β-catenin may be facilitating the stabilization and recruitment of additional transcriptional machinery to enhance transcriptional activation as it too, can directly form complexes with TIF2-AR complexes.

Bicalutamide, flutamide and cyproterone acetate (CPA) are the AR antagonists routinely used for CaP treatment. Hydroxyflutamide, the active metabolite of flutamide, are potent antagonists *in vivo*. Although these compounds can antagonize wildtype AR activation, these anti-androgens were also found to activate mutant ARs that were identified in patients. Moreover, β-catenin seemed to play a role in enhancing AR mutant transcriptional activity. The T877A mutation within the LBD is prevalent in hormone refractory CaP and *in vivo* studies have shown that T877A AR mutants could be stimulated by hydroxyflutamide but not by bicalutamide. Interestingly, Masiello et al., (2004) demonstrated that hydroxyflutamide liganded T877A AR was strongly activated by β-catenin and also stimulated interaction between the AR NTD and T877A LBD. In contrast, CPA liganded T877A mutant AR was not activated by β-catenin and neither was the CPA bound wildtype AR. While β-catenin mediated co-activation of the T877A AR was enhanced in the presence of hydroxyflutamide, T877A had no effect on β-catenin recruitment by CPA. Recently, a novel AR W741C (Tryptophan to Cysteine) mutation was isolated from bicalutamide treated LNCaP cells (Masiello et al, 2004). The significance of this mutant was that it was also identified in a patient receiving bicalutamide therapy. Interestingly, this mutation enable bicalutamide liganded W741C mutant AR to be activated by β-catenin. Such evidence shows that β-catenin is a key modulator AR structure, function and ligand sensitivity, all of which are contributing factors in prostate tumorigenesis to AI disease.

4.2 WNT/β-catenin signaling and AR

The activation of the Wnt signaling pathway results in the stabilization of β-catenin and its cytoplasmic accumulation. This requires deactivation of the destruction complex as well as β-catenin's phosphorylation at Tyrosine 142 (Tyr142). Phosphorylation at this site decreases β-catenin's interaction with α-catenin. Wang et al., (2008) used castration resistant mouse models to demonstrate consistently greater levels of Tyr142 phosphorylation of β-catenin together with increased AR expression in mouse samples. Gene expression studies also indicated that there was a decrease in Wnt transcription factors, Tcf-3 and LEF, as well as the target genes, MYC and CCND1, (Wang et al, 2008). Furthermore, β-catenin inhibitors including CSNK2B, CSK1E, GSK3B, TP53, WNT5A and PLCB4 were also decreased. Therefore, in AI disease progression, the cytoplasmic pool of β-catenin is increased while the downstream effects of β-catenin-TCF transcriptional activity are suppressed (Wang et al., 2008).

The notion that there was a direct interaction between the AR and β-catenin was first established by Truica et al., (2000), who demonstrated that β-catenin was able to enhance AR transactivation, alter the sensitivity of AR to ligands and relieve the repression of anti-androgens on AR mediated transcription. Using coimmunoprecipitation studies, Trucia et al., (2000) determined that β-catenin interacted with the AR in the absence of hormone in LNCaP cell lines which expressed the T877A mutant AR; however, upon administration of DHT, this interaction was increased. In addition, constitutive expression of a stabilized β-catenin (S33F), a mutant that increases β-catenin's half-life, potentiated luciferase reporter activity by 2.5 fold in the presence of androgen (similar results were also observed using the probasin promoter); β-catenin had no effect on reporter activity in the absence of androgen, signifying an androgen dependent mechanism. Similarly, expression of wild type AR in AR-negative cells, TSU-Pr1 and PC-3, increased AR transcriptional activity of a luciferase reporter 2-4 fold in the presence of androgen and β-catenin relative to baseline.

The modulatory role of β-catenin on AR ligand binding specificity was further confirmed by luciferase reporter assays that measured AR mediated transcription by β-catenin in the presence or absence of adrenal steroids, androstenedione and DHEA. Androstenedione and DHEA are weak androgens that mimic actions of testosterone. Transfection of S33F β-catenin and wild type AR in TSU-Pr1 cell lines showed increased AR-directed transcription with 1nM androstenedione which was comparable to the AR activation caused by 1nM testosterone. Alongside β-catenin's ability to increase AR sensitivity to ligands, β-catenin was also able to alter AR's specificity to ligand activation. Administration of R1881, an agonist of the AR, together with increasing concentrations of bicalutamide, diminished the antagonistic effects of bicalutamide in a dose dependent manner in the presence of β-catenin. Similar results were observed using estradiol. The above study by Trucia et al., (2000) was a novel development into prostate tumorigenesis as its etiology was no longer limited to AR directed transcription but now encompassed β-catenin, another oncogenic activator. β-catenin had the ability to structurally alter the AR LBD so that it may accommodate other steroids and ligands to enhance AR directed transcriptional activation. Hence, it seems as though β-catenin's role has moved beyond its functions as a co-regulator of TCF/LEF transcriptional activation to now include a greater purpose in modulating AR and/or Wnt directed prostate tumorigenesis.

The fact that β-catenin does not have a NLS make its function as a co-activator of transcriptional activity dependent on chaperones for nuclear import. β-catenin's ability to bind the AR provides β-catenin a means to enter the nucleus. Mulholland et al., (2002) provided novel evidence for ligand mediated AR-β-catenin nuclear translocation which was also accompanied by an increase in the expression of AR genes. Confocal microscopy data of LNCaP cells demonstrated that in the absence of ligand, AR was diffusely spread throughout the cells, while β-catenin was localized at the cell membrane, cytoplasm and nucleus. Upon administration of ligand, the AR and β-catenin both became strongly nuclear as observed by greater nuclear staining. There was a moderate decrease in cytoplasmic levels of β-catenin with no significant change at the cell borders (similar results were obtained from transient transfection of the AR using the AR-null PC-3 cell line). More importantly, co-localization of β-catenin and AR was present. Such evidence demonstrates that the AR mediated translocation of β-catenin was distinct from that of APC-β-catenin nuclear-cytoplasmic shuttling (Mulholland et al., 2002).

Mulholland et al., (2002) were also able to show an AR dependent binding of β-catenin to the probasin promoter and confirmed this specificity by antisense or shRNA knock down of β-catenin, which resulted in decreased PSA gene expression. This was also shown by Li et al., (2004), who demonstrated that β-catenin could be recruited to the PSA promoter. Such studies brought mechanistic insight into the co-regulatory functions of β-catenin and its role in differentially regulating AR responsive genes and downstream Wnt/AR transcription factors such as c-myc and the cyclins (Mulholland et al., 2002). Cyclin D1 is a regulator of cell cycle progression and was found to promote mitogenesis and antimitogeneic effects through activation of the cyclin dependent kinases dictated by the AF-1 domain of AR (Petre et al., 2002; Petre-Draviam et al., 2003; Mulholland et al., 2005). Interestingly, stabilization of β-catenin induced little change in cyclin D1 expression, although greatly increased the levels of c-myc (Gounari et al., 2002; Petre-Draviam et al., 2003; Mulholland et al., 2005). Currently, the relationship between cyclin D1 and β-catenin signaling activity is poorly correlated and literature agrees that increased cyclin D1 levels in prostate adenocarcinomas is a rare event and is not a clinical predictor of prognosis (Mulholland et al., 2005). On the other hand, cyclin D1 has been shown to bind the AR NTD in both ligand dependent and independent conditions, to mediate the repression of AR transcriptional activity. This interaction was also arbitrated without the requirement of an LXXLL motif (Reutens et al., 2001; Petre et al., 2002; Petre-Draviam et al., 2003; Mulholland et al., 2005). To date, cyclin D1 is well recognized as a co-repressor of the AR, however, the significance of this negative regulation conferred by cyclin D1 remains to be elucidated.

The crosstalk observed between the AR and Wnt targets, such as cyclin D1, questions whether other components of the Wnt/β-catenin pathway influence the oncogenicity of the AR. For example, Verras et al., (2004) demonstrated that cultured CaP cell lines activated by Wnt3a ligand increased AR transcriptional effects even without androgenic ligands; however, this was only observed in AR positive CaP cells. Using a PSA driven promoter luciferase assay, LNCaP cells treated with Wnt3a culture medium increased endogenous AR mediated transcription from the PSA promoter. Yang et al., (2006) further demonstrated that Wnt signaling could also increase AR mRNA expression. The AR gene is a target for Wnt signaling as TCF promoter binding elements are present within the AR promoter region. Surprisingly, even with greater levels of AR mRNA, the expression of AR protein was much reduced. Yang et al., (2006) suggested that the decrease in AR protein was likely associated with ubiquitin proteosomal degradation mediated by increased phosphorylation of MDM2 by phosphorylated AKT. Alternatively, Schweizer et al., (2008) showed that overexpression of AR in the presence of Wnt1 activation in PC-3, CWR22Rv1 and LNCaP led to an increase in luciferase reporter activity driven by a LEF-dependent promoter relative to Wnt1 stimulation alone. Based on these results, the AR seemed to have the ability to augment Wnt transcriptional activity in CaP cells. Treatment with agonists and antagonists of the AR, however, inhibited LEF reporter activity even in the presence of Wnt stimulation. Schweizer et al., (2008) reasoned that ligand bound AR may lead to interactions with other cofactors within the AR pathway thus, reducing the ability of the AR to signal through the Wnt/β-catenin pathway. Such cross regulation of the AR and TCF/LEF indicates that the Wnt and AR pathway can differentially regulate gene expression programs that can feedback onto each other. Moreover, AR signals can be potentiated under androgen ablation by Wnt or AR signal activation alone. This raises questions then, to how β-catenin, the common regulator between both pathways, contributes and divides its functions between AR and Wnt signaling.

4.3 β-catenin-TCF-AR axis

The evidence so far clearly indicates that β-catenin can interact with the AR to shuttle to the nucleus and modulate AR ligand specificity and transcriptional function (Truica et al, 2000, Chesire et al, 2002, Yang et al, 2002; Mulholland et al, 2002, Pawlowksi et al, 2002). Chesire & Isaacs, (2002) went on further to show that AR activity also had consequences for β-catenin/TCF target gene expression. Co-transfection of a luciferase reporter containing a PSA enhancer and probasin promoter (pBK-PSE-PB), and a β-catenin/TCF dependent reporter (pOT), demonstrated that AR positive cell lines (CWR22-Rv1 and LAPC-4) suppressed β-catenin/TCF signaling (CRT) in the presence of ligand. This was determined using a stabilized mutant β-catenin (identified in a hormone refractory patient) that had an interstitial deletion (Δ24-27) encompassing the entire GSK3β phosphorylation domain.

However, androgen induced suppression of CRT did not necessarily correlate with increased AR transcriptional activity. In AR dose response assays, CRT decreased as a function of total amount of liganded AR and not on AR transcriptional output. For example, overexpression of AR in CWR22-Rv1 cells reduced AR transcriptional activity; although the interference observed for ligand dependent CRT was more prominent (Chesire & Isaacs, 2002). Inhibition of CRT was also evident in cells with greater intrinsic CRT activity. Upon transient expression of AR and R1881 treatment, CRT in SW480 and HCT-116 (with loss of APC and APC mutations, respectively) was still inhibited. Alternatively, inhibition of the AR by anti-androgens such as CPA and bicalutamide alleviated androgen induced CRT repression. This suggested that AR mediated suppression of CRT was not dependent on cell specific factors (Chesire & Isaacs, 2002). Androgen dependent repression of CRT was also observed using a cyclin D1 promoter based luciferase reporter. Treatment of CWR22-Rv1 cells with AR ligand reduced the induction of cyclin D1 promoter by β-catenin. AR-negative cells did not have the same response, suggesting that AR expression was required for androgen induced CRT suppression (Chesire & Isaacs, 2002). Together with the fact that there is AR mediated repression of CRT as well as reduced CRT target gene expression of cyclin D1, it is unlikely that concentrations of cyclin D1 required to repress the AR during CaP progression would be achieved (Mulholland et al., 2005). Hence, negative regulation of cyclin D1 by the AR via the interference of CRT is likely a mechanism to counter regulate its co-repressor.

Co-factors bind liganded AR through the AR LBD, suggesting that β-catenin's modulatory function for AR and CRT activity may occur by the AR's restriction on TCF's access to β-catenin (Chesire & Isaacs, 2002). Using an AR expression construct deleted in its DBD (Δ538-614), Chesire & Isaacs, (2002) postulated that a mutant AR limited in its target gene expression capacity could retain its ability to bind to β-catenin through the LBD and inhibit CRT independent of AR target gene transcription. Despite the fact that previous studies demonstrated AR LBD alone was sufficient for β-catenin binding, Chesire & Isaacs, (2002) found that only the wildtype AR reduced CRT when compared to the mutant AR (Δ538-614). This was consistent with the fact that AR gene expression was not required for CRT interference. Further investigation showed that androgen dependent suppression of CRT was abolished with the overexpression of Tcf-4. Removing the N-terminal (ΔN) and HMG DNA binding domain (ΔHMG) of Tcf-4 (β-catenin and DNA binding sites, respectively) reduced the inhibition of CRT much less than wildtype Tcf-4. The Tcf-4 ΔNΔHMG double mutant was also unable to inhibit ligand dependent repression of CRT by the AR. Ectopic expression of Lef-1 conciliated AR signaling and potentiated CRT activity. This ultimately suggested that disruption of the AR-CRT equilibrium in CaP was likely due to a competition between Tcf-4 and AR for β-catenin.

In order to establish the mechanism by which this competition was occurring, Chesire & Isaacs, (2002) further evaluated the effects of Tcf-4 on AR transcription. Full length, ΔN, and/or ΔHMG constructs of Tcf-4 (which all fail to bind β-catenin) were able to impede AR activation of the pBK-PSE-PB promoter and block R1881 induced AR activity. Chesire & Isaacs, (2002) suggested that AR transcription by Tcf-4 likely did not involve decreased β-catenin access by TCF itself. It was more likely that CRT suppression was rather a consequence of the competition for β-catenin rather than AR target gene expression. Mulholland et al., (2003) lends further support to this hypothesis through the use of transcriptional reporter assays which demonstrated that wildtype TCF reduced the activity of AR (ARR3-Luc)-responsive reporter, while the ΔN TCF mutant did not have such an effect. Alternatively, when PC-3 cells were co-transfected with NTD/DBD or LBD/DBD AR deletion mutants and a TCF promoter luciferase reporter construct, TOPflash, the LBD/DBD mutants were capable of repressing TOPflash luciferase activity in the presence of DHT, while the NT/DBD mutant was not able to do so. TOPflash activity was repressed in a dose dependent manner and alternatively, Casodex was able to alleviate this repression. Thus, the LBD but not the NTD is required for TCF repression. Mulholland et al., (2003) went further to show that there was co-localization of TCF and AR within the nucleus. Using deconvolution microscopy, co-transfection of HcRed-Tcf and AR-EGFP constructs in LNCaP, SW480, and PC3, resulted in partial colocalization of Tcf and AR in the presence of DHT. In addition, co-expression of β-catenin-EGFP constructs with HcRed-AR or HcRed-TCF in LNCaP cells demonstrated a reduced colocalization of β-catenin with TCF upon treatment of DHT and correspondingly, increased colocalization of β-catenin and the AR; in the absence of DHT there was an increased colocalization of β-catenin with TCF. This suggested that β-catenin had the ability to shuttle between the AR and TCF androgen dependently (Mulholland et al., 2003). Treatment with Casodex reduced AR mediated depletion of TCF-β-catenin interaction and diminished androgen sensitive co-immunoprecipitation of endogenous AR and β-catenin (Mulholland et al., 2003).

It has been previously shown that steroid hormone receptor binding can be enhanced by an HMG DBD (Amir et al., 2003). For example, Yuan et al., (2001) determined that the AR can interact with sequence specific HMG box transcription factor SRY, a member of the SOX family of HMG proteins. Likewise, Tcf-4 is a sequence specific HMG transcription factor. Amir et al., (2003) demonstrated a direct interaction between Tcf-4 and AR via the AR DBD, independent of β-catenin. Using a glutathione-S-transferase (GST) fusion protein pull-down experiments, Amir et al., (2003) showed that ^{35}S-labeled Tcf-4 bound specifically to the GST-AR-DBD (aa 556-628) fusion protein (deleted in both the AR NTD and LBD). Tcf-4 did not bind the the AR hinge region (aa 634-668). Alternatively, Amir et al., (2003) confirmed that Tcf-4 repression of AR transcriptional activity was independent of β-catentin. They hypothesized that Tcf-4 repression of AR signaling may be due to the sequestration of β-catenin rather than a direct AR-Tcf-4 interaction. However, co-transfection of CV-1 (AR null) with AR expression vector, pSVARo, ARE$_4$-Luciferase reporter, and, β-catenin and Tcf-4 expression vectors only resulted in a partial reversal of Tcf-4 mediated repression of AR transcriptional activity relative to Tcf-4 expression alone. This was despite the fact that quantities of β-catenin transfected into the CV-1 cells could readily enhance AR activity. In order to confirm that the results observed were mediated by direct Tcf-4 and AR DBD interaction and not due to AR-β-catenin interactions, CV-1 cells were co-transfected with a VP16-AR DBD (aa 501-660) fusion protein and Tcf-4. Similar to wildtype AR the VP16-AR-DBD (aa 501-660) could be repressed by Tcf-4. This supported that AR transcriptional activity was not due to any negative effects of AR-β-catenin binding and was directly a result of an interaction between Tcf-4 and the AR. The fact that β-catenin could only partially reverse Tcf-4 mediated AR transcriptional activity suggested that β-catenin may lack the ability to displace a co-repressor. Co-repressor activity of Grouch/TLE proteins have been well recognized to repress Tcf-4 mediated signaling. Previously, it has been demonstrated that Groucho/TLE could bind the AR N-terminus and decrease AR transcriptional activity (Shroder, 1993; Amir et al., 2003). The limited capacity of β-catenin to alleviate Tcf-4 repression may possibly be due to its inability to compete with AR-Tcf-4-Groucho/TLE complexes (Amir et al., 2003).

Alterntively, Amir et al., (2003) went on to show that TCF could recruit β-catenin to the AR in the absence of the AR LBD. Tcf-4 binds β-catenin at its N-terminus leaving the C-terminal HMG domain free for AR binding. Thus, Amir et al., (2003) reasoned that Tcf-4 may serve to recruit β-catenin to the Tcf-4-AR complex. First, Amir et al., (2003) confirmed that β-catenin alone did not bind GST-AR-DBD. This was not surprising as it has consistently been shown that β-catenin binds to the AR LBD. Interestingly, upon co-incubation of both β-catenin and Tcf-4 with GST-AR DBD (aa 556-628), co-immunoprecipitation studies demonstrated an increase in β-catenin interaction with Tcf-4-GST-AR DBD (aa 556-628) complexes. Thus, the two β-catenin binding sites within AR-Tcf-4 complex serves as a sensitive target for β-catenin mediated transcriptional activation and also provides co-operative regulatory control over both AR and Wnt target genes (Amir et al., 2003).

The evidence for the TCF-β-catenin-AR axis is still at its infancy. However, studies strongly support the cross regulatory mechanisms that are in play between β-catenin, TCF, and AR during CaP progression. The abovementioned reports suggest that β-catenin can shift its attention between AR and TCF in an androgen dependent manner in addition to modulating AR ligand specificity, sensitivity, and transcriptional activity. Additionally, the fact that there is direct competition for β-catenin by TCF and AR transcriptional machinery further adds to the complexity of the AR-β-catenin axis and introduces another contributing factor for β-catenin mediated regulation of Wnt and AR signaling in CaP progression.

4.4 β-catenin-PI3K-AR axis

The Phosphatidylinositol-3 Kinase (PI3K) and Wnt pathway have both been implicated in the progression of CaP. Specifically, there is interplay between these two pathways through the common factor, GSK3β. Moreover, the loss of the tumor suppressor and negative regulator of the PI3K pathway, PTEN is a common occurrance in CaP causing the constitutive activation of the PI3K pathway. Consequently, there is an increased activation of the end effector protein, AKT, through its phosphorylation at key serine and threonine residues. Excessive activation of AKT results in increased cell growth, cell survival and inhibition to apoptosis. AKT has many substrates, however, for the purposes of this review we will focus on GSK3β. Activation of AKT leads to the inhibition of GSK3β through its phosphorylation at Ser9 resulting in the subsequent accumulation of β-catenin. In effect, the association between AKT-GSK3β and GSK3β-β-catenin bring the PI3K and Wnt pathways, respectively, at a junction where β-catenin's stability and nuclear availability for AR transactivation may be regulated.

Many cell lines of metastatic (LNCaP, PC-3) or AI (22RV-1) CaP have highly active PI3K/AKT activity which has also been correlated with a increased Gleason grade (Mulholland et al., 2006). To further elucidate the role of the PI3K pathway in CaP progression, Sharma et al., (2002) demonstrated that the inhibition of the PI3K pathway by LY294002 inhibited AR transactivation of the PSA gene in LNCaP cells. As expected, phosphorylation of GSK3β was reduced and nuclear levels of β-catenin correspondingly decreased 2-3 fold upon LY294002 treatment. Co-expression of a dominantly active AKT reversed this inhibition of AR activity. This suggested that repression of AR activity by LY294002 was through the inhibition of PI3K and the subsequent inactivation of AKT activity (Sharma et al, 2002). To confirm that LY294002 mediated repression was through GSK3β, Sharma et al., (2002) used a wildtype β-catenin or a β-catenin mutant containing a point mutation within the N-terminal GSK3β phosphorylation site, to demonstrate that AR transcriptional expression was only reduced by LY294002 for wildtype β-catenin and not for the β-catenin mutant. Since this mutant was void of a GSK3β binding site, the results from this study suggested that GSK3β was involved in β-catenin regulation of AR activity through the PI3K pathway (Sharma et al., 2002).

GSK3β is ubiquitously expressed within CaP cells, including LNCaP, PC-3 and DU145 (Wang et al., 2004). Wang et al., (2004) showed that GSK3β could regulate the AR through its phosphorylation. Using purified GST tagged AR N-terminal (aa 38-560), GST-AR DBD-LBD (aa 551-918) and His$_6$-AR LBD (aa 666-918), Wang et al., (2004) demonstrated that GSK3β significantly phosphorylated the AR N-terminal (aa 38-560), while only slightly phosphorylating the DBD-LBD and LBD fragments. Furthermore, the presence of GSK3β inhibited GAL4-AR-N-terminal transcriptional response to a luciferase reporter (pG5-Luc) but did not do so for the GAL4-AR LBD which contained the AF2 domain. This suggested that the inhibition of AR transactivation by GSK3β was likely mediated by the NTD AF1 domain.

In order to confirm GSK3β's regulatory role on the AR, Wang et al., (2004) examined AR activity in LNCaP cells transfected with an androgen responsive luciferase reporter (MMTV-Luc) and wildtype GSK3β. The addition of GSK3β reduced AR activity in a dose dependent manner which was then alleviated by lithium chloride (LiCl) treatment (an inhibitor of GSK3β) (Wang et al., 2004). The physical association of GSK3β to the AR was shown through GST pull down assays which demonstrated that the GSK3β interacting domain within the AR was on both the AR NTD and CTD (Wang et al., 2004, Wang et al., 2006). Thus, these results suggested that GSK3β mediates its inhibitory effects by phosphorylating the AR to diminish the interaction between the NTD and CTD, which is necessary for AR transcriptional activity (Salas et al., 2004; Wang et al, 2004; Mulholland et al., 2001).

Tyrosine 216 (Tyr216) phosphorylation of GSK3β is an activating modification that was found to be increased upon androgen stimulation (Liao et al., 2003). Phosphorylation of Tyr216 was inhibited by bicalutamide or by LY294002 suggesting that the PI3K pathway was required for androgen induced GSK3β Tyr216 phosphorylation (Salas et al., 2003). Moreover, the distribution of GSK3β was also dependent on its phosphorylation status. Using GSK3β mutants, Y216F and a GSK3β deleted at its first nine amino acids (GSK3βΔ9), the Y216F mutant was predominantly found in the cytoplasm while the GSK3βΔ9 was more dominant in the nucleus and able to co-localize with the AR in the presence of the androgens. The accumulation of the GSK3βΔ9 was also associated with the suppression of AR mediated transcription which was thought to be due to the elevated phosphorylation of the AR by GSK3β (Salas et al., 2003). Salas et al., (2003) went further to show that the AR and GSK3β were capable of co-localizing in the nucleus using immunohistochemical analysis which supported the physical interaction between these two molecules.

In contrast, some studies have reported that GSK3β was necessary for AR mediated gene expression rather than its inhibition (Liao et al., 2003; Mazor et al., 2004). Using a PSA- SEAP reporter (androgen responsive secreted alkaline phosphatase reporter; described in Ref.24 of Liao et al., 2003) transfected into LNCaP cells (known to have inactivated GSK3β due to Ser9 phosphorylation) treated with LiCl in the presence or absence of R1881 agonist, Liao et al., (2003) demonstrated that LiCl abolished androgen dependent PSA-SEAP activity; this was also evident for cells treated with PI3K inhibitor LY294002. Furthermore, LiCl treatment on LAPC-4 cell line (containing wildtype AR and PTEN) dramatically suppressed PSA expression in the presence of R1881 (Liao et al., 2003). This effect was further confirmed with siRNA knockdown of GSK3β gene. Mazor et al., (2004) also supports this hypothesis by demonstrating that overexpression of GSK3β in LNCaP cells increased AR transcriptional activity. Interestingly, there was a decrease in AR protein levels upon GSK3β inhibition (Mazor et al., 2004). Mazor et al., (2004) suggested that GSK3β's ability to phosphorylate AR may also increase AR stability as GSK3β has been shown to regulate the stability of many proteins such as Axin, and β-catenin.

Clearly there is evidence supporting PI3K/AKT/GSK3β role in AR transactivation, however, the mechanism of GSK3β activity through this pathway in CaP progression still remains elusive and conflicting. Mulholland et al., (2006) comments on this paradoxical effect and postulates that it is likely that basal activity of GSK3β is required for AR function and any increase in GSK3β activity such as the case for phosphorylated Tyr216, may result in decreased AR function directly through AR phosphorylation or indirectly by influencing β-catenin stabilization.

5. Current therapy, implications and future directions

The reciprocal interactions and interplay between the AR/Wnt-β-catenin axis suggests that the underlying mechanism potentiating CaP progression is complex and impacts the very balance of these prosurvival pathways. Current literature shows that there is indeed crosstalk between the AR and Wnt pathway occuring at various levels: a) Wnt ligands transactivate the AR, b) β-catenin interacts with the AR to increase AR mediated transcriptional activity, c) GSK3β negatively regulates AR transcription through the PI3K pathway, d) cyclin D1 (TCF/LEF target gene) can interact with AR to inhibit AR transcriptional activity, and e) competition for β-catenin occurs between AR and TCF/LEF (summarized in Wang et al., 2008). The integration of these oncogenic pathways potentiates the progression from AD-CaP to AI-CaP whereby cell growth and survival, in part, hinges on the availability of β-catenin. Furthermore, the modulatory role of β-catenin on AR expression and transactivation, and ligand specificity and sensitivity, suggests that β-catenin works through a range of intensities. Accordingly, the design of future therapeutic strategies will require the dynamic interplay between AR and β-catenin to be addressed.

The transition from AD-CaP to AI-CaP in prostate carcinogenesis provides major clinical challenges. Androgen ablation and/or anti-androgen therapies are only temporarily effective. Such therapies yield a hormone refractory tumor that is essentially untreatable with the most effective standard chemotherapeutic regimens only increasing patient survival for 2 months (Shen & Shen, 2010). The recent developments on β-catenin's regulatory function in altering the structural intergrity of the AR poses a dilemma for anti-androgens (Eg. bicalutamide, flutamide and CPA) as these agents lose their efficacy in the presence of β-catenin's modulatory effects. Moreover, the ability of β-catenin/Wnt pathway to synergistically heighten AR signaling together with non-genomic cross talk between other pro-survival factors make targetable areas for therapy difficult. Future therapies will have to be evaluated according to tumour type and be individualized to specific alterations that occur during CaP progression (Ewan & Dale, 2008). Specifically, putative chemotherapeutic agents that inhibit the shuttling of β-catenin into the nucleus (Yardy & Brewster, 2005) or those that abolish potential oncogenic AR/β-catenin interactions such as inhibitors that target AR LBD or the first six armadillo repeats may be effective (Mulholland et al, 2005). Furthermore, inhibition of upstream Wnt or PI3K signaling may pose a viable option (Mulholland et al, 2005). The caveat for such therapeutic designs is that the Wnt pathway is important for normal cell renewal; therefore, the goal is to balance therapeutic effects with minimal harm to cellular homeostasis (Ewan & Dale, 2008).

The oncogenic role of the Wnt/β-catenin pathway in CaP progression is clearly evident. However, the mechanisms underlying the interplay between Wnt and AR signaling still remains unclear. Therefore, understanding how β-catenin-AR-TCF interaction and Wnt-AR crosstalk are regulated in CaP progression will provide a means to elucidate the complexities and contexts of AI disease that are necessary for successful therapeutic intervention.

6. References

Adler, AJ., Scheller, A., Robins, DM. (1993). The stringency and magnitude of androgen-specific gene activation are combinatorial functions of receptor and nonreceptor binding site sequences. *Mol Cell Biol,* Vol 13(10), pp. 6326-6335

Amir, AL., Barua, M., McKnight, NC., Cheng, S., Yuan, X., & Balk, SP. (2003). A direct beta-catenin-independent interaction between androgen receptor and T cell factor 4. *J Biol Chem,* Vol.278, pp. 30828-30834, ISSN 0021-9258

Behrens, J., Jerchow, BA., Wurtele, M., et al. (1998). Functional interation of an axin homolog, conductin, with beta-catenin, APC, and GSK3beta. *Science,* Vol 280, pp.596-599

Behrens, J., Vakaet, L., Friis, R., Winterhager, E., van Roy, F., Mareel, MM., Birchmeier, W. (1993). Loss of epithelial differentiation and gain of invasiveness correlates with tyrosine phosphorylation of E-cadherin/β-catenin complex in cells transformed with a temperature-sensitive vsrc gen. *J cell Biol,* Vol. 120, 757-766

Bennett, NC., Gardiner, RA., Hooper, JD., Johnson, DW., & Gobe, GC. (2010). Molecular cell biology of androgen receptor signalling. *Int J Biochem Cell Biol,* Viol.42, pp. 813-827, ISSN 1357-2725

Bierie, B., Nozawa, M., Renou, JP., Shillingford, JM., Morgan, F., Oka, T., Taketo, MM., Cardiff, RD., Miyoshi, K., Wagner, KU., Robinson, GW., & Hennighausen, L. (2003). Activation of beta-catenin in prostate epithelium induces hyperplasias and squamous transdifferentiation. *Oncogene,* Vol.22, pp. 3875-3887, ISSN 0950-9232

Bienz, M., & Clevers, H. (2000). Linking colorectal cancer to Wnt signaling. *Cell,* Vol. 103, pp. 311-320

Bisson I., Prowse, D.M. (2009) Wnt signaling regulates self renewal and differentiation of prostate cancer cells with stem cell characteristics. *Cell Research,* Vol 19:683-697.

Blok, LJ., de Ruiter, PE., Brinkmann, AO. (1998). Forskolin-induced dephosphorylation of the androgen receptor impairs ligand binding. *Biochemistry,* Vol. 37(11), pp. 3850-3857

Bonfil, RD., Dong, Z., Trindade Filho, JC., Sabbota, A., Osenkowski, P., Nabha, S., Yamamoto, H., Chinni, SR., Zhao, H., Mobshery, S., Vessella, RL., Fridman, R., Cher, ML. (2007). Prostate cancer-associated membrane type1-matrix metalloproteinase: a pivotal role in bone response and intraosseous tumor growth. *Am J Pathol,* Vol. 170(6), pp. 2100-2111

Brembeck, FH S-RT., Bakkers, J., Wilhelm, S., Hammerschmidt, M., & Birchmeier, W. (2004). Essential role of BCL9-2 in the switch between beta-catenin's adhesive and transcriptional functions. *Gene Development,* Vol.18, pp. 2225-2230

Brewster, SF., Browne, S., & Brown, KW. (1994). Somatic allelic loss at the DCC, APC, nm23-H1 and p53 tumor suppressor gene loci in human prostatic carcinoma. *J Urol,* Vol.151, pp. 1073-1077, ISSN 0022-5347

Brockhausen, I., Schachter, H., & Stanley, P. (2009). O-GalNAc Glycans. In: *Essentials of Glycobiology,* pp. 115-129, n.d., Cold Spring Harbor Laboratory Press, New York

Bruxvoort, KJ., Charbonneau, HM., Giambernardi, TA., Goolsby, JC., Qian, CN., Zylstra, CR., Robinson, DR., Roy-Burman, P., Shaw, AK., Buckner-Berghuis, BD., Sigler, RE., Resau, JH., Sullivan, R., Bushman, W., & Williams, BO. (2007). Inactivation of Apc in the mouse prostate causes prostate carcinoma. *Cancer Res,* Vol.67, pp. 2490-2496, ISSN 0008-5472

Callewaert, L., Verrijdt, G., Christianens, V., Haelens, A., Classens, F. (2003). Dual function of an amino-terminal amphipatic helix in androgen receptor-mediated transactivation through specific and nonspecific response elements. *The Journal of Biological Chemistry,* Vol. 278 (10), pp. 8212-8218

Callewaert, L., Van Tilborgh, H., Claessens, F. (2006). Interplay between two hormone-independent activation domains in the androgen receptor. *Cancer Res,* Vol. 66(1), pp. 543-553

Castano, J., Raurell, I., Piedra, JA., Miravet, S., Dunach, M., & Garcia de Herreros, A. (2002). Beta-catenin N- and C-terminal tails modulate the coordinated binding of adherens junction proteins to beta-catenin. *J Biol Chem,* Vol.277, pp. 31541-31550, ISSN 0021-9258

Chamberlain, ML., Driver, ED., Miesfeld, RL. (1994). The length and location of CAG trinucleotide repeats in the androgen receptor N-terminal domain affect transactivation function. *Nucleic Acids Res,* Vol. 22(15), pp. 3181-3186

Chamberlain, NL., Whitacre, DC., Miesfeld, RL. (1996). Delineation of two distinct type 1 activation functions in the androgen receptor amino-terminal domain. *J Biol Chem,*Vol. 271(46), pp. 26772-26778

Chan, SK., & Struhl, G. (2002). Evidence that Armadillo transduces *wingless* by mediating nuclear export or cytosolic activation of Pangolin. *Cell,* Vol. 111, pp.481

Chang, CY., & McDonnell, DP. (2002). Evaluation of ligand-dependent changes in AR structure using peptide probes.*Mol Endocrinol,* Vol. 16, pp. 440-454

Cheng, S., Brzostek, S., Lee, SR., Hollenberg, AN., Balk, SP. (2002). Inhibition of the dihydrotestosterone-activated androgen receptor by nuclear receptor corepressor. *Mol Endocrinol,* Vol. 16(7), pp. 1492-1501

Chernyavsky, AI., Arredondo, J., Marubio, LM., Grando, & SA. (2004). Differential regulation of keratinocyte chemokinesis and chemotaxis through distinct nicotinic receptor subtypes. *J Cell Sci,* Vol.117, pp. 5665-5679

Chesire, DR., Ewing, CM., Sauvageot, J., Bova, GS., & Isaacs, WB. (2000). Detection and analysis of beta-catenin mutations in prostate cancer. *Prostate,* Vol.45, pp. 323-334, ISSN 0270-4137

Chesire, DR., Ewing, CM., Gage, WR., & Isaacs, WB. (2002). In vitro evidence for complex modes of nuclear beta-catenin signaling during prostate growth and tumorigenesis. *Oncogene,* Vol.21, pp. 2679-2694, ISSN 0950-9232

Chesire, DR., & Isaacs, WB. (2002). Ligand-dependent inhibition of beta-catenin/TCF signaling by androgen receptor. *Oncogene,* Vol.21, pp. 8453-8469, ISSN 0950-9232

Chien, AJ., Conrad, WH., & Moon, RT. (2009). A Wnt survival guide: from flies to human disease. *J Invest Dermatol*, Vol.129, pp. 1614-1627, ISSN 0022-202X

Choi, HJ., Huber, AH., & Weis, WI. (2006). Thermodynamics of beta-catenin-ligand interactions: the roles of the N- and C-terminal tails in modulating binding affinity. *J Biol Chem*, Vol.281, pp. 1027-1038, ISSN 0021-9258

Choong, CS., & Wilson, EM. (1998). Trinucleotide repeats in the human androgen receptor: a molecular basis for disease, *J Mol Endocrinol*, Vol. 21(3), pp. 235-257

Claessens, F., Alen, P., Devos, A., Peeters, B., Verhoeven, G., Rombauts, W. the androgen-specific probasin response element 2 interacts differentially with androgen and glucocorticoid receptors. *J Biol Chem*, Vol. 271(32), pp. 19013-19016

Clevers, H. (2006). Wnt/beta-catenin signaling in development and disease. *Cell*, Vol.127, pp. 469-480, ISSN 0092-8674

Craft, N., Shostak, ., Carey, M., Sawyer, C.. (1999). A mechanism for hormone independent prostate cancer through modulation of androgen receptor signaling by HER-2/neu tyrosine kinase. *Nature Me* Vol. 5, pp. 280-285.

Crocitto, LE., Henderson, BE., Coetzee, GA. (1997). Identification of two germline point mutations in the 5'UTR of the androgen receptor gene in men with prostate cancer. *J Urol*, Vol. 158, pp.1599-1601

Cronauer, MV., Schulaz, WA., Ackermann, R., & Burchardt, M. (2004). Effects of WNT/beta-catenin pathway activation on signaling through T-cell factor and androgen receptor in prostate cancer cell lines. *International Journal of Oncology*, Vol.26, pp. 1033-1040

Culig, Z. et al. (1999). Swith from antagonist to agonist of the androgen receptor vicalutamide is associated with proate tumour proresson in a new model system. *Br. J. Cancer*, Vol 81, pp.242-251.

Culig, Z., Hobisch, A., Cronauer, MV., Radmayr, C., Trapman, J., Hittmair, A., Bartssch, G., Klocker, H. (1994). Androgen receptor activation in prostatic tumor cell lines by insulin-like growth factor-1, keratinocyte growth factor, and epidermal growth factor. *Cancer Res*, Vol. 54(20), pp. 5474-5478

Cutress, ML., Whitaker, HC., Mills, IG, Stewart, M., Neal, DE. (2008). Structural basis for the nuclear import of the human androgen receptor. *J Cell Sci*, Vol. 121 (Part 7), pp.957-968

Dajani, R., Fraser, E., Roe, SM., Yeo, M., Good, VM., Thompson, V., Dale, TC., Pearl, LH. (2003). Structural basis for recruitment of glycogen synthase kinase 3beta to the axin-APC scaffold complex. *EMBO J*, Vol. 22(3), pp.494-501

Danguy, A., Camby, I., & Kiss, R. (2002). Galectins and cancer. *Biochim Biophys Acta*, Vol.1572, pp. 285-293, ISSN 0006-3002

Daniels, DL., & Weis, WI. (2002). ICAT inhibits beta-catenin binding to Tcf/Lef-family transcription factors and the general coactivator p300 using independent structural modules. *Mol Cell*, Vol.10, pp. 573-584, ISSN 1097-2765

Darimont, BD., Wagner, RL., Apriletti, JW, Stallcup, MR., Kushner, PJ., Baxter, JD., Fletterick, RJ., Yamamoto, KR. (1998). Structure and specificity of nuclear receptor-coactivator interactions. *Genes Dev*, Vol. 12, pp. 3343-3356

Davidson, G., Wu, W., Shen, J., Bilic, J., Fenger, U., Stannek, P., Glinka, A., & Niehrs, C. (2005). Casein kinase 1 gamma couples Wnt receptor activation to cytoplasmic signal transduction. *Nature*, Vol.438, pp. 867-872, ISSN 0028-0836

De Ferrari, GV., Papassotiropoulos, A., Biechele, T., Wavrant De-Vrieze, F., Avila, ME., Major, MB., Myers, A., Saez, K., Henriquez, JP., Zhao, A., Wollmer, MA., Nitsch, RM., Hock, C., Morris, CM., Hardy, J., & Moon, RT. (2007). Common genetic variation within the low-density lipoprotein receptor-related protein 6 and late-onset Alzheimer's disease. *Proc Natl Acad Sci U S A*, Vol. 104, pp. 9434-9439, ISSN 0027-8424

Ding, D., Xu, L., Mennon, M., Reddy, GP., Barrack, ER. (2004). Effect of a short CAG (glutamine) repeat on human androgen receptor function. *Prostate,*Vol. 58(1), pp.23-32

Drees, F., Pokutta, S., Yamada, S., Nelson, WJ., & Weis, WI. (2005). Alpha-catenin is a molecular switch that binds E-cadherin-beta-catenin and regulates actin-filament assembly. *Cell*, Vol.123, pp. 903-915

Eger, A., Stockinger, A., Schaffhauser, B., Beug. H., & Foisner, R. (2000). Epithelial mesenchymal transition by c-Fos estrogen receptor activation involves nuclear translocation of beta-catenin and upregulation of beta-catenin/lymphoid enhancer binding factor-1 transcriptional activity. *J Cell Biol*, Vol.148, pp. 173-188, ISSN 0021-9525

Eger, A., Stockinger, A., Park, J., Langkopf, E., Mikula. M., Gotzmann, J., Mikulits, W., Beug, H., Foisner, R. (2004). beta-Catenin and TGFbeta signalling cooperate to maintain a mesenchymal phenotype after FosER-induced epithelial to mesenchymal transition. *Oncogene*, Vol.23, pp. 2672-2680, ISSN 0950-9232

Ewan, KB., & Dale, TC. (2008). The potential for targeting oncogenic WNT/beta-catenin signaling in therapy. *Curr Drug Targets*, Vol.9, pp. 532-547, ISSN 1389-4501

Ewing, CM., Ru, N., Morton, RA., Rovinson, MJ., Wheelock, KR., Johnson, et al. (1995). Chromosome 5 suppresses tumorigenicity of PC3 prostate cancers: correlation with tumour invasion. *Br J Cancer*, Vol. 55, pp.4813-4817

Fang, D., Hawke, D., Zheng, Y., Xia, Y., Meisenhelder, J., Nika, H., Mills, GB., Kobayashi, R., Huntr, T., & Lu, Z. (2007). Phosphorylation of beta-catenin by AKT promotes beta-catenin transcriptional activity. *J Biol Chem*, Vol.282, pp. 11221-11229, ISSN 0021-9258

Fearon, ER. (1995). Molecular genetics of colorectal cancer. *Ann N Y Acad Sci*, Vol.768, pp. 101-110, ISSN 0077-8923

Feldman, BJ., & Feldman, D. (2001). The development of androgen-independent prostate cancer. *Nat Rev Cancer*, Vol.1, pp. 34-45, ISSN 1474-175X

Fink, CC., Bayer, KU., Myers, JW., Ferrell JE, Jr., Schulman, H., Meyer, T. (2003). Selective regulation of neurite extension and synapse formation by the beta but not the alpha isoform of CaMKII. *Neuron*, Vol.39, pp. 283-297, ISSN 0896-6273

Fu, M., Rao, M., Wu, K., Wang, C., Zhang, S., Hessien, M., Yeung, YG., Gioeli, D., Weber, ,MJ., Pestell, RG. (2004). The androgen receptor acetylation site regulates cAMP and AKT but not ERK-induced activity. *J Biol Chem*, Vol. 279(28), pp. 29436-29449

Gaddipati, JP., McLEod, DG., Heidenberg, HB., Sesterhenn, IA., Finger, MJ., Moul, JW., Srivastava, S. (1994). Frequent detection of codon 877 mutation in the androgen receptor gene in advanced prostate cancers. *Cancer Res*, Vol. 54(11), pp. 2861-2864

Gelmann, EP. (2002). Molecular biology of the androgen receptor. *J Clin Oncol*, Vol.20, pp. 3001-3015, ISSN 0732-183X

Gerstein, AV., Almeida, TA., Zhao, G., Chess, E., Shih Ie, M., Buhler, K., Pienta, K., Rubin, MA., Vessella, R., & Papadopoulos, N. (2002). APC/CTNNB1 (beta-catenin) pathway alterations in human prostate cancers. *Genes Chromosomes Cancer*, Vol.34, pp. 9-16, ISSN 1045-2257

Gewirth, DT., & Sigler, PB. (1995). The basis for half-site specificity explored through a non-cognate steroid receptor-DNA complex. *Nat Struc Biol*, Vol. 2, pp. 386-394

Gioeli, D., Ficarro, SB., Kwiek, JJ., Aaronson, D., Hancock, M., Catling, AD., White, FM., Christian, RE., Settlage, RE., Shabanowitz, J., Hunt , DF., Weber, MJ. (2002). Androgen receptor phosphorylation. Regulation and identification of the phosphorylation sites. *J Biol Chem*, Vol. 277(32), pp. 29304-29314

Glass DA., 2nd, Bialek, P., Ahn, JD., Starbuck, M., Patel, MS., Clevers, H., Taketo, MM., Long, F., McMahon, AP., Lang, RA., & Karsenty, G. (2005). Canonical Wnt signaling in differentiated osteoblasts controls osteoclast differentiation. *Dev Cell*, Vol.8, pp. 751-764, ISSN 1534-5807

Gottardi, CJ., & Gumbiner, BM. (2001). How beta-catenin interacts with its partners. *Current Biology*, Vol.11, pp. 792-794, ISSN 0960-9822

Gottardi, CJ., & Gumbiner, BM. (2004). Distinct molecular forms of beta-catenin are targeted to adhesive or transcriptional complexes. *J Cell Biol*, Vol.167, pp. 339-349, ISSN 0021-9525

Gottardi, CJ., & Peifer, M. (2008). Terminal regions of beta-catenin come into view. *Structure*, Vol.16, pp. 336-338, ISSN 0969-2126

Gounari, F., Signoretti, S., Bronson, R., Klein, L., Sellers, WR., Kum, J., Siermann, A., Taketo, MM., von Boehmer, H., KKhazaie, K. (2002). Stabilization of β-catenin induces lesions reminiscent of prostatic intraepithelial neoplasia, but terminal squamous transdifferentiation of other secretory epithelia. *Oncogene*, Vol. 21, pp. 4099-4107

Gregory, CW., Johnson, RT Jr., Mohler, JL., French, FS., Wilson, EM. (2001). Androgen receptor stabilization in recurrent prostate cancer is associated with hypersensitivity to low androgen. *Cancer Res*, Vol. 61(7), pp. 2892-2898

Graham, TA., Weaver, C., Mao, F., Kimelman, D., Xu, W. (2000). Crystal structure of a beta-catenin/Tcf complex. *Ell*, Vol 103., pp 885-896

Grossmann, ME., Huang, H., Tindall, DJ. (2001). Androgen receptor signaling in androgen-refractory prostate cancer. *J Natl Cancer Inst*, Vol 93, pp.1687-1697

Gruber, SB., Chen, H., Tomsho, LP., Lee, M., Perrone, EE., Cooney, KA. (2003). R726L androgen receptor mutation is uncommon in prostate cancer families in the united states. *Prostate*, Vol. 54(4), pp. 306-309

Guinez, C., Morelle, W., Michalski, JC., & Lefebvre, T. (2005). O-GlcNAc glycosylation: a signal for the nuclear transport of cytosolic proteins? *Int J Biochem Cell Biol*, Vol.37, pp. 765-774, ISSN 1357-2725

Haelens, A., Verrijdt. G,, Callewaert. L., Christiaens, V., Schauwaers, K., Peeters, B., Rombauts, W., & Claessens, F. (2003). DNA recognition by the androgen receptor: evidence for an alternative DNA-dependent dimerization, and an active role of sequences flanking the response element on transactivation. *Biochem J*, Vol.369, pp. 141-151, ISSN 0264-6021

Hall, CL., Daignault, SD., Shah, RB., Pienta, KJ., Keller, ET. (2008). Dickkopf-1 expression increases early in prostate cancer development and decreases during progression from primary tumor to metastasis. *Prostate*, Vol. 68(13), pp. 1396-1404

Han, G., Foster, B.A., Mistry, S., Buchanan, G., Harris., J.M., Tilley, W.D., Greenberg, N.M. (2001). Hormone statis selects for spontaneous somatic androgen receptor variant that demonstrate specific ligand and cofactor dependent activities in autochthonous prostate cancer. *The Journal of Biological Chemistry* Vol.276 (14), pp.11204-11213

Han, G., Buchanan, G., Ittmann, M., Harris, JM., Yu, X., & DeMayo, FJ. (2005). Mutation of the androgen receptor causes oncogenic transformation of the prostate. *PNAS*, Vol.102, No.4, pp. 1151-1156

Hart, G. W., & Akimoto, Y. (2009). The O-GlcNAc Modifitcation. In: *Essentials of Glycobiology*, pp. 263-292, n.d., Cold Spring Harbor Laboratory, New York

Hart, MJ, de los Santos, R., Alberta IN., et al. (1998). Downregulation of beta-catenin by human Axin and its association with the APC tumor suppressor, beta-catenin and GSK3 beta. *Curr Biol*, Vol. 8, pp. 573-581

He, B., Kemppainen, JA., Voegel, JJ., Gronemeyer, H., Wilson, EM. (1999). Activation function 2 in the human androgen receptor ligand binding domain mediates interdomain communication with the NH(2)-terminal domain. *J Biol Chem*, Vol. 274 (52), pp. 37219-37225

He, B., Lee, LW., Minges, JT., Wilson, EM.(200). Dependence of selective gene activation on the androgen receptor NH2- and COOH-terminal interaction. *J Biol Chem*, Vol. 275 (30), pp. 22986-22994

Heinlein, CA., & Chang, C. (2002). Androgen receptor (AR) coregulators: an overview. *Endocr Rev*, Vol. 23(2), pp. 175-200

Hinoi, T., Yamamoto, H., Kishida, M., et al. (200). Complex formation of adenomatous polyposis coli gene product and axin facilitates glycogen synthase kinase-3 beta-dependent phosphorylation of beta-catenin and down-regulates beta-catenin. *J Biol Chem*, Vol. 275, pp. 591-594

Henderson, BR. (2000). Nuclear-cytoplasmic shuttling of APC regulates beta-catenin subcellular localization and turnover. *Nat Cell Biol*, Vol.2, pp. 653-660, ISSN 1465-7392

Hong, H., Darimont, BD., Tang, L., Tamamoto, KR., Stallcup, MR. (1999). An additional region of coactivator GRIP1 required for interaction with the hormone-binding domains of a subset of nuclear receptors. *J Biol Chem*, Vol. 274(6), pp. 3496-3502

Honjo, Y., Inohara, H., Akahani, S., Yoshii, T., Takenaka, Y., Yoshida, J., Hattori, K., Tomiyama, Y., Raz, A., & Kubo, T. (2000). Expression of cytoplasmic galectin-3 as a prognostic marker in tongue carcinoma. *Clin Cancer Res*, Vol.6, pp. 4635-4640, ISSN 1078-0432

Horvath, LG., Lelliott, JE., Kench, JG., Lee, CS., Williams, ED., Saunders, DN., Grygiel, JJ., Sutherland, RL., & Henshall, SM. (2007). Secreted frizzled-related protein 4 inhibits proliferation and metastatic potential in prostate cancer. *Prostate*, Vol.67, pp. 1081-1090, ISSN 0270-4137

Huang, YS., & Shih, HM. (2009). Daxx positively modulates beta-catenin/TCF4-mediated transcriptional potential. *Biochem Biophys Res Commun*, Vol.386, pp. 762-768, ISSN 0006-291X

Huber, AH., Nelson, WJ., & Weis, WI. (1997). Three-dimensional structure of the armadillo repeat region of beta-catenin. *Cell*, Vol.90, pp. 871-882, ISSN 0092-8674

Huber, AH., & Weis, WI. (2001). The structure of the beta-catenin/E-cadherin complex and the molecular basis of diverse ligand recognition by beta-catenin. *Cell*, Vol.105, pp. 391-402, ISSN 0092-8674

Ingles, SA., Ross, RK., Yu, MC., Irvine, RA., La Pera, G., Haile, RW, Coetzee, GA. (1997). Association of prostate cancer risk with genetic polymorphisms in vitamin D receptor and androgen receptor. *J Natl Cancer Inst*, Vol. 89(2), pp. 166-170

Jenster, G., van der Korput, HA., Trapman, J., Brinkmann, AO. (1995). Identification of two transcription activation units in the N-terminal domain of the human androgen receptor. *J Biol Chem*, Vol. 270(13), pp. 7341-7346

Jeronimo, C., Henrique, R., Hoque, MO., Mambo, E., Ribeiro, FR., Varzim, G., Oliveira, J., Teixeira, MR., Lopes, C., & Sidransky, D. (2004). A quantitative promoter methylation profile of prostate cancer. *Clin Cancer Res*, Vol.10, pp. 8472-8478, ISSN 1078-0432

Jiang, YG., Luo, Y., He, DL., Li, X., Zhang, LL., Peng, T., Li, MC., & Lin, YH. (2007). Role of Wnt/beta-catenin signaling pathway in epithelial-mesenchymal transition of human prostate cancer induced by hypoxia-inducible factor-1alpha. *Int J Urol*, Vol.14, pp. 1034-1039 ISSN 0919-8172

Ji, J., Yamashita, T., & Wang, XW. (2011). Wnt/beta-catenin signaling activates microRNA-181 expression in hepatocellular carcinoma. *Cell Biosci*, Vol.1, pp. 4, ISSN 2045-3701

Joesting, MS., Perrin, S., Elenbaas, B., Fawell, SE., Rubin, JS., Franco, OE., Hayward, SW., Cunha, GR., & Marker, PC. (2005). Identification of SFRP1 as a candidate mediator of stromal-to-epithelial signaling in prostate cancer. *Cancer Res.* Vol.65, pp. 10423-10430, ISSN 0008-5472

Johnson, MA., Hernandez, I., Wei, Y., & Greenberg, N. (2000). Isolation and characterization of mouse probasin: An androgen-regulated protein specifically expressed in the differentiated prostate. *Prostate*, Vol.43, pp. 255-262, ISSN 0270-4137

Kalluri, R., & Weinberg, RA. (2009). The basics of epithelial-mesenchymal transition. *J Clin Invest*, Vol.119, pp. 1420-1428, ISSN 0021-9738

Kawano, Y., Diez, S., Uysal-Onganer, P., Darrington, R.S., Waxman, J., Kypta, R.(2009). Secreted Frizzled-related protein-1 is a negative regulator of androgen receptor activity in prostate cancer. *British Journal of Caner*, Vol. 100, pp. 1165-1174.

Kawano, Y., & Kypta, R. (2003). Secreted antagonists of the Wnt signaling pathway. *J Cell Sci*, Vol. 116(Pt 13), pp. 2627-2634

Kemppainen, J.S., Langley, E., Wong, C.I., Bobseine, K., Kelce, W.R., Wilson, E.M. (1999). *Mol. Endocrinol*, Vol. 13, pp. 440-454.

Kennell, J., & Cadigan, KM. (2009). APC and beta-catenin degradation. In: *APC Proteins*, Inke, SN., & Brooke, MM. pp. 1-12, Landes Bioscience and Springer Science+Business Media, ISBN 0065-2598

Kharaishvili G., Simkova, D., Makharoblidze, E., Trtkova, K., Kolar, Z., Bouchal, J. (2011). Wnt signaling in prostate development and carcinogenesis. *Biomed Pap Med Fac Univ Palacky Olomouc Czech Repub*, Vol.155(1), pp. 11-18.

Kohn, AD., & Moon, RT. (2005). Wnt and calcium signaling: beta-catenin-independent pathways. *Cell Calcium*, Vol.38, pp. 439-446, ISSN 0143-4160

Koochekpour, S. (2010). Androgen receptor signaling and mutations in prostate cancer. *Asian J Androl*, Vol.12, pp.639-657, ISSN 1008-682X

Knapp, S., Zamai, M., Volpi, D., Nardese, V., Avanzi, M., Breton, J., Plyte, S., Flocco, M., Marconi, M., Isacchi, A., Caiolfa, VR. (2001). Thermodynamics of the high-affinity interaction of TCF4 with beta-catenin. *J Mol Biol*, Vol. 306(5), 1179-1189

Krieghoff, E., Behrens, J., & Mayr, B. (2006). Nucleo-cytoplasmic distribution of beta-catenin is regulated by retention. *J Cell Sci* Vol.119, pp. 1453-1463

Krieghoff, E., Behrens, J, Mayr, B. (2006). Nucleo-cytoplasmic distribution of beta-catenin is regulated by retention. *J Cell Sci*, Vol. 119(Pt 7), pp. 1453-1463

Koivisto, P., Kononen, J., Palmberg, C., Tammela, T., Hyytinen, E., Isola, J., Trapman, J., Cleutjens, K., Noordzij, A., Visakorpi, T., Kallioniemi, OP. (1997). Androgen receptor gene amplification: a possible molecular mechanism for androgen deprivation therapy failure in prostate cancer. *Cancer Res,* Vol. 57(2), pp. 314-319

Korswagen, HC., Herman, MA., Clevers, HC. (2000). Distinct beta-catenin mediate adhesion and signaling functions in C.elegans. *Nature,* Vol. 406(6795), pp. 527-32

Kuhl, M. (2004). The WNT/calcium pathway: biochemical mediators, tools and future requirements. *Front Biosci,* Vol.9, pp. 967-974, ISSN 1093-4715

Labrie, F., Belanger, A., Simard, J., Labrie, C., Dupont A. (1993). Combination therapy for prostate cancer. Endocrine and biologic basis o(2003).f its choice as new standard first-line therapy. *Cancer (Phila.),* Vol. 71, pp. 1059-1067

Labrie, F., Dupont, A., Belanger, A., St-Arnaud, R., Giguere, M., Lacourciere, Y., Emond, J., Monfette, G. (1986). Treatment of prostate cancer with gonadotropin-releasing hormone agonists. *Endocrin Rev,* Vol. 7(1), pp. 67-74

Lemon, B., & Tjian, R. (2000). Orchestrated response: a symphony of transcription factors for gene control. *Genes Dev,* Vol. 14(20), pp. 2551-2569

Levy, L., Wei, Y., Labalette, C., Wu, Y., Renard, CA., Buendia, MA., & Neuveut, C. (2004). Acetylation of beta-catenin by p300 regulates beta-catenin-Tcf4 interaction. *Mol Cell Biol,* Vol.24, pp. 3404-3414, ISSN 0270-7306

Li , H., Kim., J.H., Koh, S.S**, Stallcup, M.R. (2004). Synergistic effects of coactivators GRIP1 and beta-catenin on gen activation: cross-talk between androgen receptor and Wnt signaling pathways. *The Journal of Biological Chemistry,* Vol 279, pp. 4212-4220.

Li, ZG., Yang, J., Vazquez, ES., Rose, D., Vakar-Lopez, F., Mathew, P., Lopez, A., Logothetis, CJ., Lin, SH., & Navone, NM. (2008). Low-density lipoprotein receptor-related protein 5 (LRP5) mediates the prostate cancer-induced formation of new bone. *Oncogene,* Vol.27, pp. 596-603, ISSN 0950-9232

Liao , G., Chen, LY., Zhang, A., Godavarthy, A., Xia F., Ghosh, JC., Li, H., Chen, JD. (2003). Regulation of androgen receptor activity by the nuclear receptor corepressor SMRT. *J Biol Chem,* Vol. 278(7), pp. 5052-5061

Liao, X., Thrasher, JB., Holzbeierlein, J., Stanley, S., & Li, B. (2004). Glycogen synthase kinase-3beta activity is required for androgen-stimulated gene expression in prostate cancer. *Endocrinology,* Vol.145, pp. 2941-2949, ISSN 0013-7227

Lilien, J., & Balsamo, J. (2005). The regulation of cadherin-mediated adhesion by tyrosine phosphorylation/dephosphorylation of beta-catenin. *Curr Opin Cell Biol,* Vol.17, pp. 459-465, ISSN 0955-0674

Lin, HK., Wang, L., Hu, YC., Altuwaijri, S., Chang, C. (2002). Phosphorylation dependent ubiquitylation and degradation of androgen receptor by Akt require Mdm2 E3 ligase. *EMBO J,* Vol. 21, pp. 4037-4048

Liu, X., Choi, R.Y., Jawad, S.M., Arnold, J.T. (2011) Androgen-induced PSA expression requires not only activation of AR but also endogenous IGF-1 or IGF-1/PI3K/AKT signaling in human prostate cancer epithelial cells. *The Prostate,* Vol.71, pp.766-777.

Liu, C., Li, Y., Semenov, M., Han C., Baeg, GH., Tan, Y., Zhang, Z., Lin, X., & He, X. (2002). Control of beta-catenin phosphorylation/degradation by a dual-kinase mechanism. *Cell*, Vol.108, pp. 837-847, ISSN 0092-8674

Liu, J., Xing, Y., Hinds, TR., Zheng, J., & Xu, W. (2006). The third 20 amino acid repeat is the tightest binding site of APC for beta-catenin. *J Mol Biol*, Vol.360, pp. 133-144, ISSN 0022-2836

Liu, YN., Liu, Y., Lee, HJ., Hsu, YH., & Chen, JH. (2008). Activated androgen receptor downregulates E-cadherin gene expression and promotes tumor metastasis. *Mol Cell Biol*, Vol.28, pp. 7096-7108, ISSN 0270-7306

Locke, J.A., Guns, E.S**, Lubik, A.A., Adomat, H.H., Hendy, S.C., Wood, C.A. (2008). Androgen levels increase by intratumoral de novo steroidogenesis during progression of castation-resistant prostate ancer. *Cancer Research*, Vol. 68(15), pp.6407-6415.

Loy, CJ., Sim, KS., Yong, EL. (2003). Filamin-A fragment localizes to the nucleus to regulate androgen receptor and coactivator functions. *Proc Natl Acad Scie USA*, Vol. 100(8), pp. 4562-4567

Lu , W., Tinsely, H.N., Keeton, A., Qu, Z., Piazza, G.A., Li, Y. (2009). Suppression of Wnt/β-catenin signaling inhibits prostate cancer cell proliferation. *European Jouranl of Pharmacology*, Vol 602, pp.8-14.

Luisi, BF., Xu, WX., Otwinoswski, Z., Freedman, LP., Yamamoto, KR**, Sigler, PB. (1991). Crystallographic analysis of the interaction of the glucocorticoid receptor with DNA. *Nature*, Vol. 352(6335), pp. 497-505

MacDonald, BT., Tamai, K., & He, X. (2009). Wnt/beta-catenin signaling: components, mechanisms, and diseases. *Dev Cell*, Vol.17, pp. 9-26, ISSN 1534-5807

Macheda, ML., & Stacker, SA. (2008). Importance of wnt signaling in the tumor stroma microenvironment. *Current Cancer Drug Targets*, Vol. 8, pp. 454-465

Maher, MT., Mo, R., Flozak, AS., Peled, ON., & Gottardi, CJ. (2010). Beta-catenin phosphorylated at serine 45 is spatially uncoupled from beta-catenin phosphorylated in the GSK3 Domain: implications for signaling. *PloS ONE*, Vol.5, No.4

Major, MB., Camp, ND., Berndt, JD., Yi, X., Goldenberg, SJ., Hubbert, C., Biechele, TL., Gingras, AC., Zheng, N., Maccoss, MJ., Angers, S., & Moon, RT. (2007). Wilms tumor suppressor WTX negatively regulates WNT/beta-catenin signaling. *Science*, Vol.316, pp. 1043-1046, ISSN 0036-8075

Marcelli, M., Ittmann, M., Mariani, S., Sutherland, R., Nigam, R., Murthy, L., Zhao, Y., Diconcini, D., Puxeddu, E., Esen, A., Eastham, J., Weigel, NL., Lamb, DJ. (2000). Androgen receptor mutations in prostate cancer. Cancer Res, Vol. 60(4), pp. 944-949

Marcias, G., Erdmann, El, Lapouge, G., Siebert, C., Barthelemy, P., Duclos, B., Bergerat, JP., Ceraline, J., Kurtz, JE. (2010). Identification of novel truncated androgen receptor (AR) mutants including unreported pre-mRNA splicing variants in the 22Rv1 hormone-refractory prostate cancer (PCa) cell line. *Hum Mutat*, Vol. 31(1), pp. 74-80

Masiello, D., Chen, SY., Xu, Y., Verhoeven, MC., Choi, E., Hollenberg, AN., & Balk, SP. (2004). Recruitment of beta-catenin by wild-type or mutant androgen receptors correlates with ligand-stimulated growth of prostate cancer cells. *Mol Endocrinol*, Vol.18, pp. 2388-2401, ISSN 0888-8809

Mazor, M., Kawano, Y., Zhu, H., Waxman, J., & Kypta, RM. (2004). Inhibition of glycogen synthase kinase-3 represses androgen receptor activity and prostate cancer cell growth. *Oncogene*, Vol.23, pp. 7882-7892, ISSN 0950-9232

McInerney, EM., Rose, DW., Flynn, SE., Westin, S., Mullen, TM., Krones, A., Inostroza, J., Torchia, J., Nolte, RT., Assa-Munt, N., Milburn, MV., Glass, CK., Rosenfeld, MG. (1998). Determinants of coactivator LXXLL motif specificity in nuclear receptor transcriptional activation. *Genes Dev*, Vol. 12, pp. 3357-3368

Megy, S., Bertho, G., Gharbi-Benarous, J., Baleux, Francoise., Benarous, R., & Girault, Jean-Pierre. (2004). Solution structure of a peptide derived from the oncogenic protein beta-catenin in its phosphorylated and nonphosphorylated states. *Peptide*, Vol.26, pp. 227-241, ISSN 0196-9781

Mercure, MZ., Ginnan, R., & Singer, HA. (2008). CaM kinase II delta2-dependent regulation of vascular smooth muscle cell polarization and migration. *Am J Physiol Cell Physiol*, Vol.294, pp. C1465-1475, ISSN 0363-6143

Miyamoto, H., & Chang, C. (2000). Antiandrogens fail to block androstenedione-mediated mutated androgen receptor transactivation in human prostate cancer cells. *Int, J Urol*, Vol. 7(1), pp. 32-34

Miyamoto, H., Yeh, S., Wilding, G., Chang, C. (1998). Promotion of agonist activity of antiandrogens by the androgen receptor coactivator, ARA70, in human prostate cancer DU145 cells. *Proc Natl Acad Sci USA*, Vol. 95(13), pp. 7370-7384

Mo, R., Chew, TL., Maher, MT., Bellipanni, G., Weinberg, ES., & Gottardi, CJ. (2009). The terminal region of beta-catenin promotes stability by shielding the Armadillo repeats from the axin-scaffold destruction complex. *J Biol Chem*, Vol.284, pp. 28222-28231, ISSN 0021-9258

Mononen, N., Syrjakoski, K., Matikainen, M., Tammela, TL., Schleutker J., Kallioniemi, OP, Trapman, J., Koivisto, PA. (2000). Two percent of Finnish prostate cancer patients have a germ-line mutation in the hormone-binding domain of the androgen receptor gene. *Cancer Res*, Vol. 60(22), pp. 6479-6481

Mulholland, DJ., Cheng, H., Reid, K., Rennie, PS., Nelson, CC. (2002). The androgen receptor can promote beta-catenin nuclear translocation independently of adenomatous polyposis coli. *J Biol Chem*, Vol.277, pp. 17933-17943, ISSN 0021-9258

Mulholland, DJ., Read, JT., Rennie, PS., Cox, ME., & Nelson, CC. (2003). Functional localization and competition between the androgen receptor and T-cell factor for nuclear beta-catenin: a means for inhibition of the Tcf signaling axis. *Oncogene*, Vol.22, pp. 5602-5613, ISSN 0950-9232

Mulholland, DJ., Dedhar, S., Coetzee, GA., & Nelson, CC. (2005). Interaction of nuclear receptors with the Wnt/beta-catenin/Tcf signaling axis: Wnt you like to know? *Endocr Rev*, Vol.26, pp. 898-915, ISSN 0163-769X

Mulholland, DJ., Dedhar, S., Wu, H., & Nelson, CC. (2006). PTEN and GSK3beta: key regulators of progression to androgen-independent prostate cancer. *Oncogene*, Vol.25, pp. 329-337, ISSN 0950-9232

Munemitsu, S., Albert, I., Souza, B., Rubinfeld, B., Polakis, P. (1995). Regulation of intracellular β-catenin levels by the adenomatous polyposis coli (APC) tumor-suppressor protein. *Proc. Natl. Acad. Sci. USA*, Vol. 92, pp. 3046-3050

Narlikar, GJ., Fan, HY., & Kingston, RE. (2002). Cooperation between complexes that regulate chromatin structure and transcription. *Cell*, Vol.108, pp. 475-487

Nathke, IS. (2004). The adenomatous polyposis coli protein: the Achilles heel of the gut epithelium. *Annu Rev Cell Dev Biol,* Vol. 20, pp. 337-366

Nazareth, LV., & Weigel, NL. (1996). Activation of the human androgen receptor through a protein kinase A signaling pathway. *J Biol Chem,* Vol. 271, pp. 19900-19907

Neufeld, KL., Zhang, F., Cullen, BR., & White, RL. (2000). APC-mediated downregulation of beta-catenin activity involves nuclear sequestration and nuclear export. *EMBO Rep,* Vol.1, pp. 519-523, ISSN 1469-221X

Neufeld, KL. (2009). Nuclear APC. In: *APC Proteins,* Inke, SN., & Brooke, MM. pp.13-29, Landes Bioscience and Springer Science+Business Media, ISBN 0065-2598

Ngan, ES., Hasimoto, Y., Ma, ZQ., Tsai, MJ., Tsai, SY. (2003). Overexperession of Cdc25B, and androgen receptor coactivator, in prostate cancer. *Oncogene,* Vol. 22, pp. 734-739

Niu, Y., Chang, TM., Yeh, S., Ma, WL., Wang, YZ., & Chang, C. (2010). Differential androgen receptor signals in different cells explain why androgen-deprivation therapy of prostate cancer fails. *Oncogene,* Vol.29, pp. 3593-3604, ISSN 0950-9232

Nolte, RT., Wisely, GB., Westin, S., Cobb, JE., Lambert, MH, Kurokawa, R., Rosenfeld, MG., WIllson, TM., Glass, CK., Milburn, MV. (1998). Ligand binding and co-activator assembly of the peroxisome proliferator-activated receptor-gamma. *Nature,* Vol. 395, pp. 137-143

Novak, A., Hsu, SC., Leung-Hagesteijn, C., Radeva, G., Papkoff, J., Montesano, R., Roskelley, C., Grosschedl, R., & Dedhar, S. (1998). Cell adhesion and the integrin-linked kinase regulate the LEF-1 and beta-catenin signaling pathways. *Proc Natl Acad Sci U S A,* Vol.95, pp. 4374-4379, ISSN 0027-8424

Ohigashi, T., Mizuno, R., Nakashima, J., Marumo, K., & Murai, M. (2005). Inhibition of Wnt signaling downregulates Akt activity and induces chemosensitivity in PTEN-mutated prostate cancer cells. *Prostate,* Vol.62, pp. 61-68, ISSN 0270-4137

O'Malley, BW., Tsai, SY., Bagchi, M., Weigel, NL., Schrader, WT., Tsai MJ. (1991). Molecular mechanism of action of a steroid hormone receptor. *Recent Prog Horm Res,* Vol. 47, pp. 1-24

Ozanne DM., Brady, ME., Cook, S., Gaughan, L., Neal, DE., Robson, CN. (2000). Androgen receptor nuclear translocation is facilitated by the f-actin cross-linking protein filamin, *Mol Endocrinol,* Vol. 14(10), pp. 1618-1626

Ozawa, M., & Kemler, R., (1998). Altered cell adhesion activity by pervanadate due to the dissociation of alpha-catenin from the E-cadherin.catenin complex. *J Biol Chem,* Vol.273, pp. 6166-6170

Palmberg, C., Koivisto, P., Kakkola., L., Tammela, TL., Kallioniemi, OP., Visakorpi, T. (2000). Androgen receptor gene amplification at primary progression predicts response to combined androgen blockade as second line therapy for advanced prostate cancer. *J Urol,* Vol 164(6), pp. 1992-1995

Pawlowski, JE., Ertel, JR., Allen, MP., Xu, M., Butler, C., Wilson, EM., & Wierman, ME. (2002). Liganded androgen receptor interaction with beta-catenin: nuclear co-localization and modulation of transcriptional activity in neuronal cells. *J Biol Chem,* Vol.277, pp. 20702-20710, ISSN 0021-9258

Petre, CE., Wetherill, YB., Danielsen, M., Knudsen KE. (2002). Cyclin D1: mechanism and consequence of androgen receptor co-repssor activity. *J Biol Chem,* Vol. 277, pp. 2207-2215

Petre-Draviam, CE., Cook, SL., Burd, CJ., Marshall, TW., Wetherill, YB., Knudsen KE. (2003). Specificity of cyclin D1 for androgen receptor regulation. *Cancer Res*, Vol. 63, pp.4903-4913

Piedra,.J., Martinez, D., Castano, J., Miravet, S., Dunach, M., & de Herreros, AG. (2001). Regulation of beta-catenin structure and activity by tyrosine phosphorylation. *J Biol Chem*, Vol.276, pp. 20436-20443, ISSN 0021-9258

Piedra, J., Miravet, S., Castano, J., Palmer, HG., Heisterkamp, N., Garcia de Herreros, A., & Dunach, M. (2003). p120 Catenin-associated Fer and Fyn tyrosine kinases regulate beta-catenin Tyr-142 phosphorylation and beta-catenin-alpha-catenin Interaction. *Mol Cell Biol*, Vol.23, pp. 2287-2297, ISSN 0270-7306

Pinarbasi, E., Gunes, EG., Pinarbasi, H., Donmez, G., & Silig, Y. (2010). AXIN2 polymorphism and its association with prostate cancer in a Turkish population. *Med Oncol*, ISSN 1357-0560

Polakis, P. (1995). Mutations in the APC gene and their implications for protein structure and function. *Curr Opin Genet Dev*, Vol. 5, pp. 1053-1057

Poukka, J., Karvonen, U., Janne, OA., Palvimo, JJ. (2000). Covalent modification of the androgen receptor by small ubiquitin-like modifier 1 (SUMO-1). *Proc Natl Acad Sci USA*, Vol. 97, pp.14145-14150

Poy, F., Lepourcelet, M., Shivdasani, RA., & Eck, MJ. (2001). Structure of a human Tcf4-beta-catenin complex. *Nat Struct Biol*, Vol.8, pp. 1053-1057, ISSN 1072-8368

Quyn, AJ., Steele, RJ., Carey, FA., Nathke, IS. (2008). Prognostic and therapeutic implications of Apc mutations in colorectal cancer. *Surgeon*, Vol.6, pp. 350-356, ISSN 1479-666X

Railo, A., Nagy, II., Kilpelainen, P., & Vainio, S. (2008). Wnt-11 signaling leads to down-regulation of the Wnt/beta-catenin, JNK/AP-1 and NF-kappaB pathways and promotes viability in the CHO-K1 cells. *Exp Cell Res*, Vol.314, pp. 2389-2399, ISSN 0014-4827

Rahmann, M., Miyamoto, H., Chang, C. (2004). Androgen receptor coregulators in prostate cancer: mechanisms and clinical implications. *Clin Cancer Res*, Vol. 10(7), pp. 2208-2219

Rastinejad, F., Perlmann, T., Evans, RM., Sigler, PB. Structural determinants of nuclear receptor assembly on DNA direct repeats. *Nature*, Vol. 375(6528), pp. 203-211

Ravindranath, A., O'Connell, A., Johnston, PG., & El-Tanani, MK. (2008). The role of LEF/TCF factors in neoplastic transformation. *Curr Mol Med*, Vol.8, pp. 38-50, ISSN 1566-5240

Rennie, PS., Bruchovsky, M., Leco, KJ., Sheppard, PC., McQueen, SA., Cheng, H., Snoek, R., Hamel, A., Bock, ME**, MacDonald, BS., et al. (1993). Characterization of two cis-acting DNA elements involved in the androgen regulation of the probasin gene. *Mol Endocrinol*, Vol. 7(1), pp. 23-26

Reutens, AT., Fu, M., Wang, C., Albanese C., McPhaul, MJ., Sun Z., Balk, SP., Janne, OA., Palvimo, JJ., Pestell, RG. (2001). Cyclin D1 binds the androgen receptor and regulates hormone-dependent signaling in a p300/CBP-associated factor (P/CAF)-dependent manner. *Mol Endocrinol*, Vol. 15, pp.797-811

Richmond, PJ., Karayiannakis, AJ., Yagafuchi, A., Kaisary, AV., Pignatelli, M. (1997). Aberrant E-cadherin and alpha-catenin expression in prostate cancer: correlation with patient survival. *Cancer Res*, Vol 57(15), pp. 3189-3193

Rosin-Arbesfeld, R., Townsley, F., Bienz, M. (2000). The APC tumour suppressor has a nuclear export function. *Nature,* Vol. 406, pp. 1009-1012

Roura, S., Miravet, S., Piedra, J., Garcia de Herreros, A., & Dunach, M. (1999). Regulation of E-cadherin/Catenin association by tyrosine phosphorylation. *J Biol Chem,* Vol.274, pp. 36734-36740, ISSN 0021-9258

Rubinfeld, B., Souza, B., Alberta, I., Muller, O., Chamberlain, SH., Masiarz, FR., Munemitsu, S., Polakis, P. (1993). Association of the APC gene product with β-catenin. *Science,* Vol. 272, pp.39037-39045

Sampietro, J., Dahlberg, CL., Cho, US., Hinds, TR., Kimelman, D., & Xu, W. (2006). Crystal structure of a beta-catenin/BCL9/Tcf4 complex. *Mol Cell,* Vol.24, pp. 293-300 ISSN 1097-2765

Salas, TR., Kim, J., Vakar-Lopez, F., Sabichi, AL., Troncoso, P., Jenster, G., Kikuchi, A., Chen, SY., Shemshedini, L., Suraokar, M., Logothetis, CJ., DiGiovanni, J., Lippman SM., & Menter, DG. (2004). Glycogen synthase kinase-3 beta is involved in the phosphorylation and suppression of androgen receptor activity. *J Biol Chem,* Vol.279, pp. 19191-19200, ISSN 0021-9258

Sasaki C.Y.,Lin, H., Morin, P.J., Longo, J.L. (2000). Tructation of the extracellular region abrogrates cell contact but retains the growth-supporessive activity of E-cadherin. *Cancer Research,* Vol 60, pp.7057-7065.

Sayat, R., Leber, B., Grubac, V., Wiltshire, L., & Persad, S. (2008). O-GlcNAc-glycosylation of beta-catenin regulates its nuclear localization and transcriptional activity. *Exp Cell Res,* Vol.314, pp. 2774-2787, ISSN 0014-4827

Schaufele, Fl, Carbonell, X., Guerbadot, M., Borngraeber, S., Chapman, MS., Ma, AA., Miner, JN., Diamond, MI. (2005). The structural basis of androgen receptor activation: intramolecular and intermolecular amino-carboxy interactions. *Proc Natl Acad Sci USA,* Vol. 102 (28), pp. 9802-9807

Schneider, SQ., Finnerty, JR., & Martindale, MQ. (2003). Protein evolution: structure-function relationships of the oncogene beta-catenin in the evolution of multicellular animals. *J Exp Zool B Mol Dev Evol,* Vol.295, pp. 25-44, ISSN 1552-5007

Schwabe, JW., Chapman, L., Finch, JT., Rhodes, D. (1993). The crystal structure of the estrogen receptor DNA-binding domain bound to DNA: How receptors discriminate between their response elements. *Cell,* Vol. 75, pp. 567-578

Schweizer, L., Rizzo, CA., Spires, TE., Platero, JS., Wu, Q., Lin, TA., Gottardis, MM., & Attar, RM. (2008). The androgen receptor can signal through Wnt/beta-Catenin in prostate cancer cells as an adaptation mechanism to castration levels of androgens. *BMC Cell Biol,* Vol.9, pp. 4, ISSN 1471-2121

Shaffer, PL., Jivan, A., Dollins, DE., Claessens, F., & Gewirth, DT. (2004). Structural basis of androgen receptor binding to selective androgen response elements. *Proc Natl Acad Sci U S A,* Vol.101, pp. 4758-4763, ISSN 0027-8424

Sharma, M., Chuang, WW., & Sun, Z. (2002). Phosphatidylinositol 3-kinase/Akt stimulates androgen pathway through GSK3beta inhibition and nuclear beta-catenin accumulation. *J Biol Chem,* Vol.277, pp. 30935-30941, ISSN 0021-9258

Shen, MM., & Abate-Shen, C. (2011). Molecular genetics of prostate cancer: new prospects for old challenges. *Gene Dev,* Vol.24, pp. 1967-2000

Shen, HC., Buchanan, G., Butler, LM., Prescott, J., Henderson, M., Tilley, WD., Coetzee, GA. (2005). GRIP1 mediates the interaction between the amino- and carboxyl-termini of the androgen receptor. *Biol Chem*, Vol.286(1), pp. 144-150

Shiau, A.K., Barstad, D., Loria, P.M., Cheng, L., Kushner P.J., Agard, A., Green G.L. (1998) Crstallographic structures of the ligand-binding domains of the androgen receptor and its T877A mutant complexed with the natural agonist dihdrotestosterone. *Proc. Natil. Acad. Sci.*, Vol. 98, pp. 4904-4909.

Shiau, AK., Barstad, D., Loria, PM., Cheng, L., Kushner, PJ., Agard DA., Greene, GL. (1998). The structural basis of estrogen receptor/coactivator recognition and the antagonism of this interaction by tamoxifen. *Cell*, Vol. 95, 927-937

Shih, HM., Chang, CC., Kuo, HY., & Lin, DY. (2007). Daxx mediates SUMO-dependent transcriptional control and subnuclear compartmentalization. *Biochem Soc Trans*, Vol.35, pp. 1397-1400, ISSN 0300-5127

Shimura, T., Takenaka, Y., Tsutsumi, S., Hogan, V., Kikuchi, A., & Raz, A. (2004). Galectin-3, a novel binding partner of beta-catenin. *Cancer Res*, Vol.64, pp. 6363-6367 ISSN 0008-5472

Simental, JA., Sar., M., Lane, MV., French, RS., Wilson, EM. (1991). Transcriptional activation and nuclear targeting signals of the human androgen receptor. *J BiolChem*, Vol. 266(1), pp. 510-518

Staal, FJ., Noort Mv, M., Strous, GJ., & Clevers, HC. (2002). Wnt signals are transmitted through N-terminally dephosphorylated beta-catenin. *EMBO Rep*, Vol.3, pp. 63-68, ISSN 1469-221X

Stadeli, R., Hoffmans, R., & Basler, K. (2006). Transcription under the control of nuclear Arm/beta-catenin. *Curr Biol*, Vol.16, pp. R378-385, ISSN 0960-9822

Sokol, SY. (2011). Wnt signaling through T-cell factor phosphorylation. *Cell Research*, Vol.21, pp. 1002-1012, ISSN 1001-0602

Song, DH., Dominguez, I., Mizuno, J., Kaut, M., Mohr, SC., & Seldin, DC. (2003) CK2 phosphorylation of the armadillo repeat region of beta-catenin potentiates Wnt signaling. *J Biol Chem*, Vol.278, pp. 24018-24025, ISSN 0021-9258

Song, LN., Herrell, R., Byers, S., Shah, S., Wilson, EM., & Gelmann, EP. (2003). Beta-catenin binds to the activation function 2 region of the androgen receptor and modulates the effects of the N-terminal domain and TIF2 on ligand-dependent transcription. *Mol Cell Biol*, Vol.23, pp. 1674-1687, ISSN 0270-7306

Southwell, J., Chowdhury, SF., Gottlieb, B., Beitel, LK., Lumbroso, R., Purisima, EO., & Trifiro, M. (2008). An investigation into CAG repeat length variation and N/C terminal interactions in the T877A mutant androgen receptor found in prostate cancer. *J Steroid Biochem Mol Biol*, Vol.111, pp. 138-146, ISSN 0960-0760

Spink, EK., Fridman, SG., Weis, WI. (2001). Molecular mechanisms of β-catenin recognition by adenomatous polyposis coli revealed by the structure of an APC-β-catenin complex. *EMBO J*, Vol. 20, pp. 6203-6212

Su, LK., Vogelstein, B., Kinzler, KW. (1993). Association of the APC tumor suppressor protein with catenins. *Science*, Vol 262(5140), pp. 1734-1737

Tago, K., Nakamura, T., Nishita, M., Hyodo, J., Nagai, S., Murata, Y., Adachi, S., Ohwada, S., Morishita, Y., Shibuya, H., & Akiyama, T. (2000). Inhibition of Wnt signaling by ICAT, a novel beta-catenin-interacting protein. *Genes Dev*, Vol.14, pp. 1741-1749, ISSN 0890-9369

Takahashi, S., Watanabe, R., Okada, M., Inoue, K., Ueda, T., Takada, I., Watabe, R., et al. (2011).Noncanonical Wnt signalin mediates androgen-dependent tumor growth in a mouse model of prostate cancer. *PNAS,* Vol 108(12), pp.4938-4943.

Talpin, M.E., et al. (1999). Selection for androgen receptor mutation in prostate cancers treated with androgen antagonists. *Cancer Research,* Vol.59, pp. 2511-2515

Taplin, ME., Bubley, GJ., Shuster, TD., Frantz, ME., Spooner, AE., Ogata, GK., Keer, HN., Balk, SP. (1995). Mutation of the androgen-receptor gene in metastatic androgen-independent prostate cancer. *N Engl J Med,* Vol. 332(21), pp. 1393-1398

Terry, S., Yang, X., Chen, MW., Vacherot, F., & Buttyan, R. (2006). Multifaceted interaction between the androgen and Wnt signaling pathways and the implication for prostate cancer. *J Cell Biochem,* Vol.99, pp. 402-410, ISSN 0730-2312

Thiele, S., Rauner, M., Goettsch, G., Rachner T.D., Benad, P., Fuessel, S., Erdmann, K., Hamann, C., Baretton, G.B., With, M.P., Jakob, F., Hofbauer, L.C. (2011). Expression profile of wnt molecules in prostate cancer and its regulation by aminobisphosphonates. *Journal of Cellular Biochemistry,* Vol. 112, pp. 1593-1600.

Thompson, J., Saatciogl, F., Janne, O.S., Palvimo, J.J. (2001). Disrupted amino-and carboxyl-terminal interactions of the androgen receptor are linked to androgen insensitivity. *Molecular Endocrinology,* Vol. 15 (6), pp. 923-935.

Thudi, N.K., Martin, C.K., Murahari, S., Shu, S.T., Lanigan, L.G., Werbeck, J.L., Keller, E.T., McCauley L.K., Pinzone, J.J., Rosol, T.J. (2011). Dickkopf-1 (DKK-1) stimulated prostate cancer growth and metastasis and inhibited bone formation in osteoblastic bone metastases. *The Prostate,* Vol. 71,pp. 615-625.

Tilley, WD., Buchanan, G., Hickey, TE., Bentel, JM. (1996). Mutations in the androgen receptor gene are associated with progression of human prostate cancer to androgen independence. *Clin Cancer Res,* Vol. 2(2), pp. 277-285

Tolwinski, NS., & Wieschaus, E. (2004). A nuclear function for armadillo/beta-catenin. *PLoS Biology,* Vol.2, pp. E95, ISSN 1544-9173

Topol, L., Jiang, X., Choi, H., Garrett-Beal, L., Carolan, PJ., & Yang, Y. (2003). Wnt-5a inhibits the canonical Wnt pathway by promoting GSK-3-independent beta-catenin degradation. *J Cell Biol,* Vol.162, pp. 899-908, ISSN 0021-9525

Truica, CI., Byers, S., & Gelmann, EP. (2000). Beta-catenin affects androgen receptor transcriptional activity and ligand specificity. *Cancer Res,* Vol.60, pp. 4709-4713, ISSN 0008-5472

Tutter, AV., Fryer, CJ., & Jones, KA. (2001). Chromatin-specific regulation of LEF-1-beta-catenin transcription activation and inhibition in vitro. *Genes Dev,* Vol.15, pp. 3342-3354, ISSN 0890-9369

Uysal-Onganer, P., Kawano, Y., Car, M., Walker, M.M., Diez, S., Siobhan Darrington, R., Waxman, J., Kypta, R.M. (2010). Wnt-11 promotes neuroendocrine like differentiation, survival and migrationof prostate cancer cells. *Molecular Cancer,* Vol.9, pp.55.

van den Brule, FA., Waltregny, D., Liu, FT., & Castronovo, V. (2000). Alteration of the cytoplasmic/nuclear expression pattern of galectin-3 correlates with prostate carcinoma progression. *Int J Cancer,* Vol.89, pp. 361-367, ISSN 0020-7136

Veeman, MT., Axelrod, JD., Moon, RT. (2003). A second canon. Functions and mechanisms of beta-catenin-independent Wnt signaling. *Dev Cell,* Vol. 5, pp.367-377

Veldscholte, J., Berrevoets, CA., Zegers, ND., van der Kwast, TH., Grootegoed, J.S., Mulder, E. (1992). Hormone-induced dissociation of the androgen receptor-heat-shock protein comples: use of a new monoclonal antibody to distinguish transformed from nontransformed receptors. *Biochemistry,* Vol. 31(32), pp. 7422-7430

Verras, M., Brown, J., Li, X., Nusse, R., & Sun, Z. (2004). Wnt3a growth factor induces androgen receptor-mediated transcription and enhances cell growth in human prostate cancer cells. *Cancer Res,* Vol.64, pp. 8860-8866, ISSN 0008-5472

Verras, M., & Sun, Z. (2006). Roles and regulation of Wnt signaling and beta-catenin in prostate cancer. *Cancer Lett,* Vol.237, pp. 22-32, ISSN 0304-3835

Verrijdt, G., Schoenmakers, E.., Alen, P., Haelens, A., Peeters, B., Rombauts, W., Claessens, F. (1999). Androgen specificity of a response unit upstream of the human secretory component gene is mediated by differential receptor binding to an essential androgen response element. *Mol Endocrinol,* Vol. 13(9), pp. 1558-1570

Verrijdt, G., Schoenmakers, E., Haelens, A., Peeters, B., Verhoeven, G., Rombauts, W., Claessens, F. Change of specificity mutations in androgen-selective enhances. Evidence for a role of differential DNA binding by the androgen receptor. *J Biol Chem,* Vol. 275(16), pp. 12298-12305

Westin, SR., Kurokawa, R., Nolte, RT., Wisely, GB., McInerney, EM., Rose, DW., Milburn, MV., Rosenfeld, MG., Glass, CK. (1998). Iinteractions controlling the assembly of nuclear-receptor heterodimers and co-activators. *Nature,* Vol. 395, pp. 199-202

Visakorpi, T., Hyytinen,E., Koivisto, P., Tanner, M., Keinanen, R., Palmberg., C., Palotie, A., Tammela, T., Isola, J., Kallioniemi, O.P. (1995). In vivo amplification of the androgen receptor gene and progression of human prostate cancer. *Nat. Genet,* Vol. 9, pp.401-406.

Wang, G., Wang, J., & Sadar, MD. (2008). Crosstalk between the androgen receptor and beta-catenin in castrate-resistant prostate cancer. *Cancer Res,* Vol.68, pp. 9918-9927, ISSN 0008-5472

Wang, L., Lin, HK., Hu, YC., Xie, S., Yang, L., & Chang, C. (2004). Suppression of androgen receptor-mediated transactivation and cell growth by the glycogen synthase kinase 3 beta in prostate cells. *J Biol Chem,* Vol.279, pp. 32444-32452, ISSN 0021-9258

Wang, Q., Symes, A.J., Kane, C.A., Freeeman,A., Nariculam, J., Munson, P., Thrasivoulou, C., Masters, J.R.W., Ahmed, A. (2010). A novel role for Wnt/CA2+ signaling in actin cytoskeleton remodeling and cell motility in prostate cancer. *Plos One,* Vol. 5 (5), pp.1-11

Wang, Y., Kreisberg, JI., & Ghosh, PM. (2007). Cross-talk between the androgen receptor and the phosphatidylinositol 3-kinase/Akt pathway in prostate cancer. *Curr Cancer Drug Targets,* Vol.7, pp. 591-604, ISSN 1568-0096

Weeraratna, AT., Jiang, Y., Hostetter, G., Rosenblatt, K., Duray, P., Bittner, M., & Trent, JM. (2002). Wnt5a signaling directly affects cell motility and invasion of metastatic melanoma. *Cancer Cell,* Vol.1, pp. 279-288, ISSN 1535-6108

Wissmann, C., Wild, PJ., Kaiser, S., Roepcke, S., Stoehr, R., Woenckhaus, M., Kristiansen, G., Hsieh, JC., Hofstaedter, F., Hartmann, A., Knuechel, R., Rosenthal, A., & Pilarsky, C. (2003). WIF1, a component of the Wnt pathway, is down-regulated in prostate, breast, lung, and bladder cancer. *J Pathol,* Vol.201, pp. 204–212

Wu, G., Xu, G., Schulman, BA., Jeffrey, PD., Harper, JW., & Pavletich, NP. (2003). Structure of a beta-TrCP1-Skp1-beta-catenin complex: destruction motif binding and lysine specificity of the SCF(beta-TrCP1) ubiquitin ligase. *Mol Cell,* Vol.11, pp. 1445-1456, ISSN 1097-2765

Wuebken, A., Schmidt-Ott, KM. (2011). WNT/beta-catenin signaling in polycystic kidney disease. *Kidney Int,* Vol.80, pp. 135-138, ISSN 0085-2538

Xing, Y., Clements, WK., Kimelman, D., & Xu, W. (2003). Crystal structure of a beta-catenin/axin complex suggests a mechanism for the beta-catenin destruction complex. *Genes Dev,* Vol.17, pp. 2753-2764, ISSN 0890-9369

Xing, Y., Clements, WK., Le Trong, I., Hinds, TR., Stenkamp, R., Kimelman, D., & Xu, W. (2004). Crystal structure of a beta-catenin/APC complex reveals a critical role for APC phosphorylation in APC function. *Mol Cell,* Vol.15, pp. 523-533, ISSN 1097-2765

Xing, Y., Takemaru, K., Liu, J., Berndt, JD., Zheng, JJ., Moon, RT., & Xu, W. (2008). Crystal structure of a full-length beta-catenin. *Structure,* Vol.16, pp. 478-487, ISSN 0969-2126

Xu, W., & Kimelman, D. (2007). Mechanistic insights from structural studies of beta-catenin and its binding partners. *J Cell Sci,* V.120, pp. 3337-3344, ISSN 0021-9533

Yang, F., Li, X., Sharma, M., Sasaki, CY., Longo, DL., Lim, B., & Sun, Z. (2002). Linking beta-catenin to androgen-signaling pathway. *J Biol Chem,* Vol.277, pp. 11336-11344, ISSN 0021-9258

Yang, X CM., Terry, S., Vacherot, F., Chopin, DK., Bemis, DL., Kitajewski, J., Benson, MC., Guo, V., Buttyan, R. (2005). A Human- and Male-Specific Protocadherin that Acts through the Wnt Signaling Pathway to Induce Neuroendocrine Transdifferentiation of Prostate Cancer Cell. *Cancer Research,* Vol.65, pp. 5263-5271

Yang, X., Chen, MW., Terry, S., Vacherot, F., Bemis, DL., Capodice, J., Kitajewski, J., de la Taille, A., Benson, MC., Guo, Y., & Buttyan, R. (2006). Complex regulation of human androgen receptor expression by Wnt signaling in prostate cancer cells. *Oncogene,* Vol.25, pp. 3436-3444, ISSN 0950-9232

Yang, CS., Vitto, MJ., Busby, SA., Garcia, BA., Kesler, CT., Gioeli, D., Shabanowitz, J., Hunt, DF., Rundell, K., Brautigan, DL., Paschal, BM. (2005). Simian virus 40 small t antigen mediates conformation-dependent transfer of protein phosphatase 2A onto the androgen receptor. *Mol Cell Biol,* Vol. 25(4), pp.1298-1308

Yamamoto, H., Oue, N., Sato, A., Hasegawa, Y., Yamaoto, H., Matsubara, A., Yasui, W., Kikuchi, A. (2010). Wnt5a signaling is involved in the aggressiveness of prostate cancer and expression of metalloproteinase. *Oncogene,* Vol. 29(14), pp. 2036-2046

Yardy, GW., & Brewster, SF. (2005). Wnt signalling and prostate cancer. *Prostate Cancer Prostatic Dis,* Vol.8, pp. 119-126, ISSN 1365-7852

Yardy, GW., Bicknell, DC., Wilding, JL., Bartlett, S., Liu, Y., Winney, B., Turner, GD., Brewster, SF., & Bodmer, WF. (2009). Mutations in the AXIN1 gene in advanced prostate cancer. *Eur Urol,* Vol.56, pp. 486-494, ISSN 0302-2838

Yaun, S., Lu, ML., Li, T., Balk, SP. (2001). SRY interacts with and negatively regulates androgen receptor transcriptional activity. *J Biol Chem,* Vol. 276(49), pp. 46647-46654

Yee, DS., Tang, Y., Li, X., Liu, Z., Guo, Y., Ghaffar, S., McQueen, P., Atreya, D., Xie, J., Simoneau, AR., Hoang, BH., & Zi, X. (2010) The Wnt inhibitory factor 1 restoration in prostate cancer cells was associated with reduced tumor growth, decreased capacity of cell migration and invasion and a reversal of epithelial to mesenchymal transition. *Mol Cancer,* Vol.9, pp. 162, ISSN 1476-4598

Yeh, S., et al. (1999). From Her2.Neu signal cascade to androgen receptor and its co-activators: a novel pathway by induction of androgen targen genes through MAK kinase in prostate cancer cell. *Proc. Natl Acad. Sci*, Vol. 95, pp. 5458-5463.

YL, JHZ., Jiang, YG., He, DL., Wu, CT. (2011). Knockdown of β-Catenin Through shRNA Cause a Reversal of EMT and Metastatic Phenotypes Induced by HIF-1α. *Cancer Investigation*, pp. 377-382

Yu, X., Wang, Y., Jiang, M., Bierie, B., Roy-Burman, P., Shen, MM., Taketo, MM., Wills, M., & Matusik, RJ. (2009). Activation of beta-Catenin in mouse prostate causes HGPIN and continuous prostate growth after castration. *Prostate*, Vol.69, pp. 249-262, ISSN 0270-4137

Yu, X., Wang, Y., DeGraff, DJ., Wills, ML., & Matusik, RJ. (2011). Wnt/beta-catenin activation promotes prostate tumor progression in a mouse model. *Oncogene*, Vol.30, pp. 1868-1879, ISSN 0950-9232

Zhao, XY., Boyle, B., Krishnan, AV., Navone, NM., Peehl, DM, Feldman, D. (1999). Two mutations identified in the androgen receptor of the new human prostate cancer cell line MDA PCa 2a. *J Urol*, Vol. 162(6), pp. 2192-2199

Zhao, JH., Luo, Y., Jiang, YG., He, DL., Wu, CT. (2011). Knockdown of β-catenin through shRNA cause a reversal of EMT and metastatic phenotypes induced by HIF-1α. *Cancer Invest*, Vol. 29(6), pp. 377-382

Zhao, XY., Malloy, PJ., Krishnan, AV., Swami, S., Navone, NM., Peehl, DM., Feldman, D. (2000). Glucocorticoids can promote androgen-independent growth of prostate cancer cells through a mutated androgen receptor. *Nat Med*, Vol 6(6), pp. 703-706

Zhu, H., Mazor, M., Kawano, Y., Walker, MM., Leung, HY., Armstrong, K., Waxman, J., & Kypta, RM. (2004). Analysis of Wnt gene expression in prostate cancer: mutual inhibition by WNT11 and the androgen receptor. *Cancer Res*, Vol.64, pp.7918-7926, ISSN 0008-5472

Zhu, ML., & Kyprianou, N. (2010). Role of androgens and the androgen receptor in epithelial-mesenchymal transition and invasion of prostate cancer cells. *FASEB J*, V.24, pp. 769-777, ISSN 0892-6638

Zi, X., Guo, Y., Simoneau, AR., Hope, C., Xie, J., Holcombe, RF., & Hoang, BH. (2005). Expression of Frzb/secreted Frizzled-related protein 3, a secreted Wnt antagonist, in human androgen-independent prostate cancer PC-3 cells suppresses tumor growth and cellular invasiveness. *Cancer Res*, Vol.65, pp. 9762-9770, ISSN 0008-5472.

2

Prostate Carcinoma and Hot Flashes

Santiago Vilar-González and Alberto Pérez-Rozos
Instituto de Medicina Oncológica y Molecular de Asturias.IMOMA
Spain

1. Introduction

In prostate cancer patients, the use of hormonal-deprivation (HD) therapies, such as the gonadotrophin-releasing hormone analogues (GnRHa) or luteinizing hormone releasing hormone analogues (LHRHa), antiandrogens, or bilateral orchiectomy, induces a range of hormone-related symptoms. Hot flashes (HF) are one of most common and distressing symptoms that can occur. Other signs and symptoms caused by estrogen and androgen deprivation are metabolic syndrome, increased cardiovascular risk, loss of libido, erectile dysfunction, accelerated osteopenia/osteoporosis, increased bone fractures, neurocognitive dysfunction, weight gain, decreased muscle mass, etc.

Since the pioneering studies by Huggins and Hodges (Huggins & Hodges, 1941), hormonal manipulation in which tumor cells are deprived of hormonal steroids has gained increasing relevance in the treatment of some types of cancer. They reported episodes of HF in 9 of 21 castrated patients 2 to 3 weeks after surgery (Huggins & Hodges, 1941).

Surgical castration, the most commonly used procedure to obtain HD a few years ago, has been gradually replaced by medical castration with the addition of LHRHa. After orchiectomy, approximately 50% of the patients experienced HF within months (Charig & Rundle, 1989; Maatman et al., 1985; Aksel et al., 1976; Buchholz & Matarelli, 1994).

The incidence of HF is 60-75% with the use of LHRHa (Harvey et al., 1985; Leuprolide Study Group, 1984; Sarosdy et al., 1999; Parmar et al., 1987). The reason why this incidence rate is higher than that observed with surgical removal is not well understood. As is the case with orchiectomy, HF occur over several months and may persist, although with less intensity, for many years.

Hot flashes are a major clinical problem in many cancer patients undergoing HD (Charig & Rundle, 1989; Nishiyama et al., 2004; J. S. Carpenter et al., 2004), as demonstrated by the quality of life studies.

While HF are not considered a serious adverse effect, their frequency and severity may be bothersome and can impair patients' quality of life. Thus we need to understand the mechanism of hot flashes and use this information to develop patient-tailored therapies to address these symptoms.

The purpose of this chapter is to discuss theories, to observe how they are reflected in the pathophysiology of HF, and to describe current treatments.

2. Pathophysiology

Hot flashes are characterized by a subjective sensation of heat perceived mainly in the upper part of the chest, followed by excessive perspiration. The major symptom is the subjective feeling of heat which may last several (4 to 10) minutes, and may be associated with other clinical complaints such as anxiety, irritability, palpitations, blushing, panic, and a sensation of loss of control, along with significant physical and emotional distress (Albertazzi, 2006). A mean rise of 0.9° C in body temperature is detected between 7 and 20 minutes before the hot flashes, with an ensuing increase in both the energy expenditure and the respiratory quotient (J. S. Carpenter et al., 2004).

Generalized peripheral vasodilatation typically appears within the first seconds of the episode (Molnar, 1975; F. L. Kronenberg et al., 1984). In addition, an increase in sweating and electric conductance are observed, with a strong correlation between both parameters (Molnar, 1975). During a HF a 30-second rise of 2-μS in skin conductance occurs (Robert R Freedman, 2005; J. S. Carpenter et al., 1999). Independently of the patient's perception, the measurement of skin conductance might be used for the clinical monitoring of HF, since it can be recorded on an outpatient basis by means of a Holter-like system. In such cases, a close correlation exists between these recordings and those obtained from daily data-collection questionnaires (Robert R Freedman, 2005; J. S. Carpenter et al., 1999).

There are many hypotheses about the mechanism of HF (**Figure 1**). We will proceed to explain the most important ones.

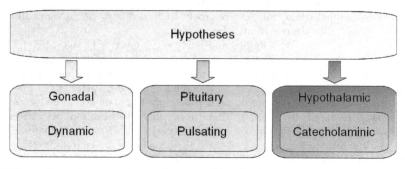

Fig. 1. Different hypotheses on the mechanism of hot flashes

2.1 Gonadal hypothesis

Since HF are commonly associated with orchiectomy in men and with menopause and ovarian failure in women, it may be assumed that they are causally related to low sex hormone levels.

It is necessary to remember that estrogens come from androgens. Aromatase cytochrome P450 is the enzyme that is responsible for estradiol biosynthesis from testosterone.

The hormone deprivation theory applied to prostate and breast carcinoma patients seems appealing and is based on the occurrence of HF following both medical and surgical castration. The responses to hormone replacement therapy and the effects following its withdrawal further support this hypothesis. However, an argument against this hypothesis is the absence of HF in patients with congenital hypogonadism (Turner and Kallman syndromes) as well as in prepubertal children (Kouriefs et al., 2002). These scenarios suggest that HF result from the dynamic reduction or sudden deprivation of sex hormones rather than their absolute plasma concentration. The **Dynamic hypothesis** is currently the most widely accepted theory (Kouriefs et al., 2002).

2.2 Pituitary hypothesis

In 1976, Alksel (Aksel et al., 1976) argued against the deprivation hypotheses. After suggesting that HF occurred due to a rise in gonadotrophin levels, he postulated a pituitary rather than a gonadal cause for this phenomenon. His theory is supported by studies performed on premenopausal women in whom a correlation was found between HF and the levels of both luteinizing hormone (LH) and follicle-stimulating hormone (FSH) (Melldrum et al., 1984). Casper (Casper et al., 1979) and Tataryn (Tataryn et al., 1979) demonstrated a synchrony between LH peaks and HF, which led them to propose a **pulsating hypothesis**. However, it must be noted that LH surges are not consistently associated with HF, although all hot flash episodes do coincide with an LH peak.

2.3 Hypothalamic hypothesis

In postmenopausal women, no correlation has been seen between gonatropin levels and HF (Linsell & Lightman, 1983). Also to be noted is the absence of HF in patients with Klinefelter syndrome in whom constitutively high gonadotrophin levels are found, and in other treated patients with high induced gonadotrophin levels (such as those used in ovulation-inducing protocols). HF does appear, however, after a hypophysectomy and during the LHRHa therapy for prostate cancer.

As a result of these findings, many investigators have suggested a potential role for the hypothalamus in the pathophysiology of HF (Kouriefs et al., 2002).

The similarities between HF and adrenergic symptoms have led to theories regarding the potential involvement of catecholamines (Albertazzi, 2006) in the hypothalamic hypothesis. After failing to show a correlation between HF and peripheral catecholamine levels, Casper (Casper et al., 1979) postulated the involvement of central pathways. On the other hand, some evidence points to noradrenaline (NA) as the hypothalamic neurotransmitter responsible for HF. Animal experiments have shown that the intrahypothalamic administration of NA affected thermoregulation (Albertazzi, 2006). Furthermore, high peripheral concentrations of MHPG (3-methoxy-4-hydroxiphenylglycol) − the major brain NA metabolite− during HF were found, while no changes in VMA (vanilmandelic acid) −a peripherally produced NA metabolite− were seen (R R Freedman, 2001).

Additional evidence to support this **catecholaminic hypothesis (Figure 1)** is the finding that the administration of yohimbine (an α_2-adrenergic antagonist) to symptomatic women increases hypothalamic NA concentrations and induces HF that subside after administration of clonidine (an α_2-agonist) (R R Freedman et al., 1990). The increased sympathetic activation, mediated by the α_2-adrenergic receptor, plays a major role in the occurrence of HF. Since α_2 receptors are modulated by estrogens, abrupt estrogen deprivation is likely to contribute to the development of HF via this pathway (Etgen et al., 2001). Exposure to high temperatures and hot drinks generates a reduction in the number of α_2 receptors, which is followed by a further release of additional amounts of NA and the appearance of HF (Kouriefs et al., 2002).

On the other hand, the hypothalamic thermoregulatory center is anatomically very close to the LHRH producing center (de Boer et al., 2009). **(Figure 2)**

Increases in hypothalamic NA caused by HD are thus likely to both stimulate LHRH producing neurons and activate the heat-losing mechanisms controlled by the adjacent thermoregulatory center (R R Freedman & Krell, 1999; Dacks & Rance, 2010). It has also been observed that high NA levels trigger HF by lowering the sweat-flash threshold in symptomatic postmenopausal women (Albertazzi, 2006).

The relation between sex steroids and hypothalamic cathecolamines remains unclear. The catecholestrogen (2-hydroxiestrogen) theory is based on the fact that the chemical structure of catecholestrogens, the most common estrogen metabolites, is similar to that of catecholamines (Paul & Axelrod, 1977).

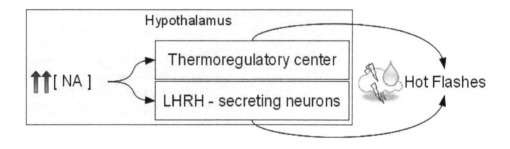

Fig. 2. Direct effect of noradrenaline on hypothalamic nucleus to trigger hot flash mechanism

Hypothalamic catecholestrogen concentrations are ten times greater than those of estrogens. Catecholestrogens act on the enzymes catecholmethyltranspherase and tyrosinhydroxilase which, in turn, influence the synthesis and breakdown of catecholamines, thus reducing NA levels. Therefore, low hypothalamic catecholestrogen concentrations will result in an increase of NA levels and the onset of HF. (**Figure 3**)

Opioids are also implicated in the pathogenesis of HF. Stubbs et al. (Stubbs et al., 1978) induced HF with the administration of opioids to healthy volunteers. Naloxone, an opioid antagonist, causes vasomotor symptoms when administered to opioid-dependent animals (Tulandi et al., 1985). Sex steroids induce the hypothalamic production of β-endorphins, which are endogenous hypothalamic opioids that inhibit catecholamine synthesis by reducing the activity of the estrogen-2-hydroxilase (Fishman et al., 1980). Peripheral sex hormones promote the formation of catecholestrogens as well, which in turn block the hypothalamic synthesis of NA (Robert R Freedman, 2005). (**Figure 3**) Therefore, a sudden deprivation of sex hormones will result in decreased endorphin levels and loss of negative feedback (R R Freedman & Krell, 1999).

The ensuing rise in hypothalamic NA levels eventually enhances the release of LHRH by the LHRH-secreting neurons. NA also acts on the thermoregulatory center by shortening its response range, lowering its temperature tolerance thresholds, and generating HF, which in turn enhances heat loss (Robert R Freedman, 2005; R R Freedman & Krell, 1999). (**Figure 2**) At the regulatory center, there is a zone for the control of body temperature. At the lower threshold, a shivering mechanism is triggered, leading to a rise in temperature. At the upper threshold, heat loss is induced through skin vasodilatation and profuse sweating. Between these two thresholds is a thermoneutral zone (Savage & Brengelman, 1996). (**Figure 4**)

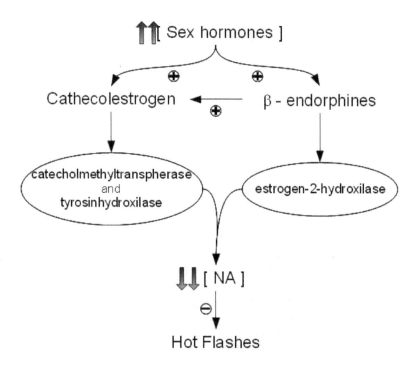

Fig. 3. Negative impact of sex hormones on noradrenaline production

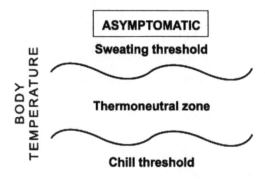

Fig. 4. Body temperature control range in an asymptomatic patient

In patients with HF, the thermoneutral zone is quite narrow, which is why small changes may influence the thermoregulatory center (Robert R Freedman, 2005; Dacks & Rance, 2010). (**Figure 5**) The increase in body temperature after a rise in ambient temperature or the intake of excessively hot food exceeds the upper threshold of the thermoneutral zone and triggers the heat-dissipating mechanisms (Dacks & Rance, 2010; Savage & Brengelman, 1996).

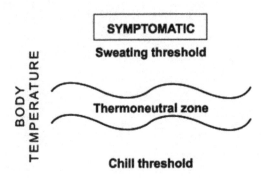

Fig. 5. Body temperature control range in symptomatic patient

The increase in hypothalamic levels of certain substances, such as noradrenaline, tends to narrow this zone, while other agents such as serotonin and dopamine have the opposite effect (Berendsen, 2000). (**Figure 6**) It has been concluded that the thermoneutral zone is 0.4 °C in asymptomatic and 0.0 °C in symptomatic patients (Robert R Freedman, 2005).

Serotonin (5-hydroxytryptamine or 5-HT) levels are reduced in postmenopausal women, even though they normalize following replacement therapies.

A sudden deprivation of sex hormones results in a reduction of circulating serotonin, with a parallel increase in its 5-HT2A hypothalamic receptors. These receptors may also play a role in the pathogenesis of HF (Albertazzi, 2006).

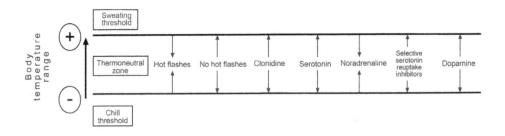

Fig. 6. Effect on thermoneutral zone of various substances

To sum up, a basic feature in the pathogenesis of HF is the negative effect of plasma sex hormones on the hypothalamic secretion of noradrenaline, as well as its balance with serotonin and dopamine. (**Figure 7**)

Other information supports the hypothalamic hypothesis. It has recently been demonstrated that serum IL-8 concentrations were significantly higher in women with HF than without HF. IL-8 could play an important role in the pathophysiology of HF (Yasui et al., 2006; Noguchi et al., 2008).

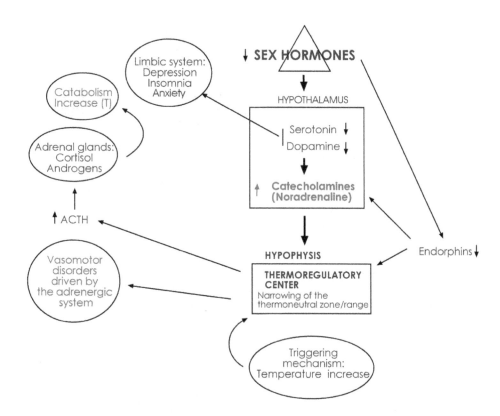

Fig. 7. Negative effect of sex hormones on hypothalamic noradrenaline

The rat ortholog of the human IL-8 receptor has been identified (Dunstan et al., 1996), and the functions of IL-8 appear to be performed by cytokine-induced neutrophil chemoattractant (CINC) in rodents (Guex-Crosier et al., 1996). It has been shown that CINC stimulates the secretion of prolactin, GH, and ACTH but suppresses the secretion of LH and FSH from the anterior pituitary cells (Koike et al., 1994). In animal models HF could be triggered by intracerebroventricular injection (i.c.v.) of LHRH analogues (Noguchi et al., 2008; Noguchi et al., 2003). After that, an increase of CINC around the periventricular area in the hypothalamus is observed in ovariectomized rats.

Hypothalamic thermoregulation by CINC and LHRH may, therefore, be a reciprocal relationship. However, changes in CINC concentration and skin temperature after i.c.v. injection of LHRHa were reversed by replacement of estradiol. Therefore, there may be a feedback regulation mechanism involving LHRH and CINC through the hypothalamus-pituitary-gonadal axis (Noguchi et al., 2008).

Consequently, LHRH and CINC play a key role in the homeostasis of body temperature in HD situations (Noguchi et al., 2008). All these finding support the **hypothalamic hypothesis**.

New aspects of hot flash research, including neuroimaging and the study of genetic polymorphisms, when combined with increasingly nuanced ways of asking questions of culturally distinct populations, pose challenges, but at the same time offer a rich complexity from which a better understanding of hot flashes will emerge (F. Kronenberg, 2010).

Other parts of the brain can be seen to be involved in the development of hot flashes. Magnetic resonance imaging has shown activation of the insula and anterior cingulated cortex during hot flash episodes (F. Kronenberg, 2010).

Finally, genetic variation in CYP19 and sex hormone binding globulin contributes to variance in circulating hormone levels between postmenopausal women, and it could potentially have an influence on hot flashes (Dunning et al., 2004).

3. Current treatment of hot flashes

As is to be expected, the great majority of published studies were carried out in menopausal women or in breast cancer survivors, but more and more trials are being conducted in patients undergoing hormone deprivation for prostate cancer.

In view of their pathophysiology, the regulatory mechanisms on negative feedback should be taken into account as causes of these hot flashes.

3.1 Hormone replacement

Hormone replacement with estrogens was the first treatment used in the 20th century. Other forms of replacement included progesterones and androgens, but because of the hormone sensitivity of prostate cancer, the latter would be contraindicated.

As for estrogens, it should be noted that despite their high efficacy even at low doses, they have negative side effects. These include thromboembolic phenomena, cardiovascular morbidity and painful gynecomastia (J. A. Smith, 1994; J. I. Miller & Ahmann, 1992; Atala et al., 1992).

The most widely used estrogen, both orally and transdermally, is estradiol (Shanafelt et al., 2002), which requires at least a month to obtain benefits. Higher doses provide better control of symptoms than lower doses but also have more side effects, though these are fewer when transdermal formulations are used. The usual oral doses are ≥ 0.25 mg/day, whereas the daily amount required for patches is less than 0.05 mg/day.

In summary, estrogen therapy shows a dose-dependent response, with a balance in favor of transdermal therapy and an efficacy of 80-90%, reducing the number of hot flashes by 2.5 to 3 hot flashes daily (Rossouw et al., 2002; Nelson, 2004), but with undesirable side effects that need to be considered (Kouriefs et al., 2002; Rossouw et al., 2002). Its effectiveness was confirmed in a 2002 meta-analysis from the Cochrane Library, in an extensive review published in JAMA in 2004 (Nelson, 2004), and in a more recent systematic review in Lancet Oncology (Frisk, 2010).

Progesterones, like estrogens, stimulate the production of hypothalamic β-endorphins. Their use is also not free from undesirable side effects (C L Loprinzi et al., 1994; Quella et al., 1998; C L Loprinzi et al., 1992). There is experience in both men and women, and the most used is megestrol acetate, with starting doses of 20 mg twice daily and subsequent reduction to the lowest effective dose, with response rates of 80-90% (Frisk, 2010; J. W. Goodwin et al., 2008; Quella et al., 1998; C L Loprinzi et al., 1994).

As a second drug in use, cyproterone acetate is a steroidal antiandrogen with progestogenic action. It shows response rates comparable to megestrol acetate but with risk of hepatoxicity, fatigue, painful gynecomastia and galactorrhea (Frisk, 2010). Treatment for hot flashes should be started at 50 mg/day, and not exceed 300 mg/day (Moon, 1985; Irani et al., 2010).

Lastly, we need to mention medroxyprogesterone acetate given in 20-40 mg oral doses daily with equal or superior efficacy to megestrol or a single 400 mg i.m. depot dose with an effect sustained over at least 6 months (Irani et al., 2010; Prior et al., 1995). Although some experts consider 400 mg to be a very high dose, it is a small dose if we compare it to the 500 mg intramuscular or oral doses used daily during months for the treatment of breast cancer. It was found to be correctly tolerated and weight gain was the only undesirable effect.

There have been reservations regarding the use of progesterones in prostate cancer because it has been reported in some articles to be related to increases in PSA levels (Dawson & McLeod, 1995; Wehbe et al., 1997). Clarification is still required before these results can be extrapolated to support the use of low-dose progesterones in the treatment of prostate cancer, although their antitumor activity has also been reported in breast, endometrium and prostate cancer (Wentz, 1985; Bonomi et al., 1985).

The effect of estrogens and progesterones can persist for extended periods after their withdrawal (C L Loprinzi et al., 1994; Haas et al., 1988).

The problems of the use of hormone replacement therapy in menopausal women have acquired a certain prominence as a result of the publication of the results of the Women´s Health Initiative randomized controlled trial, which reveal the increased risk of developing breast cancer, cognitive disorders, cardiovascular and thromboembolic disease. Alternative treatments are therefore desirable.

The absolute risks per 10,000 person-years were 7 more coronary events, 8 more strokes, 8 more pulmonary embolisms, and 8 more invasive breast cancers, while absolute risk reductions per 10,000 person-years were 6 fewer colorectal cancers and 5 fewer hip fractures. They also reduced vasomotor symptoms and vulvovaginal atrophy (G. L. Anderson et al., 2004).

3.2 Non-hormonal therapies

The current availability of non-hormonal therapies is a major advance both for women who have survived breast cancer and for men with a prostate adenocarcinoma undergoing hormone deprivation, in whom hormone replacement therapy may be contraindicated due to adverse effects.

Several drugs have been tested for the management of vasomotor symptoms. A 2006 meta-analysis of well-designed studies (Nelson et al., 2006) showed that the only effective therapies are, in increasing order of effectiveness: gabapentin, selective serotonin-reuptake inhibitors, and clonidine. A brief description of these therapies is discussed below. Their efficacy is slightly less than with hormone replacement, but their effectiveness has been widely demonstrated.

Since noradrenaline is the neurotransmitter involved in the control of the thermoregulatory center, the blockade of both α- and β-adrenoceptors may provide symptomatic relief. On this basis, the α_2 agonist clonidine (Clayden et al., 1974) has been tested in both men and women (Pandya et al., 2000). Alpha$_2$ receptors have been identified at both hypothalamic and peripheral levels. Their presynaptic activation brings about a decrease of NA release (R R Freedman & Dinsay, 2000). They are also peripherally active by reducing vasodilatation, which contributes to improved control of hot flashes (Kouriefs et al., 2002). Although higher doses are associated with a more significant symptomatic relief, they also involve a greater toxicity. Transdermal administration (Nagamani et al., 1987) results in equivalent absorption to oral administration, but is associated with more common skin reactions. Recommended doses are between 25 to 400 µg. Its efficacy is lower than that of hormonal therapy (20-55%), and side effects are common. Two recent double-blind randomized-controlled clinical trials and a systematic review, comparing clonidine to venlafaxine, have reported conflicting results (Frisk, 2010; Buijs et al., 2009; Loibl et al., 2007). The drug may be potentially useful when other therapies are contraindicated (Kouriefs et al., 2002).

Response rates of 44-60% have been achieved with gabapentin 300 mg every 8 hours, with the main side effects being somnolence, dizziness, fatigue, skin rash, palpitations, and peripheral edema (Charles L Loprinzi et al., 2007; C L Loprinzi et al., 2009). In a recent open-label, randomized, cross-over trial gabapentin is worse tolerated than Venlafaxine (Bordeleau et al., 2010).

Its mechanism of action, although at present unclear, may involve the modulation of calcium channels (T. J. Guttuso, 2000). In a recent study, gabapentin has been shown to be useful in patients with an inadequate response to antidepressants (Charles L Loprinzi et al., 2007).

Some serotonin-acting antidepressants may be of value in the management of hot flashes. As mentioned above, serotonin levels, which are decreased in postmenopausal women, tend to normalize after replacement therapies. Thus, an abrupt fall in sex hormones is likely to produce a decrease in circulating serotonin along with an up-regulation of their $5-HT_{2A}$ hypothalamic receptors (Albertazzi, 2006; Curcio et al., 2005), which may be involved in the pathogenesis of hot flashes.

The potency of $5-HT_{2A}$ antagonists varies widely among the first generation (tricyclic) antidepressants, although the resulting impact on the therapeutic activity of these drugs has not yet been defined. Another class of antidepressants, known as phenylpiperazines, has been shown to be more selective than tricyclics and to possess more potent $5HT_{2A}$ receptor-blocking activity.

Newer antidepressants, mainly venlafaxine, desvenlafaxine and paroxetine, play an important role in the non-hormonal therapy of hot flashes (Albertazzi, 2006). Observed response rates are approximately 50-69 %, somewhat lower than those achieved with hormonal therapies; however, their improved safety profile in cancer survivors makes them an appealing option for this group of patients. Serious side effects are rare, since the doses used are lower than those normally given for the treatment of depression, and a withdrawal syndrome has not been associated with such doses (Irani et al., 2010; Buijs et al., 2009; Loibl et al., 2007; C L Loprinzi et al., 2000; Archer et al., 2009).

There is little data regarding the use of new-generation antidepressants for the treatment of hot flashes in prostate cancer patients undergoing hormone deprivation. Venlafaxine has been shown to produce symptomatic relief in a study involving 16 patients (Quella et al., 1999). Another small study with 24 patients reported symptomatic relief of hot flashes in men who received paroxetine for 5 weeks (Charles L Loprinzi et al., 2004). **(Table 1)**

However, the use of selective reuptake inhibitors such as paroxetine during tamoxifen treatment must be evaluated with caution, as it is associated with an increased risk of death from breast cancer. This could be due to the inhibition of the cytochrome P450 2D6 (CYP2D6) pathway (Kelly et al., 2010).

Another interesting antidepressant is trazodone, a triazolopiridine-derived phenylpiperazine. Trazodone is a potent and selective postsynaptic antagonist of the $5-HT_{2A}$ receptor as well as a moderate inhibitor of serotinin reuptake (Pansini et al., 1995). It belongs to a class of antidepressants called SARI (serotonin 2A agonist and reuptake inhibitors). Trazodone shows a high affinity for 5-HT$_{2A}$ receptors, along with a moderate affinity for 5-HT$_{1A}$ receptors. **(Figure 8)**

Paroxetine	doses between 10 and 25 mg/day, with 60-65 % response rates
Venlafaxine	25 or 37,5 mg/day increased to 75 mg/day after 1 week, with response rates of 50-65 %.
Desvenlafaxine	150 mg/day, with response rates of 51-69 %.
Fluoxetine	doses of 20 mg/day, with an effectiveness of about 50%.
Citalopram	20 mg/day, with an effectiveness of about 50%. (Suvanto-Luukkonen et al., 2005; Debra L Barton et al., 2010)
Veralipride	antidopaminergic drug
Sertraline	50 mg/day, with a response rate of 36 % (Kimmick et al., 2006).

Table 1. Dosages and response rates for selected antidepressants

Conversely, a traditional selective serotonin reuptake inhibitor (SSRI), such as fluoxetine, has little affinity for 5-HT$_{1A}$ and 5-HT$_{2A}$ receptors, even though its potency to inhibit serotonin reuptake is greater than that of trazodone. In fact, the concentration of drug needed to produce a 50% inhibition (IC$_{50}$) of reuptake is only 6 nmol/l for fluoxetine and 115 nmol/l for trazodone (Owens et al., 1997).

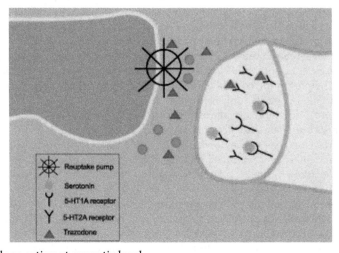

Fig. 8. Trazodone action at synaptic level.

SSRIs stimulate all types of serotonin receptors because they increase free 5-HT levels without blocking any receptors. Although these drugs have been useful in the treatment of depression, they cause adverse reactions, such as agitation, anxiety, and sexual dysfunction, due to the stimulation of 5-HT$_{2A}$ receptors in other tissues (e. g., brainstem and spinal cord) (Stahl, 1998). It is worth noting that 5-HT$_{2A}$ receptors are the main receptors associated with hot flashes and are inhibited by trazodone.

Since trazodone does not cause a clinical blockade of acetylcholine receptors, the potential anticholinergic effects (blurred vision, cardiac alterations, mouth dryness, intestinal disorders, urinary retention, and increased intraocular pressure) are negligible. Moreover, since it lacks any clinical effects on NA inhibition, other potential side effects such as apathy, lack of motivation, anhedonia, and difficulty concentrating are minimal.

Nevertheless, trazodone shows an interesting affinity for α-receptors. The high and moderate activity of trazodone for α_1- and α_2- adrenergic receptors, respectively, might contribute to the beneficial effects described on erectile dysfunction (Krege et al., 2000). On the other hand, this same property could also lead to orthostatic hypotension.

Trazodone also blocks H_1-histamine receptors (H_1) and, probably due to its histamine-blocking properties and potent 5-HT_{2A} antagonist activity (Stahl, 1998; Marek et al., 1992), also exhibits a sedative activity that has been shown to be useful for the treatment of elderly patients with agitation and insomnia.

Because of its pharmacological profile, this antidepressant may be valuable in the treatment of hot flashes in prostate cancer patients undergoing hormone deprivation.

As mentioned above, NA acts on the thermoregulatory center by shortening its response range and lowering its tolerance threshold, which in turn results in cutaneous vasodilation and profuse sweating. Drugs with noradrenergic properties, which could trigger the onset of hot flashes, should thus not be used in prostate cancer patients undergoing hormone deprivation. Furthermore, while NA shortens the thermoregulatory response range, serotonin and dopamine have an opposite effect. (**Figure 6**)

The use of serotonergic antidepressants may be warranted and, in fact, a few of them have already been tested with encouraging results.

In addition, considering that hormone deprivation is associated with low serotonin concentrations and stimulation of 5-HT_{2A} receptors, some drugs, such as trazodone, whose pharmacological profile is characterized by a high affinity for these 5-HT_{2A} receptors and a moderate effect on serotonin reuptake, might be beneficial in the management of hot flashes, unlike serotonergic antidepressants (SSRIs), which lack this property. This profile might also be significantly helpful in the control of anxiety, sleep and erectile dysfunction, all of which would result in a quality of life improvement.

To date there are few studies examining the use of trazodone in hormonally deprived patients. One pilot study assessed the management of hot flashes in 25 menopausal women. No objective effect was seen after doses of 75 mg/day for 3 months, although anxiety, insomnia and irritability were reduced (Pansini et al., 1995). Further studies are required to elucidate the potential efficacy of trazodone against hot flashes by using validated scales to ascertain such effect.

It should be mentioned that the placebo effect can improve hot flashes in 20-40 % of patients, with perceived efficacy rates of 50-75 % for initialuse (J A Sloan et al., 2001; Moyad, 2002).

Other drugs have been shown to be either less effective or ineffective, or have been disregarded for the management of hot flashes because of their high incidence of side effects. (**Table 2**)

Some dietetic measures can be helpful, namely: cold water irrigations or the application of cold; avoiding excessively hot food and very hot environments; limiting the consumption of spicy food, coffee and alcohol; following a diet rich in soy protein-containing products (the use of phytoestrogens, although recommended by some authors, is to be avoided because of its potential effect on hormonal-dependent cancer) (J A Sloan et al., 2001; Carmignani et al., 2010); reducing stress by means of relaxation techniques like yoga ; engaging in non -

strenuous physical exercise to maintain an appropriate weight (being overweight can increase both the frequency and severity of hot flashes) (Sideras & Charles L Loprinzi, 2010; Robert R Freedman, 2005); and quitting smoking.

• Bellergal (phenobarbital + ergotamine + belladonna alkaloids), with a 30 % withdrawal rate from therapy due to toxicity (Bergmans et al., 1987). • Dietary supplements. • High-dose supplements of isoflavones/phytoestrogens (both estrogenic and antiestrogenic effects). • Medicinal plants (Moyad, 2002). • Vitamin E (Moyad, 2002). • Methyldopa (M. G. Hammond et al., 1984). • Relaxation techniques, physical exercise, acupuncture. • L-Isoleucine and L-Valine (T. Guttuso et al., 2008).

Table 2. Some commonly used measures for hot flash management

Drug or Action	Dosage and Actions	Percentage of Response
Estrogens	Estradiol p.o. (0.25 mg/day) or transdermal (0.05 mg/day)	80-90 %
Progesterones	Megestrol acetate 20 mg/12 h Cyproterone acetate 50-100 mg/day Medroxyprogesterone acetate p.o. 20-40 mg/day or single 400 mg i.m. depot dose	80-90 %
Clonidine	25-400 mcg/day	20-55 %
Antidepressants	Paroxetine 10-25 mg/day Venlafaxine 25-75 mg/day Desvenlafaxine 150 mg/day Fluoxetine 20 mg/day Sertraline 50 mg/day Trazodone 50-150 mg/day	60-65 % 55-65 % 51-69 % 50 % 36 %
Gabapentin	300 mg/8 h	44-60 %
Placebo effect		20-40 %
Others	Bellegard Isoflavones/phytoestrogens Vitamin E Cimifuga Racemosa Acupuncture L-Isoleucine and L-Valine Methyldopa Physical exercise Relaxation techniques	

Table 3. Summary of all data presented

Acupuncture has been studied for alleviation of hot flashes in patients with prostate carcinoma (Harding et al., 2009) and in postmenopausal women (E. M. Walker et al., 2010). However more studies are needed to confirm any benefit (Sideras & Charles L Loprinzi, 2010).

A correlation between body mass index and the frequency of hot flashes, as determined by insulin metabolism in fat tissues and an increase in body temperature, has been shown in recent studies, (Robert R Freedman, 2005; Gold et al., 2000). A relationship has also been reported with tobacco consumption, which might be explained by an effect on estrogen metabolism or a thermogenic action of nicotine, (Robert R Freedman, 2005; Whiteman et al., 2003; Jessen et al., 2003)

4. Acknowledgments

We want to thank Ms. Marian Torres Berruezo for helping with the pictures and Mr. Garth Stobbs and Murat Yilmaz to help translate this manuscript.

5. References

Aksel, S., Schomberg, D. W., Tyrey, L., & Hammond, C. B. 1976. Vasomotor symptoms, serum estrogens, and gonadotropin levels in surgical menopause. *Am J Obstet Gynecol* 126: 165-169.

Albertazzi, P. 2006. Noradrenergic and serotonergic modulation to treat vasomotor symptoms. *J Br Menopause Soc* 12: 7-11.

Anderson, G. L., Limacher, M., Assaf, A. R., Bassford, T., Beresford, S. A. A., Black, H., Bonds, D., Brunner, R., Brzyski, R., Caan, B., Chlebowski, R., Curb, D., Gass, M., Hays, J., Heiss, G., et al. 2004. Effects of conjugated equine estrogen in postmenopausal women with hysterectomy: the Women's Health Initiative randomized controlled trial. *JAMA* 291: 1701-1712.

Archer, D. F., Dupont, C. M., Constantine, G. D., Pickar, J. H., & Olivier, S. 2009. Desvenlafaxine for the treatment of vasomotor symptoms associated with menopause: a double-blind, randomized, placebo-controlled trial of efficacy and safety. *Am J Obstet Gynecol* 200: 238.e1-238.e10.

Atala, A., Amin, M., & Harty, J. I. 1992. Diethylstilbestrol in treatment of postorchiectomy vasomotor symptoms and its relationship with serum follicle-stimulating hormone, luteinizing hormone, and testosterone. *Urology* 39: 108-110.

Barton, Debra L, LaVasseur, Beth I, Sloan, Jeff A, Stawis, A. N., Flynn, K. A., Dyar, M., Johnson, D. B., Atherton, Pamela J, Diekmann, B., & Loprinzi, Charles L. 2010. Phase III, placebo-controlled trial of three doses of citalopram for the treatment of hot flashes: NCCTG trial N05C9. *J Clin Oncol* 28: 3278-83.

Berendsen, H. H. G. 2000. The role of serotonine in hot flushes. *Maturitas* 36: 155-164.

Bergmans, M. G., Merkus, J. M., Corbey, R. S., Schellekens, L. A., & Ubachs, J. M. 1987. Effect of Bellergal Retard on climacteric complaints: a double-blind, placebo-controlled study. *Maturitas* 9: 227-234.

Boer, H. de, Gastel, P. van, & Sorge, A. van. 2009. Luteinizing hormone-releasing hormone and postmenopausal flushing. *N Engl J Med* 361: 1218-9.

Bonomi, P., Pessis, D., Bunting, N., Block, M., Anderson, K., Wolter, J., Rossof, A., Slayton, R., & Harris, J. 1985. Megestrol acetate used as primary hormonal therapy in stage D prostatic cancer. *Semin Oncol* 12: 36-39.

Bordeleau, L., Pritchard, Kathleen I, Loprinzi, Charles L, Ennis, M., Jugovic, O., Warr, D., Haq, R., & Goodwin, P. J. 2010. Multicenter, randomized, cross-over clinical trial of venlafaxine versus gabapentin for the management of hot flashes in breast cancer survivors. *J Clin Oncol* 28: 5147-5152.

Buchholz, N. P., & Matarelli, G. 1994. Hot flushes after orchidectomy in treatment of prostate cancer – a serious effect. *Z Gerontol* 27: 334-336.

Buijs, C., Mom, C. H., Willemse, P. H. B., Marike Boezen, H., Maurer, J. M., Wymenga, A. N. M., Jong, R. S. de, Nieboer, P., Vries, E. G. E. de, & Mourits, M. J. E. 2009. Venlafaxine versus clonidine for the treatment of hot flashes in breast cancer patients: a double-blind, randomized cross-over study. *Breast Cancer Res Treat* 115: 573-580.

Carmignani, L. O., Pedro, A. O., Costa-Paiva, L. H., & Pinto-Neto, A. M. 2010. The effect of dietary soy supplementation compared to estrogen and placebo on menopausal symptoms: a randomized controlled trial. *Maturitas* 67: 262-269.

Carpenter, J. S., Andrykowski, M. A., Freedman, R R, & Munn, R. 1999. Feasibility and psychometrics of an ambulatory hot flash monitoring device. *Menopause* 6: 209-215.

Carpenter, J. S., Gilchrist, J. M., Chen, K., Gautam, S., & Freedman, R R. 2004. Hot flashes, core body temperature and metabolic parameters in breast cancer survivors. *Menopause* 11: 375-381.

Casper, R. F., Yen, S. S., & Wilkes, M. M. 1979. Menopausal flushes: a neuroendocrine link with pulsatile luteinizing hormone secretion. *Science* 205: 823-825.

Charig, C. R., & Rundle, J. S. 1989. Flushing. Long-term side effects of orchidectomy in treatment of prostatic cancer. *Urology* 33: 175-178.

Clayden, J. R., Bell, J. W., & Pollard, P. 1974. Menopausal flushing: double-blind trial of a non-hormonal medication. *Br Med J* 1: 409-412.

Curcio, J. J., Kim, L. S., Wollner, D., & Pockaj, B. A. 2005. The potential of 5-hydryoxytryptophan for hot flash reduction: a hypothesis. *Altern Med Rev* 10: 216-221.

Dacks, P. A., & Rance, N. E. 2010. Effects of estradiol on the thermoneutral zone and core temperature in ovariectomized rats. *Endocrinology* 151: 1187-1193.

Dawson, N. A., & McLeod, D. G. 1995. Dramatic prostate specific antigen decrease in response to discontinuation of megestrol acetate in advanced prostate cancer: expansion of the antiandrogen withdrawal syndrome. *J urol* 153: 1946-1947.

Dunning, a M., Dowsett, M., Healey, C. S., Tee, L., Luben, R. N., Folkerd, E., Novik, K. L., Kelemen, L., Ogata, S., Pharoah, P. D. P., Easton, D. F., Day, N. E., & Ponder, B. a J. 2004. Polymorphisms Associated With Circulating Sex Hormone Levels in Postmenopausal Women. *J Natl Cancer Inst* 96: 936-945.

Dunstan, C. A., Salafranca, M. N., Adhikari, S., Xia, Y., Feng, L., & Harrison, J. K. 1996. Identification of two rat genes orthologous to the human interleukin-8 receptors. *J Biol Chem* 271: 32770-32776.

Etgen, A. M., Ansonoff, M. A., & Quesada, A. 2001. Mechanisms of ovarian steroid regulation of norepinephrine receptor-mediated signal transduction in the hypothalamus: implications for female reproductive physiology. *Horm Behav* 40: 169-177.

Fishman, J., Norton, B. I., & Hahn, E. F. 1980. Opiate regulation of estradiol-2-hydroxylase in brains of male rats: mechanism for control of pituitary hormone secretion. *Proc Natl Acad Sci U S A* 77: 2574-6.

Freedman, R R. 2001. Physiology of hot flashes. *Am J Hum Biol* 13: 453-464.

Freedman, R R, & Dinsay, R. 2000. Clonidine raises the sweating threshold in symptomatic but not in asymptomatic postmenopausal women. *Fertil Steril* 74: 20-23.

Freedman, R R, & Krell, W. 1999. Reduced thermoregulatory null zone in postmenopausal women with hot flashes. *Am J Obstet Gynecol* 18: 66-70.

Freedman, R R, Woodward, S., & Sabharwal, S. C. 1990. α2–Adrenergic mechanism in menopausal hot flushes. *Obstet Gynecol* 76: 573-578.

Freedman, Robert R. 2005. Hot flashes: behavioral treatments, mechanisms, and relation to sleep. *Am J Med* 118 Suppl: 124-130.

Frisk, J. 2010. Managing hot flushes in men after prostate cancer--a systematic review. *Maturitas* 65: 15-22.

Gold, E. B., Sternfeld, B., Kelsey, J. L., Brown, C., Mouton, C., Reame, N., Salamone, L., & Stellato, R. 2000. Relation of demographic and lifestyle factors to symptoms in a multi-racial/ethnic population of women 40-55 years of age. *Am J Epidemiol* 152: 463-473.

Goodwin, J. W., Green, S. J., Moinpour, C. M., Bearden, James D, Giguere, J. K., Jiang, C. S., Lippman, S. M., Martino, S., & Albain, K. S. 2008. Phase III randomized placebo-controlled trial of two doses of megestrol acetate as treatment for menopausal symptoms in women with breast cancer: Southwest Oncology Group Study 9626. *J Clin Oncol* 26: 1650-1656.

Guex-Crosier, Y., Wittwer, A. J., & Roberge, F. G. 1996. Intraocular production of a cytokine (CINC) responsible for neutrophil infiltration in endotoxin induced uveitis. *Br J Ophthal* 80: 649-653.

Guttuso, T. J. 2000. Gabapentin's effects on hot flashes and hypothermia. *Neurology* 54: 2161-2163.

Guttuso, T., McDermott, M. P., Su, H., & Kieburtz, K. 2008. Effects of L-isoleucine and L-valine on hot flushes and serum homocysteine: a randomized controlled trial. *Obstet Gynecol* 112: 109-115.

Haas, S., Walsh, B., Evans, S., Krache, M., Ravnikar, V., & Schiff, I. 1988. The effect of transdermal estradiol on hormone and metabolic dynamics over a six-week period. *Obstet Gynecol* 71: 671-676.

Hammond, M. G., Hatley, L., & Talbert, L. M. 1984. A double blind study to evaluate the effect of methyldopa on menopausal vasomotor flushes. *J Clin Endocrinol Metab* 58: 1158-1160.

Harding, C., Harris, A., & Chadwick, D. 2009. Auricular acupuncture: a novel treatment for vasomotor symptoms associated with luteinizing-hormone releasing hormone agonist treatment for prostate cancer. *BJU Int* 103: 186-190.

Harvey, H., Lipton, A., Max, D., Pearlman, H., Diaz-Perches, R., & Garza, J. D. L. 1985. Medical castration produced by the GnRH analogue leuprolide to treat metastatic breast cancer. *J Clin Oncol* 3: 1068-1072.

Huggins, C., & Hodges, G. V. 1941. Studies on prostate cancer. I. The effect of castration, estrogen and androgen injections on serum phosphatases in Metastatic carcinoma of the prostate. *Cancer Res* 1: 293-295.

Irani, J., Salomon, L., Oba, R., Bouchard, P., & Mottet, N. 2010. Efficacy of venlafaxine, medroxyprogesterone acetate, and cyproterone acetate for the treatment of vasomotor hot flushes in men taking gonadotropin-releasing hormone analogues for prostate cancer: a double-blind, randomised trial. *Lancet Oncol* 11: 147-154.

Jessen, A. B., Toubro, S., & Astrup, A. 2003. Effect of chewing gum containing nicotine and caffeine on energy expenditure and substrate utilization in men. *Am J Clin Nutr* 77: 1442-1447.

Kelly, C. M., Juurlink, D. N., Gomes, T., Duong-Hua, M., Pritchard, K. I, Austin, P. C., & Paszat, L. F. 2010. Selective serotonin reuptake inhibitors and breast cancer mortality in women receiving tamoxifen: a population based cohort study. *BMJ* 340: c693-c693.

Kimmick, G. G., Lovato, J., McQuellon, R., Robinson, E., & Muss, H. B. 2006. Randomized, double-blind, placebo-controlled, crossover study of sertraline (Zoloft) for the treatment of hot flashes in women with early stage breast cancer taking tamoxifen. *Breast J* 12: 114-122.

Koike, K., Sakamoto, Y., Sawada, T., Ohmichi, M., Kanda, Y., Nohara, A., Hirota, K., Kiyama, H., & Miyake, A. 1994. The production of CINC/gro, a member of the interleukin-8 family, in rat anterior pituitary gland. *Biochem Biophys Res Commun* 202: 161-167.

Kouriefs, C., Georgiou, M., & Ravi, R. 2002. Hot flushes and prostate cancer: pathogenesis and treatment. *BJU Int* 89: 379-383.

Krege, S., Goepel, M., Sperling, H., & Michel, M. C. 2000. Affinity of trazodone for human penile alpha1- andalpha2-adrenoceptors. *BJU Int* 85: 959-61.

Kronenberg, F. L., Cote, L. J., Linkie, D. M., Dyrenfurth, I., & Downey, J. A. 1984. Menopausal hot flashes: thermoregulatory, cardiovascular and circulating catecholamine and LH changes. *Maturitas* 6: 31-43.

Kronenberg, F. 2010. Menopausal hot flashes: a review of physiology and biosociocultural perspective on methods of assessment. *J Nut* 140: 1380S-1385S.

Leuprolide Study Group. 1984. Leuprolide versus diethylstilbestrol for metastatic prostate cancer. *N Engl J Med* 311: 1281-1286.

Linsell, C. R., & Lightman, S. L. 1983. Postmenopausal flashes: studies of chronological organisation. *Psychoneuroendocrinology* 8: 435-440.

Loibl, S., Schwedler, K., Minckwitz, G. von, Strohmeier, R., Mehta, K. M., & Kaufmann, M. 2007. Venlafaxine is superior to clonidine as treatment of hot flashes in breast cancer patients--a double-blind, randomized study. *Ann Oncol* 18: 689-693.

Loprinzi, C L, Dueck, A C, Khoyratty, B. S., Barton, D L, Jafar, S., Rowland, K. M., Atherton, P J, Marsa, G. W., Knutson, W. H., Bearden, J D, Kottschade, L., & Fitch, T. R. 2009. A phase III randomized, double-blind, placebo-controlled trial of gabapentin in the management of hot flashes in men (N00CB). *Ann Oncol* 20: 542-549.

Loprinzi, C L, Johnson, P. A., & Jensen, M. 1992. Megestrol acetate for anorexia and cachexia. *Oncology* 49 Suppl 2: 46-49.

Loprinzi, C L, Kugler, J W, Sloan, J A, Mailliard, J. A., LaVasseur, B I, Barton, D L, Novotny, P J, Dakhil, S. R., Rodger, K., Rummans, T. A., & Christensen, B J. 2000. Venlafaxine in management of hot flashes in survivors of breast cancer: a randomised controlled trial. *Lancet* 356: 2059-2063.

Loprinzi, C L, Michalak, J. C., Quella, S. K., O'Fallon, J. R., Hatfield, A. K., Nelimark, R A, Dose, A. M., Fischer, T., Johnson, C., & Klatt, N. E. 1994. Megestrol acetate for the prevention of hot flashes. *N Engl J Med* 331: 347-352.

Loprinzi, Charles L, Barton, Debra L, Carpenter, L. A., Sloan, Jeff A, Novotny, Paul J, Gettman, M. T., & Christensen, Bradley J. 2004. Pilot evaluation of paroxetine for treating hot flashes in men. *Mayo Clin Proc* 79: 1247-1251.

Loprinzi, Charles L, Kugler, John W, Barton, Debra L, Dueck, Amylou C, Tschetter, L. K., Nelimark, Robert A, Balcueva, E. P., Burger, K. N., Novotny, Paul J, Carlson, M. D., Duane, S. F., Corso, S. W., Johnson, D. B., & Jaslowski, A. J. 2007. Phase III trial of gabapentin alone or in conjunction with an antidepressant in the management of hot flashes in women who have inadequate control with an antidepressant alone: NCCTG N03C5. *J Clin Oncol* 25: 308-312.

Maatman, T. J., Gupta, M. K., & Montie, J. E. 1985. Effectiveness of castration vs intravenous estrogen in producing rapid endocrine control of metastatic cancer of prostate. *J Urol* 133: 620-621.

Marek, G. J., McDougle, C. J., Price, L. H., & Seiden, L. S. 1992. A comparison of trazodone and fluoxetine: implications for a serotonergic mechanism of antidepressant action. *Psychopharmacology* 109: 2-11.

Melldrum, D. R., Defazio, J. D., Erlik, Y., Lu, J. K. H., Wolfsen, A. F., Carlson, H. E., HershmanN, J. M., & Judd, H. L. 1984. Pituitary hormones during the menopausal hot flash. *Obstet Gynecol* 64: 752-756.

Miller, J. I., & Ahmann, F. R. 1992. Treatment of castration-induced menopausal symptoms with low dose diethylstilbestrol in men with advanced prostate cancer. *Urology* 40: 499-502.

Molnar, G. W. 1975. Body temperature during menopausal hot flashes. *J Appl Physiol* 38: 499-503.

Moon, T. D. 1985. Cyproterone acetate for treatment of hot flashes after orchiectomy. *J Urol* 134: 155-156.

Moyad, M. A. 2002. Complementary/alternative therapies for reducing hot flashes in prostate cancer patients: reevaluating the existing indirect data from studies of breast cancer and postmenopausal women. *Urology* 59: 20-33.

Nagamani, M., Kelver, M. E., & Smith, E. R. 1987. Treatment of menopausal hot flashes with transdermal administration of clonidine. *Am J Obstet Gynecol* 156: 561-565.

Nelson, H. D. 2004. Commonly used types of postmenopausal estrogen for treatment of hot flashes: scientific review. *JAMA* 291: 1610-1620.

Nelson, H. D., Vesco, K. K., Haney, E., Nedrow, A., Miller, J., Nicolaidis, C., Walker, M., & Humphrey, L. 2006. Nonhormonal therapies for Menopausal hot flashes. Systematic Review and Meta-analysis. *JAMA* 295: 2057-2071.

Nishiyama, T., Kanazawa, S., Watanabe, R., Terunuma, M., & Takahashi, K. 2004. Influence of hot flashes on quality of life in patients with prostate cancer treated with androgen deprivation therapy. *Int J Urol* 11: 735-741.

Noguchi, M., Ikarashi, Y., Yuzurihara, M., Kase, Y., Takeda, S., & Aburada, M. 2003. Significance of measured elevation of skin temperature induced by calcitonin gene-related peptide in anaesthetized rats. *J Pharm Pharmacol* 55: 1547-1552.

Noguchi, M., Yuzurihara, M., Kase, Y., Yasui, T., & Irahara, M. 2008. Involvement of cytokine-induced neutrophil chemoattractant in hypothalamic thermoregulation of luteinizing hormone-releasing hormone. *Endocrinology* 149: 2899-2906.

Owens, M. J., Morgan, W. N., Plott, S. J., & Nemeroff, C. B. 1997. Neurotransmitter receptor and transporter binding profile of antidepressants and their metabolites. *J Pharmacol Exp Ther* 283: 1305-1322.

Pandya, K. J., Raubertas, R. F., Flynn, P. J., Hynes, H. E., Rosenbluth, R. J., Kirshner, J. J., Pierce, H. I., Dragalin, V., & Morrow, G. R. 2000. Oral clonidine in postmenopausal patients with breast cancer experiencing tamoxifen-induced hot flashes: a University of Rochester Cancer Center Community Clinical Oncology Program study. *Ann Intern Med* 132: 788-793.

Pansini, F., Albertazzi, P., Bonaccorsi, G., Zanotti, L., Porto, S., Dossi, L., Campobasso, C., & Mollica, G. 1995. Trazodone: a non-hormonal alternative for neurovegetative climacteric symptoms. *Clin Exp Obstet Gynecol* 22: 341-344.

Parmar, H., Edwards, L., Phillips, R. H., Allen, L., & Lightman, S. L. 1987. Orchiectomy versus long-acting D-Trp-6-LHRH in advanced prostatic cancer. *Br J Urol* 59: 248-54.

Paul, S. M., & Axelrod, J. 1977. Catechol estrogen – presence in brain and endocrine tissues. *Science* 197: 657-659.

Prior, J. C., McKay, D. W., Vigna, Y. M., & Barr, S. I. 1995. Medroxyprogesterone increases basal temperature: a placebo-controlled crossover trial in postmenopausal women. *Fertil Steril* 63: 1222-1226.

Quella, S. K., Loprinzi, C L, Sloan, J A, Vaught, N. L., DeKrey, W. L., Fischer, T., Finck, G., Pierson, N., & Pisansky, T. 1998. Long term use of megestrol acetate by cancer survivors for the treatment of hot flashes. *Cancer* 82: 1784-1788.

Quella, S. K., Loprinzi, C L, Sloan, J., Novotny, P., Perez, E. A., Burch, P. A., Antolak, S. J., & Pisansky, T. M. 1999. Pilot evaluation of venlafaxine for the treatment of hot flashes in men undergoing androgen ablation therapy for prostate cancer. *J Urol* 162: 98-102.

Rossouw, J. E., Anderson, G. L., Prentice, R. L., LaCroix, A. Z., Kooperberg, C., Stefanick, M. L., Jackson, R. D., Beresford, S. A. A., Howard, B. V., Johnson, K. C., Kotchen, J. M., & Ockene, J. 2002. Risks and benefits of estrogen plus progestin in healthy postmenopausal women: principal results From the Women´s Health Initiative randomized controlled trial. *JAMA* 288: 321-333.

Sarosdy, M. F., Schellhammer, P. F., Soloway, M. S., Vogelzang, N. J., Crawford, E. D., Presti, J., Chodak, G. W., Mitchell, P., & Porter, L. 1999. Endocrine effects, efficacy and tolerability of a 10.8-mg depot formulation of goserelin acetate administered every 13 weeks to patients with advanced prostate cancer. *BJU Int* 83: 801-6.

Savage, M. V., & Brengelman, G. L. 1996. Control of skin blood flow in the neutral zone of human body temperature regulation. *J Appl Physiol* 80: 1249-1257.

Shanafelt, T. D., Barton, Debra L, Adjei, A. A., & Loprinzi, Charles L. 2002. Pathophysiology and treatment of hot flashes. *Mayo Clin Proc* 77: 1207-1218.

Sideras, K., & Loprinzi, Charles L. 2010. Nonhormonal management of hot flashes for women on risk reduction therapy. *J Natl Compr Canc Netw* 8: 1171-1179.

Sloan, J A, Loprinzi, C L, Novotny, P J, Barton, D L, Lavasseur, B. I., & Windschitl, H. 2001. Methodologic lessons learned from hot flash studies. *J Clin Oncol* 19: 4280-4290.

Smith, J. A. 1994. A prospective comparison of treatments for symptomatic hot flushes following endocrine therapy for carcinoma of the prostate. *J Urol* 152: 132-134.

Stahl, S. M. 1998. Basic psychopharmacology of antidepressants, part 1: Antidepressants have seven distinct mechanisms of action. *J Clin Psychiatry* 59 Suppl 4: 5-14.

Stubbs, W. A., Jonesa, A., Edwards, C. R. W., Delitala, G., Jeffcoate, W. J., Ratter, S. J., Besser, G. M., Bloomb, S. R., & Albertic, K. G. M. M. 1978. Hormonal and metabolic responses to an enkephalin analogue in normal man. *Lancet* 2: 1225-1227.

Suvanto-Luukkonen, E., Koivunen, R., Sundström, H., Bloigu, R., Karjalainen, E., Häivä-Mällinen, L., & Tapanainen, J. S. 2005. Citalopram and fluoxetine in the treatment of postmenopausal symptoms: a prospective, randomized, 9-month, placebo-controlled, double-blind study. *Menopause* 12: 18-26.

Tataryn, I. V., Meldrum, D. R., Lu, K. H., Frumar, A. M., & Judd, H. C. 1979. LH, FSH and skin temperature during the menopausal hot flush. *J Endocrinol Metab* 49: 152-154.

Tulandi, T., Kinch, R. A., Guyda, H., Maiolo, L. M., & Lal, S. 1985. Effect of naloxone on menopausal flushes, skin temperature, and luteinizing hormone secretion. *Am J Obstet Gynecol* 151: 277-280.

Walker, E. M., Rodriguez, A. I., Kohn, B., Ball, R. M., Pegg, J., Pocock, J. R., Nunez, R., Peterson, E., Jakary, S., & Levine, R. a. 2010. Acupuncture versus venlafaxine for the management of vasomotor symptoms in patients with hormone receptor-positive breast cancer: a randomized controlled trial. *J Clin Oncol* 28: 634-640.

Wehbe, T. W., Stein, B. S., & Akerley, W. L. 1997. Prostate-specific antigen response to withdrawal of megestrol acetate in a patient with hormone-refractory prostate cancer. *Mayo Clin Proc* 72: 932-934.

Wentz, W. B. 1985. Progestin therapy in lesions of the endometrium. *Semin Oncol* 12: 23-27.

Whiteman, M. K., Staropoli, C. A., Langenberg, P. W., McCarter, R. J., Kjerulff, K. H., & Flaws, J. A. 2003. Smoking, body mass, and hot flashes in midlife women. *Obstet Gynecol* 101: 264-272.

Yasui, T., Uemura, H., Tomita, J., Miyatani, Y., Yamada, M., Kuwahara, A., Matsuzaki, T., Maegawa, M., Tsuchiya, N., Yuzurihara, M., Takeda, S., & Irahara, M. 2006. Association of interleukin-8 with hot flashes in premenopausal, perimenopausal, and postmenopausal women and bilateral oophorectomized women. *J Clin Endocrinol Metab* 91: 4805-4808.

3

Evaluation of Phyllanthus, for Its Anti-Cancer Properties

Yin-Quan Tang and Shamala Devi Sekaran
University of Malaya
Malaysia

1. Introduction

1.1 Cancer

Cancer is a name given to a group of diseases that arise from a single cell when it starts to grow abnormally in an uncontrollable manner to form a group of undifferentiated cells, known as tumour. Tumour can be classified into two categories; benign and malignant. Not all benign tumours are cancerous but all malignant tumours are (Hanahan & Weinberg, 2000). The main difference between these tumours is benign tumour lack the metastatic ability, grows locally and is less harmful. However, some benign tumours can transform into malignant tumours that possess the metastatic ability to invade and spread to other parts of the body via the blood or lymphatic circulation and form secondary tumour and eventually lead to death (Vincent & Gatenby, 2008).

1.2 Development of cancer (carcinogenesis)

Cancer develops through a multistep process known as carcinogenesis (Fig 1), which includes initiation, promotion and progression (Pitot, 2006). An initiation stage is a permanent and irreversible event, which involves one or more cellular changes arising upon exposure to carcinogens, which leads to alteration in DNA and may result in a mutated cell to divide rapidly (hyperplasia). These transformed (initiated) cells can remain harmless, unless exposed to a stimulator, which enhances the tumour to grow into a larger mass. This is a reversible process and is known as the promotion stage. The progression stage is an irreversible conversion of a benign tumour to become a malignant tumour. This carcinogenesis process usually takes 10 years or more to develop and usually depends on the internal (life style) and external (environmental) factors of the patient (Pitot, 2002).

1.3 Hallmarks of cancer

A transformed cell has to acquire six hallmarks in order to be developed into cancer (Fig 2) (Hanahan & Weinberg, 2000). Each of these hallmarks is derived upon changes in the normal cell's physiology and interacts with each other to promote malignant growth. The conversion from a normal cell to become a transformed cell usually starts from mutations in DNA which cause the cells no longer depend on growth signals, thus gaining uncontrolled growth and proliferation. The irresponsiveness or insensitivity to anti-growth signals in cancer cells, enables them to evade apoptosis. The mutations in cancer cells can also change the normal function of the telomerase, thus give rise to cancer cell a limitless replicative potential (Bree et al. 2002; Kim et al. 1994). Tumour invasion, metastasis and angiogenesis play important roles in allowing the progression of a malignant tumour, by escaping the primary site, invading into blood or lymph circulation, migration to a distant site and finally establishing a secondary tumour.

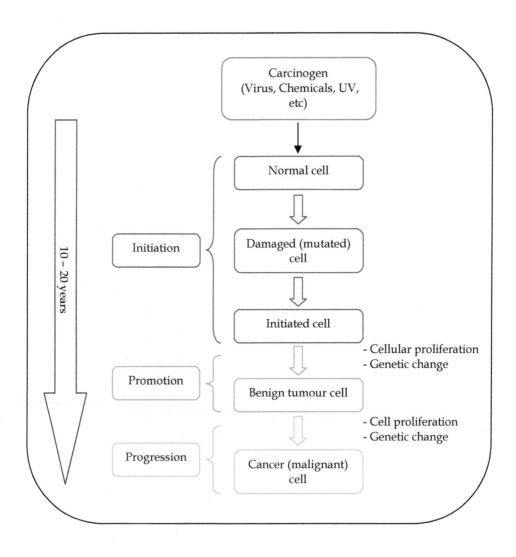

Fig. 1. Three stages of carcinogenesis

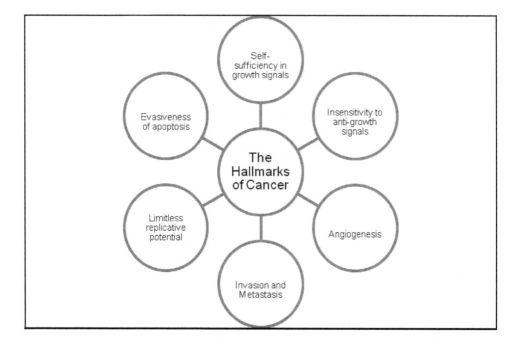

Fig. 2. The Hallmarks of Cancer (Hanahan & Weinberg, 2000)

2. Prostate cancer

Prostate is a gland in the male reproductive system that is responsible for the production and storage of seminal fluid. The normal adult human prostate is about the walnut size and is located at the neck of the urinary bladder and surrounds part of the urethra. Prostate cancer develops when its semen-secreting prostate gland cells are transformed into cancer cells, and has been classified as adenocarcinoma. Prostate cancer is one of the most commonly diagnosed cancers in men and it is the second leading cause of cancer death after lung cancer worldwide. The incidence and mortality rates of prostate cancer are increasing in Asia as well as in the United States over the past few decades (National Cancer Institute [NCI], 2011).

2.1 Symptoms & diagnosis

Prostate cancer will cause male patients to experience difficulties during urination such as nocturia, hematuria, dysuria, and will also interfere with sexual functions and performance. The high mortality rate in prostate cancer patients is due to late detection as prostate cancer is usually asymptomatic or the symptoms appear only during the advanced stage of disease. About 50% of prostate cancer patients are usually diagnosed with bone metastasis. Table 1 shows several tests for prostate cancer diagnosis in male patients by doctor (NCI, 2011).

Test	Description
Biopsy	Removal of small pieces of prostate tissue through rectum (transrectal) or skin between scrotum and rectal (transperineal) for microscopic examination by urologist, oncologist and/or pathologist
Digital rectal examination	Detect prostate gland abnormalities such as lumps
Transrectal ultrasonography	High energy ultrasound from probe in the rectum is enable to create a picture (sonogram) of the prostate gland to examine its abnormalities
Prostate tumour markers	Detection the abnormal levels of prostate specific antigen (PSA) in blood

Table 1. List of test for the diagnosis of prostate cancer (Source: NCI, USA)

2.2 Stages
It is important to determine the stage of prostate tumour in order to plan an effective treatment in patient (Table 2). This is because there is a differential response to treatment in the different stages of this cancer. To determine accurately the stage of prostate tumour in patients, different tests are conducted and all information will be gathered from CT (computerised tomography) scan, MRI (magnetic resonance imaging), PSA (prostate-specific antigen) test and tumour biopsy (NCI, 2011).

Stage	Description
I	Cancer cells are found in prostate gland only and PSA < 10
II	Divided to 2 categories;
IIA IIA	Found in one half or less than one lobe and PSA < 20 Found in both lobes of prostate gland and PSA < 20
III	Spread beyond the outer layer of prostate gland and may spread to seminal vesicle, PSA value is ranging from 2-10.
IV	Spread to nearby or other organs such as rectum, bladder and bone, any level in PSA

Table 2. Stages of prostate tumour (Source: NCI, USA)

2.3 Treatments
Currently, there are four standard treatments for prostate cancer; watchful waiting, surgery, radiation therapy and hormone therapy. In watchful waiting, a patient will be closely monitored by doctors and no treatment will be given until symptoms start to appear. While

in surgery, prostate gland from patients will be removed before the cancer cells are able to spread to other organs. In radiation therapy, high energy X-rays will be used to kill cancer cells. Antiandrogens, estrogens and luteinizing hormone-releasing hormone agonists, are the few examples used in hormone therapy to stop the cancer cells by disrupt their growth and/or kill them. While other treatment includes chemotherapy and proton-beam radiation therapy which are used in conjunction with other standard treatments (NCI, 2011).

2.4 Problems

Prostate cancer is extremely hard to treat due to several distinct classes of tumour that exhibit different responses to treatment. Most of the synthetic anticancer agents such as doxorubicin mainly affect the fast-dividing cells of the body and cause side effects such as pain, nausea, vomiting, alopecia, and anaemia (CancerBackup, 2003). Nevertheless, prostate cancer cells are derived from normal cells and thus, cancer cells have the ability to maintain the usual physiological functions to protect themselves from anything that can cause cell destruction. Estramustine and mitoxantrone are the only two drugs approved by the US FDA for prostate cancer treatment; however, neither showed to increase lifespan of patients (NCI, 2011).

Therefore, the development of resistance to anticancer drugs by cancer cells is a major problem in cancer therapies and has resulted in a high mortality rate in prostate cancer patients. About 50% of male prostate cancers patients are diagnosed at advanced stage with metastasis into their bone (Uehara et al. 2003; Koeneman et al. 1999). Thus, tumour metastasis is a major cause of morbidity and has become a major challenge for a successful treatment (Hung et al. 2009). Currently, there is no effective treatment for prostate cancer, so intense research is required to obtain new anticancer agents for this cancer.

3. Natural products

Herbs and plants-derived medicines have a long history of use in the various treatments and now, they still remain as important sources for the development of anticancer drugs. More than 3000 plants species have been reported to be involved in the development of anticancer drugs (Shoeb, 2006). The exploration of anticancer agents from plant sources has started since the 1950s. Since then, extensive research and investigations have been conducted and lead to the discovery and development of several anticancer agents derived from plant such as taxol, vinblastine and vincristine (Cragg & Newman, 2005). From 1940-2006, more that 40% of drugs in the market are anticancer agents and 65% of these anticancer drugs mimic natural compounds.

The development of chemoresistant of cancer cells to anticancer drugs have resulted high mortality in prostate cancer patients. Thus, scientists have begun to focus on natural-product as alternative to produce new therapeutic agents in prostate cancer treatments. Although, no new plant derived clinical anticancer agents have been launched in market recently, but a number of agents are being tested in the preclinical stage such as thapsigargin (Cragg & Newman, 2005).

3.1 Thapsigargin (TG)

Thapsigargin is a plant-derived anti-tumour agent, isolated from Thapsia garganica L (Familly Apiaceae), collected in Mediterranean island of Ibiza. TG can evoke apoptosis in prostate cancer cells through the disruption of Ca^{2+} intracellular levels. In addition, TG can completely inhibit tumour growth in prostate tumour bearing nude mouse without causing significant toxicity signs. Currently, TG is tested in preclinical stage against prostate cancer (Cragg & Newman, 2005).

3.2 Turmeric (curcumin)

Turmeric or known as curcumin is derived from the dried root of a plant (Curcuma longa L.) of the ginger family. It possesses a variety of pharmacological effects including anti-oxidant and anti-inflammatory activities. It has also been reported to possess anti-cancer effects through its inhibition on proliferation and apoptosis induction in wide variety of cancer cell lines including breast, lung and prostate cancer cells. The apoptosis induction is due to activation of pro-apoptotic proteins (Bax and Bak) and caspases involved in prostate cancer cells by turmeric. Currently in human clinical trials, turmeric is administered at dose up at 10g/day without causing any toxicity signs (Cragg & Newman, 2005; Kuttan et al. 1987).

4. Phyllanthus

The plant of the genus *Phyllanthus* is a small annual plant and is widely distributed throughout the tropical and subtropical regions of world (Lee et al. 1996). This plant has a long history in medical herbalism system to treat kidney and urinary bladder disturbances. Thus, substantial studies on *Phyllanthus* regarding their chemistry, pharmacological activity and clinical effectiveness have been carried out. The extracts of these plants have been reported to have pharmacological effects such as antiviral activity against hepatitis B and related hepatitis viruses, anti-bacterial activity, anti-hepatotoxic or liver-protecting activity, and hypoglycaemia properties (Etta, 2008; Mazumder et al. 2006; Kloucek et al. 2005; Ott et al. 1997; Lee et al. 1996; Blumberg et al. 1990; Venkatswaran et al. 1987).

The anticancer effects of the genus *Phyllanthus* has been reported in a few papers, for instance *P. amarus* protects the liver from hepatocarcinogenesis and the root extract of *P. acuminatus* exerts growth inhibition in murine P-388 lymphocytic leukemia and B-16 melanoma cell lines (Pettit et al. 1990; Powis & Moore, 1985). Thus, it is believed that the plant genus *Phyllanthus* might possess anticancer properties against prostate cancer as well.

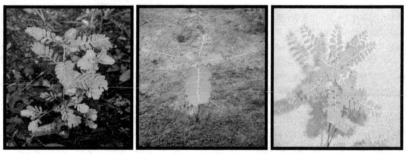

Fig. 3. *P.urinaria* (Fito Pharma 2011), *P.amarus* (Siddha Global, 2010) and *P.niruri* (Nova Laboratories Sdn Bhd, 2011).

4.1 Bioactive compounds

"Bioactive compound" is a general term to describe the nutritional constituents that are contained in plants. These compounds are intensively studied and various reports from numerous types of epidemiological and case controlled studies have linked their effects on health such as cardiovascular disease and cancer. Many bioactive compounds have been discovered and classified in different groups based on their chemical structure and function (Kris-Etherton et al. 2002). For example, phenolic and flavonoid compounds are found in all plants such as vegetables and fruits.

For the detection of bioactive compounds contained in *Phyllanthus*, HPLC (High Performance Liquid Chromatography) and MS-MS (Tandem mass spectrometry) are often used. These methods allow the separation and identification of compound from in *Phyllanthus* extracts. Various bioactive compounds have been identified from different species of *Phyllanthus* and are listed in Table 3. Most of these bioactive compounds such as gallic acid, gereniin and rutin, possess antioxidant and anticancer effects.

4.2 Anti-proliferative effects

One of the hallmarks of cancer is uncontrolled proliferation. Thus, the anti-proliferative effect of a substance is referring to the ability of the substance to halt cancer growth by inhibiting/killing cancer cells. The anti-proliferative effects of *Phyllanthus* have been detected in different cancer cell lines including breast, lung, melanoma, liver, lung, leukemia and prostate (Lee et al. 2011; Tang et al. 2010; Huang et al. 2006, 2004, 2003; Sureban et al. 2006). The water extract of *P.urinaria* have been found to possess a selective anti-proliferative effect on leukemia cells without showing cytotoxicity on normal cells (Huang et al. 2004). Similar findings have also been reported by Lee et al (2011) and Tang et al (2010), where four plant species of *Phyllanthus* (*P.amarus, P.niruri, P.urinaria* and *P.watsonii*) does possesses selective anti-proliferative effects on four different cancer cells; MeWo, A549, MCF-7 and PC-3 cell lines, without cytotoxic effects on their respective normal cells. In addition, the methanolic extracts of these plants were proven to have better anti-proliferative effects on cancer cells than aqueous extracts as their effects were exhibited at a relatively low dose. Several studies reported that the effectiveness of organic-soluble compounds in inhibiting or being lethal to cancerous cells is because most bioactive compounds are more likely to dissolve in organic solvents such as ethanol and methanol and only partially dissolve in polar solvents such as water (Wu et al. 2009; Saetung et al. 2005; Ojala et al. 2000). The anti-proliferative effects of *Phyllanthus* could be due to the presence of different bioactive compounds such as galic acid, rutin, geraniin and quercetin. Majority of polyphenol compounds found in *Phyllanthus* plant possesses anti-proliferative effects. One such example is gallic acid being found to have anti-proliferative effects on several cancer cells (Huang et al. 2009; Zhong et al.2009). Their anti-proliferative effects are always associated with their naturally antioxidant activity. The role of these polyphenol compounds on cancer have well documented as their can reduces the chance of cancer development by prevent mutation to occur in normal cells, which cause from free radicals. Due to their protective role on normal cells, the anti-proliferative effects on these cells are diminished.

4.3 Cell cycle inhibitor

Cell is the building block of all living things in this world. The cell cycle is a critical regulator that controls proliferation and growth of a cell. Cell cycle is the series of events that leads the cells to divide and replicate. This biological process involves a sequence of molecular events to ensure correct transmission of the genetic material to subsequent generations. Error in this transmission will lead the cells to either undergo checkpoints to correct the error or cause cell death. Defects in regulation of cell cycle will lead modification (mutation) in genetics of the cell and cells which leads to tumorigenesis. An uncontrolled proliferation and the ability to evade of apoptosis by mutated (cancer) cells are the hallmarks for the development of cancer.

Compound	*Phyllanthus* species	References
Gallic acid	*P.amarus, P.niruri, P.urinaria, P.watsonii, P.emblica*	Lee et al. 2011; Tang et al. 2010; Zhong et al.2009; Huang et al. 2009
Corilagen	*P.amarus, P.niruri, P.urinaria, P.watsonii*	Lee et al. 2011; Tang et al. 2010; Zhang et al. 2004
Geraniin	*P.amarus, P.niruri, P.urinaria, P.watsonii*	Lee et al. 2011; Tang et al. 2010; Zhang et al. 2004
Caffeolquinic acid	*P.amarus, P.niruri, P.urinaria, P.watsonii*	Lee et al. 2011; Tang et al. 2010;
Rutin	*P.amarus, P.niruri, P.urinaria, P.watsonii*	Lee et al. 2011; Tang et al. 2010
Quercetin	*P.amarus, P.niruri, P.urinaria, P.watsonii, P.orbiculatus*	Tang et al. 2010; Huang et al. 2009; Nara et al., 1977
Galloylglucopyronoside	*P.amarus, P.niruri, P.urinaria, P.watsonii*	Lee et a. 2011; Tang et al. 2010
Phyllaemblic acid	*P.emblica*	Zhang et al. 2004
Chebulagic acid	*P.emblica*	Zhang et al. 2004
7V-hydroxy-3V,4V,5,9,9V-pentamethoxy-3,4-methylene dioxy lignan	*P.urinaria*	Giridharan et al. 2002
Astragalin	*P.niruri, P.urinaria, P.orbiculatus*	Nara et al., 1977
Phyllanthine and hypophyllanthine	*P.amarus*	Islam et al. 2008; Figueira et al.2006
Ellagic acid	*P.urinaria*	Huang et al. 2011, 2009

Table 3. Bioactive compounds in *Phyllanthus* species

Targeting the cell cycle could be an approach for anticancer agents to halt the uncontrolled proliferation of cancer cells and initiate them to undergo apoptosis (Sharpio & Harper, 1999). The cytotoxic effects of *Phyllanthus* extracts on growth inhibition against skin melanoma and prostate cancer cells in their cell cycle could partially explain their mode of activity.

Phyllanthus have been found to inhibit cancer growth by arresting the cancer cells at different cell cycle phases which later initiates them to undergo apoptosis. *Phyllanthus* had been found to arrest of different type of cancer cells in different phases. Both the aqueous and methanolic extracts of four different species of *Phyllanthus* (*P.amarus, P.niruri, P.urinaria* and *P.watsonii*) have been reported to induce G1-phase arrest in PC-3 cells (Tang et al. 2010). Arrested in G1 phase indicated that *Phyllanthus* extracts might disrupt the protein synthesis that required for PC-3 cells to enter next phase of cell cycle. In addition, these *Phyllanthus* species also disrupt the DNA synthesis on malignant melanoma MeWo cells by arrested them in S-phase during their cell cycle (Tang et al. 2010). Besides that, these findings reveal that the growth arrest of *Phyllanthus* treated PC-3 and MeWo cancer cells is accompanied by an accumulation of apoptotic cells. When the cells are arrested at a particular phase, they lose their uncontrolled proliferation properties and the cells will be initiated to undergo apoptosis. Although there are different polyphenol compounds contained in *Phyllanthus*, but they are believed to exhibits similar effects on cell cycle and led to apoptosis induction in treated cancer cells. For example, gallic acid and quercetin induces G1 phase cell cycle arrest and apoptosis in cancer cells by inactivate the phosphorylation of cdc25A/cdc25C-cdc2 via ATM-Chk2 activation, reduces cyclin D production and activate caspase-3 activity (Suh et al. 2010; Agarwal et al. 2006).

4.4 Apoptosis inducer

There are two main cell deaths; necrotic and apoptotic processes. Apoptosis is one of the main types of programmed cell death (PCD) that occurs only in multicellular organisms to eliminate damaged or unneeded cells without local inflammation from leakage of cell contents. It does provide a balance between cell proliferation and elimination, as a part of homeostasis. Apoptosis involves a series of biochemical events, which leads to distinct characteristics of cell morphology and death such as cell shrinkage and membrane blebbing. Necrotic cell death is characterized by cellular swelling, plasma membrane rupture, cell lysis and induction of inflammation around the necrotic cells due to leakage of the intracellular contents (Chen and Wang, 2002).

Dysregulation of the apoptotic process in human body can disrupt the equilibrium between cell's growth and death and this dysregulation implicated in a variety of diseases states. Acquired immunodeficiency syndrome (AIDS) and neurodegenerative diseases such as Alzheimer's disease are examples of diseases due to acceleration of cell death rates. Conversely, an inappropriate low rate of apoptotic process can give rise to autoimmune disorders or cancer (Fadeel & Orrenius, 2005). The genetic abnormalities of cancer cells are able bypass the apoptosis and escape from cell death. Thus, evasiveness of apoptosis is a hallmark of cancer and is critical for cancer development and the survival of a tumour cell (Vincent & Gatenby, 2008).

The regulations of apoptosis on cancer cells are always associated with caspases activation. Caspases (cysteine-aspartic proteases or cysteine-dependent aspartate-directed proteases) are a family of cysteine proteases that play essential roles in apoptosis. There are two types of apoptotic caspases: initiator and effector caspases. Initiator caspases (caspase-2, -8, -9 and -10) are responsible to activate the effector caspases which initially are in an inactive pro-form. The active effector caspases (caspase-3, -6 and -7) will in turn cleave other proteins to initiate the apoptotic process to occur. In addition, these caspases will also activate other degradative enzymes such as DNases, which cleave the DNA into fragments in an apoptotic cell.

The apoptotic inducer ability of *Phyllanthus* plant on various types of cancer cells has been identified (Lee et al. 2011; Tang et al. 2010; Huang et al. 2009; Zhong et al. 2009). Different species of *Phyllanthus* plant has been shown to trigger activation of caspase-3 and -7, which later lead to apoptosis induction in treated cancer cells. These reveals that *Phyllanthus* can restore the apoptosis function of different cancer cells besides halting the uncontrolled proliferation of cell (Lee et al. 2011; Abhyankar et al. 2010; Ngamkitidechakul et al. 2010; Tang et al., 2010; Huang et al. 2009, 2004, 3003).

Different species of *Phyllanthus* induce apoptosis in human cancer cells in different ways are noticed. This could be due to various bioactive compounds contained in *Phyllanthus* and might use different pathways to induce apoptosis in cancer cells. For example, *P.amarus* induces apoptosis in human breast cancer cell line, MCF-7, by increasing their levels of intracellular reactive oxygen species (ROS) and decreased mitochondrial membrane potential (MMP). Besides that, *P.amarus* induces expression of caspase-3 and down-regulates expression of Bcl-2 to allow apoptosis in treated cancer cells. The down-regulation of the antiapoptotic family, Bcl-2 was also noticed in Lewis lung carcinoma cells after being treated with a different species of *Phyllanthus*, *P.urinaria*. In addition, *Phyllanthus* was also shown to induce TNF-α production and inhibit expression of other antiapoptotic genes including IL-8 and COX-2 in human hepatocarcinoma cells. Various bioactive compounds contained in *Phyllanthus* extract are believed to increase efficiency of *Phyllanthus* to induce apoptosis in cancer cells.

4.5 Anti-metastatic effect

Once cancer cells have transformed into malignant, they would have acquire metastatic in which the cells can detach from primary tumour and spread to other parts of the human body. Metastasis of cancer cells involves multistep processes and various cytophysiological changes, including disruption to adhesion interaction between cancer cells and the extracellular matrix (ECM) components. It also involves an over expression of proteolytic enzymes, such as matrix metalloproteinases (MMPs), which have the capability to degrade ECM components in the basal membrane of blood vessels. This allows the cancer cells to migrate and invade via the blood or lymphatic system into target organs and lead to the development of secondary tumours (Auerbach, 2000).

Therapeutic intervention strategies to prevent metastasis have an impact on cancer mortality. However, development of these therapies are requires a better understanding and knowledge in the biology and molecular events of the metastasis process. To achieve this, various of assays been conducted based on molecular events of tumour metastasis in human body.

The anti-metastatic properties of a compound can be defined by its inhibition on cancer cells' invasion and migration. *Phyllanthus* have shown reduced migration ability of treated cancer cells by reducing the number of treated cancer cells migrating through a 8-μm pore size transwell filter culture plate towards a growth factor (Lee et al. 2011; Ho et al. 2010; Ngamkitidechakul et al. 2010). The anti-migration effect of *Phyllanthus* was identified when gallic acid showed disruption on cancer cell-cell interaction in a mechanical scratch-wound cellular monolayer healing assay (Lee et al. 2011; Ho et al. 2010). In addition, *Phyllanthus* inhibited the invasion ability of cancer cells in a dose-dependent manner through the ECM as matrix barrier, which mimics the *in vivo* basement membrane of blood vessel (Lee et al. 2011; Ngamkitidechakul et al. 2010). All these indicate that *Phyllanthus* possess anti-metastatic effects by decrease cancer cells' migration and invasion abilities in dose-dependent manner.

The anti-metastatic effect of *Phyllanthus* was further noticed when *Phyllanthus* showed inhibition effects on different MMPs in different type of cancer cells. Table 4 below shows the inhibition effects of *Phyllanthus* on different MMPs.

MMP	*Phyllanthus*	References
MMP-1	*P.emblica*	Fujii et al. 2008; Chaudhuri et al. 2004
MMP-2	*P.urinaria*	Huang et al. 2010
MMP-3	*P.emblica*	Chaudhuri et al. 2004

Table 4. Inhibition on MMP members by different *Phyllanthus* species

4.6 Anti-angiogenesis effects

Angiogenesis is a process by where a new blood vessel is formed from pre-existing blood vessels. It is a normal and vital process in humans' growth and development, such as wound healing. In cancer, angiogenesis plays an essential role to its growth and development. In normal circumstances, solid tumour's size is around 1 to 2 mm^2 and not vascularized. However, when this tumour reaches beyond the 2 mm^2, oxygen and nutrients are hardly diffuse to the tumour and cause cellular hypoxia. This condition will lead to the onset of tumour angiogenesis (Folkman, 1971).

The balance between proangiogenic and antiangiogenic molecules is essential to maintain normal homeostasis in human body. Disruption of this balance would implicate to a variety of diseases states such as excessive (e.g. cancer and psoriasis) or inadequate (e.g. chronic wounds and stroke) angiogenesis. To date, angiogensis inhibitors have been reported to have less toxicity to normal cells and no development of drug resistance of cancer cells was notice such as bevacizumab, which been proven to improve the overall response including cancer time to progression, and survival rate. This makes the anti-angiogenic drugs highly advantageous over the conventional cytotoxic drugs. In addition, limited effectiveness of chemotherapy on advanced cancer has turn attention to these anti-angiogenic drugs and it is believed that these drugs will substitute the standard therapy (e.g. surgery, radiotherapy and chemotherapy).

Endothelial cells are involved in tumour angiogenesis by forming the linings of blood vessels, however, these tumour vessels have abnormal morphologies and are in immature forms. Thus, targeting these tumour vessels can be a promising target for antiangiogenic therapy (Auerbach, 2003). Tumour angiogenesis is critically important for tumour growth and metastasis with formation of new blood vessels to supply oxygen and nutrients to cancer cells and also to eliminate metabolic waste products (Auerbach, 2003). Thus, both tumour metastasis and angiogenesis are major cause of morbidity and they remain a challenge in cancer treatments.

Since the relationship between angiogenesis and cancer is clearly related where inhibition of angiogenesis could suppress/restrict tumour growth, this had attracted a strong interest from researchers worldwide to search for potential compounds that could inhibit angiogenesis. Although there are some successful anti-angiogenic drugs that have been commercialized and used in clinical and some in pre-clinical testing stage, but more effective and safer approaches are still required. The identification of new anticancer compounds from nature has a long and successful history. Interestingly, there are some plants that possess proangiogenic (e.g. β-sitosterol and resveratrol) and antiangiogenic (e.g. camptothecin and combretastatin) properties and have been used in Traditional Chinese Medicine (TCM) from thousands of years. A wide range of plants contains compounds with angiogenesis modulating properties including pacific yew tree (e.g. Taxol) and Chinese tree *camptotheca acuminate* (e.g. camptothecin).

The anti-angiogenesis properties of *Phyllanthus* were supported by various scientific assays. *Phyllanthus* showed no cytotoxic effect on HUVECs (human umbilicial vein endothelial cells) as the cells' viability did not change. *Phyllanthus* also decrease the migration and invasion ability of HUVECs (Huang et al. 2006). The anti-angiogenic effect of *Phyllanthus* was noticeable where it inhibited capillary tube formation of endothelial cells on extracellular matrix, which mimics the *in vivo* lining of blood vessel. The anti-angiogenic effect of *Phyllanthus* was further proven by other *in vivo* studies where it could decrease the vessel density in a lung cancer animal model. Besides that, *ex vivo* studies using chick chorioallantoic membrane (CAM) assay also indicated the present of anti-angiogenesis in *Phyllanthus* (Huang et al. 2011).

4.7 Antitumour effects

The antitumour effects of *Phyllanthus* were reported in different cancer animal model including skin, liver and lung (Huang et al. 2006, 2003; Sancheti et al. 2005; Jeena et al. 1999). Currently, there are no toxicity of *Phyllanthus* on different experimental animal mice model were reported. Instead, *Phyllanthus* been found that possesses radioprotective activity by inhibit the myelosuppression and elevated the levels of antioxidant enzymes in the blood, liver and intestine and decrease the lipid peroxidation levels (Harikumar & Kuttan, 2007) in treated mice.

All studies indicate that *Phyllanthus* do possess antitumour effects on different tumour by reducing the tumour size and increase the lifespan of cancer animal models. The antitumour properties of *Phyllanthus* should be conducted in other cancer animal models such as prostate cancer to prove its antitumour properties to various cancers.

5. Conclusion

These findings revealed that *Phyllanthus* plants do possess anticancer activity in a selective manner towards cancer cells and initiate them to undergo apoptosis. The anticancer activity of *Phyllanthus* plant on prostate cancer cells was through its regulation on cancer cell cycle and apoptosis induction mediated via caspases activation. The anti-metastatic and anti-angiogenesis effects observed in *Phyllanthus* plant, indicate their potential in inhibiting the development of secondary tumour. Further investigations into the mechanism of anti-carcinogenic, anti-metastatic, anti-angiogenesis and apoptotic regulation properties of the herbal plant, *Phyllanthus* against prostate cancer cells is required. This may create an opportunity for the plants to not only be designed and developed as anticancer agents, but also as a dietary supplement for the prevention of cancer development. However, the preliminary *in vitro* data is insufficient and less convincing due to its limitation as all experiments are done in an artificial environment outside a human body. Thus, an *in vivo* study using experimental prostate cancer animal model is needed to determine the pharmacological and toxicological data as well as anti-tumour effect of *Phyllanthus*, to provide more information on the safe use and effectiveness of this plant.

6. Acknowledgment

We would like to thank Ms. Anusyah Rathakrishnan and Ms. Thamil Vaani for their assistance in editing the manuscript.

7. References

[1] Abhyankar, G., Suprasanna, P., Pandey, B.N., Mishra, K.P., Rao, K.V. & Reddy, V.D. (2010). Hairy root extract of *Phyllanthus amarus* induces apoptotic cell death in human breast cancer cell. *Innovative Food Science Emerging Technologies*, Vol. 11, No. 3, (July 2010), pp. 526-532, ISSN 1466-8564

[2] Agarwal, C., Tyagil, A. & Agarwal, R. (2006). Gallic acid causes inactivating phosphorylation of cdc25A/cdc25C-cdc2 via ATM-Chk2 activation, leading to cell cycle arrest, and induces apoptosis in human prostate carcinoma DU145 cells. *Molecular Cancer Therapeutics*, Vol. 5, No. 12, (December 2006), pp. 3294-3302, ISSN 1535-7163

[3] Auerbach, R., Lewis, R., Shinners, B., Kubai, L. & Akhtar, N. (2003). Angiogenesis assay: A critical overview. *Clinical Chemistry*, Vol. 49, No. 1, (October 2002), pp. 32-40, ISSN 0009-9147

[4] Blumberg, B.S., Millman, I., Venkeateswaran, P.S. & Thyagarajan, S.P. (1990). Hepatitis B virus and primary hapatocellular carcinoma: treatment of HBV carriers with *Phyllanthus amarus. Vaccine*, (March 1990), S86-S92, ISSN 0264-410X

[5] Bree, R.T., Stenson-Cox, C., Grealy, M., Byrnes, L., Gorman, A.M. & Samali, A. (2002). Cellular longevity: role of apoptosis and replicative senescence. *Biogerontology*. Vol. 3, No.4, (December 2001), pp. 195–206, ISSN 1389-5729

[6] Chaudhuri, R.K., Guttierez, G. & Serrar, M. (2004). Low Molecular-Weight Tannins of *Phyllanthus emblica*: A New Class of Anti-Aging Ingredients. *Proceedings Active Ingredients Conference, Paris.*

[7] Chen, M. & Wang, J. (2007). Initiator caspases in apoptosis signaling pathways. *Apoptosis*. Vol. 7, No. 4, pp. 313-319, ISSN 1360-8185

[8] Cragg, G.M. & Newman, D.J. (2005). Plants as a source of anti-cancer agents. *Journal of Ethnopharmacology*, Vol. 100, (July 2005), pp. 72–79, ISSN 0378-8741

[9] Etta, H. (2008). Effects of *Phyllanthus amarus* on litter traits in albino rats. *Scientific Research and Essay*. Vol. 3, No. 8, (August 2008), pp. 370-372, ISSN 1992-2248

[10] Fadeel, B. & Orrenius, S. (2005). Apoptosis: a basic biological phenomenon with wide-ranging implications in human disease. *Journal of Internal Medicine*, Vol. 258, No. 6, (December 2005), pp. 479–517, ISSN 1365-2796

[11] Giridharan, P., Somasundaram, S.T., Perumal, K., Vishwakarma, R.A., Karthikeyan, N.P., Velmurugan, R. & Balakrishnan, A. (2002). *British Journal of Cancer*. Vol. 87, (June 2002), pp. 98–105, ISSN 0007-0920.

[12] Figueira, G.M., de Magalhães, P.M., Rehder, V.I.G., Sartoratto, A. & Vaz, A.P.A. (2006). Chemical preliminary evaluation of selected genotype of *Phyllanthus amarus* Schumach. grown in four different counties of São Paulo State. *Revista Brasileira de Plantas Medicinais*, Vol. 8 (esp), pp. 43-45, ISSN 1516-0572

[13] Hanahan, D. & Weinberg, R.A. (2000). The Hallmarks of Cancer. *Cell*. Vol. 100, No. 1, (January 2000), pp. 57–70, ISSN 0092-8674

[14] Harikumar, K.B.N. & Kuttan. (2007). An Extract of Phyllanthus amarus Protects Mouse Chromosomes and Intestine from Radiation Induced Damages. *Journal of Radiation Research*. Vol. 48, (July 2007), pp. 469-476, ISSN 1349-9157

[15] Ho, H.H., Chang, C.S., Ho, W.C., Liao, S.Y., Wu, C.H., & Wang, C.J. (2010). Anti-metastasis effects of gallic acid on gastric cancer cells involves inhibition of NF-kappaB activity and downregulation of PI3K/AKT/small GTPase signals. *Food and Chemical Toxicology*, Vol. 48, No. 8-9, pp. 2508-2516, ISSN 0278-6915

[16] Huang, S.T., Yang, R.C., Yang, L.J., Lee, P.N. & Pang, J.H.S. (2003). *Phyllanthus urinaria* triggers the apoptosis and Bcl-2 down-regulation in Lewis carcinoma cells. *Life Sciences*, Vol. 72, No. 15, (February 2003), pp. 1705-1716, ISSN 0024-3205

[17] Huang, S.T., Yang, R.C., Chen, M.Y. & Pang, J.H.S. (2004). Phyllanthus urinaria induces the Fas receptor/ligand expression and ceramide-mediated apoptosis in HL-60 cells. *Life Sciences*, Vol. 75, No. 3, (June 2004), pp. 339–351, ISSN 0024-3205

[18] Huang, S.T., Yang, R.C., Lee, P.N., Yang, S.H., Liao, S.K., Chen, T.Y. & Pang, J.H.S. (2006). Anti-tumor and anti-angiogenic effects of Phyllanthus urinaria in mice bearing Lewis lung carcinoma. *International Immunopharmacology*, Vol. 6, No. 6, (June 2006), pp. 870–879, ISSN 1567-5769

[19] Huang, S.T., Wang, C.Y., Yang, R.C., Chu, C.J., Wu, H.T. & Pang, J.H.S. (2009). Phyllanthus urinaria increases apoptosis and reduces telomerase activity in human nasopharyngeal carcinoma cells. *Forsch Komplementmed*, Vol. 16, No. 1, (February 2009), pp. 34-40, ISSN 1661-4119

[20] Huang, S.T., Wang, C.Y., Yang, R.C., Wu, H. T., Yang, S.H., Cheng, Y.C. & Pang, J.H.S. (2011). Ellagic Acid, the Active Compound of *Phyllanthus urinaria*, Exerts *In Vivo* Anti-Angiogenic Effect and Inhibits MMP-2 Activity. *Evidence-Based Complementary and Alternative Medicine*. Vol. 2001, (October 2009), ISSN 1533-2101

[21] Hung S.H, Shen, K.H., Wu, C.H, Liu, C.L. & Shih, Y.W. (2009). α–Mangostin suppresses PC-3 human prostate carcinoma cell metastasis by inhibiting matrix metalloproteinase-2/9 and urokinase-plasminogen expression through the JNK signaling pathway. *Journal of Agricultural and Food Chemistry*, Vol. 57, No. 4, (February 2009), pp. 1291-1298, ISSN 0021-8561

[22] Islam, A., Selvan, T., Mazumder, U.K., Gupta, M., & Ghosal, S. (2008). Antitumour effect of Phyllanthin and hypophyllanthin from *Phyllanthus amarus* against Ehrlich Ascites carcinoma in mice. *Pharmacologyonline* Vol. 2, pp. 796-807, ISSN 1827-8620

[23] Kim, N.W., Piatyszek, M.A., Prowse, K.R., Harley, C.B., West M.D., Ho, P.L., Coviello, G.M., Wright, W.E., Weinrich, S.L. & Shay, J.W. (1994). Specific association of human telomerase activity with immortal cells and cancer. *Science*. Vol. 266, No. 5193, (December 1994), pp. 2011-2015, ISSN 0036-8075

[24] Kloucek, P., Polesny, Z., Svobodova, B., Vlkova, E. & Kokoska, L. (2005). Antibacterial screening of some Peruvian medicinal plants used in Calleria District. *Journal of Ethnopharmacology*. Vol. 99, No. 2, (June 2005), pp. 309-312, ISSN 0378-8741

[25] Koeneman, K.S., Fan, Y. & Chun, L.W.K. (1999). Osteomimetic properties of prostate cancer cells: A hypothesis supporting the predilection of prostate cancer metastasis and growth in the bone environment. *The Prostate*, Vol. 39, No. 4, (June 1999), pp. 246-261, ISSN 0270-4137

[26] Kris-Etherton, P.M., Hecker, K.D., Bonanome, A., Coval, S.M., Binkoski, A.E., Hilpert, K.F., Griel, A.E. & Etherton, T.D. (2002). Bioactive compounds in foods: their role in the prevention of cardiovascular disease and cancer. *The American Journal of Medicine*. Vol. 113, No. 9, (December 2002), pp. 71-88, ISSN 0002-9343

[27] Kuttan, R., Sudheeran, P.C. & Josph, C.D. (1987). Turmeric and curcumin as topical agents in cancer therapy. *Tumori*, Vol. 73, No. 1, (February 1987), pp. 29-31, ISSN 0300-8916

[28] Lee, C.D., Ott, M., Thygarajan, S.P., Shfritz, D.A., Burk, R.D. & Gupta, S. (1996). *Phyllanthus amarus* down-regulates hepatitis B virus mRNA transcription and translation. *European Journal of Clinical Investigation.* Vol. 26, No. 12, (December 2006), pp. 1069-1076. ISSN 1365-2362

[29] Lee, S.H., Jaganath, I.B., Wang, S.M. & Sekaran, S.D. (2011). Antimetastatic Effects of Phyllanthus on Human Lung (A549) and Breast (MCF-7) Cancer Cell Lines. *PLoS ONE,* Vol. 6, No. 6, (June 2011), pp. e20994. doi:10.1371/journal.pone.0020994.

[30] Mazumder, A., Mahato, A. & Mazumder, R. (2006). Antimicrobial potentially of *Phyllanthus amarus* against drug resistant pathogens. *Natural Product Research,* Vol. 20, No. 4, (April 2006), pp. 323-326, ISSN 1478-6427

[31] Nara, T.K., Gleye, J., Cerval, E.L., Stanistan, E. (1977). Flavonoids of *Phyllanthus niruri, Phyllanthus urinaria, Phyllanthus orbiculatus. Plantes Medicinales et Phytotherapie,* Vol. 11, pp. 82-86

[32] Ngamkitidechakul, C., Jaijoy, K., Hansakul, P., Soonthornchareonnon, N. & Sireeratawong, S. (2010). Antitumour effects of *Phyllanthus emblica* L.: induction of cancer cell apoptosis and inhibition of *in vivo* tumour promotion and *in vitro* invasion of human cancer cells. *Phytotherapy research,* Vol. 24, No. 9, (September 2010), pp. 1405-1413, ISSN 0951-418X

[33] Ojala, T., Remes, S., Haansuu, P., Vuorela, H., Hiltunen, R., Haahtelab, K. & Vuorela, P. (2000) Antimicrobial activity of some coumarin containing herbal plants growing in Finland. *The Journal of Ethnopharmacology,* Vol. 73, No. 1-2, (November 2000), pp. 299-305, ISSN 0378-8741

[34] Ott, M., Thyarajan, S.P. & Gupta, S. (1997). *Phyllanthus amarus* suppress hepatitis B virus interrupting interactions between HBV enhancer I and cellular transcription factors. *European Journal of Clinical Investigation.* Vol. 27, No. 11, (November 1997), pp. 908-915. ISSN 1365-2362

[35] Pettit, G. R., Schaufelberger, D. E., Nieman, R. A., Dufresne, C. & Saenz-Renauld, J. A. (1990). Antineoplastic agents, 177. Isolation and structure of phyllantostatin 6. *Journal of Natural Products.* Vol. 53, No. 6, (November – December 1990), pp. 1406-1413, ISSN 0163-3864

[36] Phyllanthus amarus, In: *Siddha Global.* 2.05.2011. Available from: http://siddhaglobal.blogspot.com/2010_03_01_archive.html

[37] Phyllanthus niruri, In: *Nova Laboratories Sdn Bhd.* 2.05.2011. Available from: http://www.hepar-p.com.my/phyllanthus_botanical_info.htm

[38] *Phyllanthus urinaria* L. – Chamber Bitter, In: *Fito Pharma.* 2.05.2011. Available from: http://www.fitoco.com/ru/informatsija/lekarstvennye-rastenija/158-fillantus-filantija-phyllanthus-urinariae.html

[39] Pitot, H.C. (2006). The molecular biology of carcinogenesis. *Cancer.* Vol. 72, No. 3, (August 1993), pp. 962-970, ISSN 1097-0142

[40] Powis, G. & Moore, D.J. (1985). High-performance liquid chromatographic assay for the antitumor glycoside phllanthoside and its stability in plasma of several species. *Journal of Chromatography B: Biomedical Sciences and Application,* Vol. 342, (December 1984), pp. 129-134, ISSN 1570-0232

[41] Prostate cancer, In: *National Institute Cancer (NCI).* 3.05.2011, Available from: http://www.cancer.gov/cancertopics/types/prostate

[42] Saetung, A., Itharat, A., Dechsukum, C., Wattanapiromsakul, C., Keawpradub, N. & Ratanasuwan, P. (2005) Cytotoxic activity of Thai medicinal plants for cancer treatment. *Songklanakarin Journal of Science and Technology,* Vol. 2 (Suppl. 2), pp. 469-478, ISSN 01253395

[43] Sancheti, G., Jindal, A., Kumari, R., & Goyal, P.K. (2005). Chemopreventive action of emblica officinalis on skin carcinogenesis in mice. *Asian Pacific Journal of Cancer Prevention*, Vol. 6, No. 2, (April – June 2005), pp. 197-201, ISSN 1513-7368

[44] Sharpiro, G.I. & Harper, J.W. (1999). Anticancer drug targets: cell cycle and checkpoint control. *The Journal of Clinical Investigation*, Vol. 104, No. 12, (December 1999), pp. 1645-1653, ISSN 0021-9738

[45] Shoeb, M. (2006). Anticancer agents from medicinal plants. *Bangladesh Journal of Pharmacology*, Vol. 1 (November 2006), pp.35-41, ISSN 1991-0088

[46] Suh, D.K., Lee, E, J., Kim, H.C. & Kim, J.H. (2010). Induction of G1/S phase arrest and apoptosis by quercetin in human osteosarcoma cell. *Archives of Pharmacal Research*, Vol. 33, No. 5, (May 2010), pp. 781-785, ISSN 0253-6269

[47] Sureban, S.M., Subramaniam, D., Rajendran, P., Ramanujam, R.P., Dieckgraefe, B.K., Houchen, C.W. & Anant, S. (2006). Therapeutic effects of *Phyllanthus* species: anti-proliferative activity in HepG2 a hepatocellular carcinoma cells. *American Journal of Pharmacology and Toxicology*, Vol. 1, No. 4, pp. 65-71, ISSN 1557-4962

[48] Tang, Y.Q., Jaganath, I.B. & Sekaran, S.D. (2010). Phyllanthus spp. induces selective growth inhibition of PC-3 and MeWo human cancer cells through modulation of cell cycle and induction of apoptosis. *PLoS ONE*, Vol. 5, No. 9, (September 2010), pp. e12644. doi:10.1371/journal.pone.0012644

[49] Taxol, In: *Cancerbackup*. (3.03.2011). Available from: http://www.cancerbackup.org.uk/Treatment/Chemotherapy/Individualdrugs/Paclitaxol

[50] Uehara, H., Sun, J.K., Karashima, T., Shepherd, D.L., Dominic, F., Rachel, T., Killion, J.J., Logothetis, C., Mathew, P. & Fidler, I.J. (2003). Effects of Blocking Platelet-Derived Growth Factor-Receptor Signaling in a Mouse Model of Experimental Prostate Cancer Bone Metastases. *Journal of the National Cancer Institute*, Vol. 95, No. 6, (March 2003), pp. 458-490, ISSN 0027-8874

[51] Venkateswaran, P.S., Millman, I. & Blumberg, B.S. (1987). Effects of an extracts from *Phyllanthus niruri* on hepatitis B and woodchuck hepatitis virus: *in vitro* and *in vivo* studies. *Proceedings of National Academy of Science, USA*. Vol. 84, No. 1, (January 1987). pp. 274-278, ISSN 0027-8424

[52] Vincent, T.L. & Gatenby, R.A. (2008). An evolutionary model for initiation, promotion, and progression in carcinogenesis. *International Journal of Oncology*. Vol. 32, (April 2008), pp. 729-737, ISSN 1019-6439

[53] Wu, S.J., Chang, S.P., Lin, D.L., Wang, S.S., Hou, F.F. & Ng, L.T. (2009) Supercritical carbon dioxide extract of *Physalis peruviana* induced cell cycle arrest and apoptosis in human lung cancer H661 cells. *Food and Chemical Toxicology*, Vol. 47, No. 6, (June 2000), pp. 1132-1138, ISSN 0278-6915

[54] Zhang, Y.J., Nagao, T., Tanaka, T., Yang, C.R., Okabe, H. & Kouno, I. (2004). Antiproliferative Activity of the Main Constituents from Phyllanthus emblica. *Biological & Pharmaceutical Bulletin*. Vol. 27, (October 2003), pp. 251-255

[55] Zhong, Z.G., Huang, J.L., Liang, H., Zhong, Y.N., Zhang, W.Y., Wu, D.P., Zeng, C.L., Wang, J.S. & Wei, Y.H. (2009). The effect of gallic acid extracted from leaves of *Phyllanthus emblica* on apoptosis of human hepatocellular carcinoma BEL-7404 cells. *Zhong Yao Cai*, Vol. 32, No. 7, pp. 1097-1101, ISSN 1001-4454

4

Paradigm Shift in the Concept of Hormonal Milieu of Prostate Cancer

Tsutomu Nishiyama

Division of Urology, Department of Regenerative and Transplant Medicine
Niigata University Graduate School of Medical and Dental Sciences, Niigata
Japan

1. Introduction

Androgens and the androgen receptor have been implicated in a number of human diseases and conditions, most notably prostate cancer. [1] Huggins and Hodges in 1941 demonstrated that bilateral orchiectomy or estrogen treatment is an effective treatment for prostate cancer.[2] Based upon their findings, androgen deprivation therapy (ADT) has remained the main therapeutic option for patients with advanced prostate cancer for about 70 years. Different therapeutic approaches, including surgical or medical castration with gonadotropin-releasing hormone (GnRH) agonists, and an antiandrogen therapy, have become the gold standard for prostate cancer treatment with metastases. ADTs are quite successful, leading to regression of tumors in a majority of cases; however, 12-18 months later, most prostate cancers recur in a more aggressive, castration-resistant form (castration-resistant prostate cancer (CRPC)) that is incurable. Median survival for these patients after recurrence is 24-36 months.[3, 4] New ADTs and other promising therapies for CRPC have been actively developed.[5] This review will provide an overview of prostate cancer aggressiveness and the androgen levels in blood and prostatic tissues, androgen milieu during ADT, androgen milieu during CRPC, and the prospects of ADT on the ground of the androgen milieu in the prostate.

2. Androgen milieu in blood

Biosynthetic pathway for androgen synthesis is the Δ-5 pathway in primates like humans. [6] (Fig. 1) As a result, a large amount of dehydroepiandrosterone (DHEA) and DHEA sulfate (DHEA-S) are in the blood in humans. In rodents, biosynthetic pathway for androgen synthesis is the Δ-4 pathway. In human males, testosterone is the major circulating androgen. More than 95% of testosterone is secreted by the Leydig cells, situated in the testicular interstitium, while the adrenal cortex also contributes to this production. [7, 8] The Leydig cells produce testosterone in response to hormonal stimulation by the pituitary gonadotropin luteinizing hormone (LH). Testosterone plays a key role in health and well-being as well as in sexual functioning. Testosterone effects can be classified as virilizing and anabolic effects including growth of muscle mass and strength, increased bone density and strength. Serum testosterone levels decline with advancing age. [9] Recently, a pooled analysis of moderately sized prospective studies including 3886 cases of prostate cancer and 6438 matched controls reported no association of circulating androgens and risk of prostate cancer, either overall or for subgroups according to tumor stage or grade. [10] Prostate cancer risk and tumour aggressiveness are not related to serum levels of total and free testosterone. [11] However, this negative result does not deny the role of androgens for the prostate cancer, rather emphasizes the importance of the androgen metabolism in the prostate. It is not clear to what extent the testosterone and dihydrotestosterone (DHT) in the prostate derive from adrenal androgens or other steroid precursors.

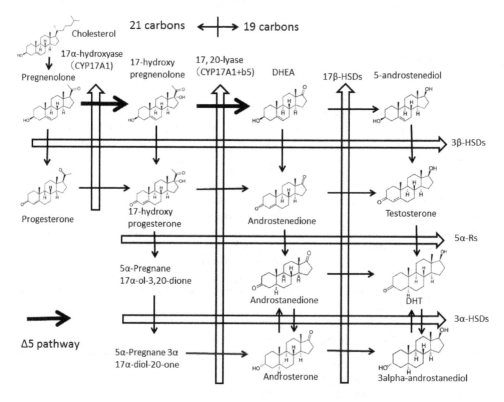

*b5: cytochrome-b5 reductase
CYP17A1: Cytochrome P450, family 17, subfamily A, polypeptide 1
DHEA: dehydroepiandrosterone
DHT: dihydrotestosterone
HSD: hydroxysteroid dehydrogenase
5α-Rs: 5-α-reductases

Fig. 1. The androgen metabolic pathway and enzyme related products of human being. Biosynthetic pathway for androgen synthesis is the Δ-5 pathway in primates like humans. As a result, a large amount of DHEA and DHEA-S is in the serum in humans.

3. Androgen milieu in the prostate

Testosterone and DHT can be synthesized from DHEA with various androgen synthetic enzymes in the human prostate. The conversion of testosterone from 17-ketosteroid, androstenedione, is said to be catalyzed by the 17β-hydroxysteroid dehydrogenase (HSD) type 1, 3, 5, 12. [12] 17β-HSD type3 is mainly expressed to convert into testosterone from androstenedione in the testis. Aldo-keto reductase family 1, member C3 (AKR1C3) , known as 17β-HSD type5, is mainly expressed to convert into testosterone from androstenedione in the prostate. [13] Humans have three isoenzymes of 5-α-reductase. Both type 1 and type 2 5-α-reductase catalyze the conversion of testosterone to DHT. [14, 15] Type 1 enzyme (encoded by SRD5A1) is expressed mostly in skin and hair, while type 2 enzyme (encoded by SRD5A2) is located primarily in androgen target tissues, including genital skin and prostate. Recently, the existence of 5-α-reductase type 3 (encoded by SRD5A3) is identified. [16] Godoy et al. showed that expression of 5α-reductase type 3 in "classical" as well as "non-classical" androgen-regulated tissues is consistent with 5α-reductase type 3 enzyme having functions other than converting testosterone to DHT in human tissues, such as participation in the N-glycosylation process. [17] They also showed that over-expression of 5α-reductase type 3 in breast, testis, lung, thyroid, and particularly prostate cancer, compared to their benign counterparts, suggests a potential role for 5α-reductase type 3 as a biomarker of malignancy, and over-expression of 5α-reductase type 3 in androgen sensitive prostate cancer and CRPC suggests a potential role for this enzyme in synthesizing DHT in both an androgen-stimulated and an androgen-deprived human prostate microenvironment. Therefore, the prostate is not only the androgen dependent organ but also the androgen productive organ. Recently, DHT mainly synthesizes via testosterone as stated above, but also synthesizes without testosterone biosynthesis, 'backdoor' pathway. [14, 18, 19] An alternate 'backdoor' pathway to DHT was elucidated in the tammar wallaby pouch young, and studies in knockout mice showed that this pathway uses 5-α-reductase type 1 to convert 17-hydroxyprogesterone to 5-α-reduced androgen precursors.[20] The role of 'backdoor' pathway to DHT in human androgen metabolism, however, is not clear yet. The traditional belief that prostate cancer growth is dependent on the serum testosterone level has been challenged by recent negative studies in non-castrated men.[21, 22] The evidence clearly indicates that there is a limit to the ability of androgens to stimulate prostate cancer growth. A Saturation Model based on androgen-AR binding provides a satisfactory conceptual framework to account for the dramatic effects seen with castration as well as the minor impact of testosterone administration in non-castrated men.[23]

4. Prostate cancer aggressiveness and the androgen milieu in the prostate and in blood

Sex hormones in serum have been hypothesized to influence the risk of prostate cancer. Large prospective study and a pooled analysis of moderately sized prospective studies did not show convincing evidence of a relationship between serum sex hormones and prostate cancer. [10, 24] However, these negative results do not deny the role of androgens for the prostate cancer, rather emphasizes the importance of the androgen metabolism in the prostate. It is not clear to what extent the testosterone and DHT in the prostate derive from adrenal androgens or other steroid precursors. The 90-95% decrease in serum testosterone is observed after castration; however, the prostate efficiently transforms the adrenal androgen precursors DHEA-S, DHEA, and androstenedione into the active androgens, testosterone and DHT. All the enzymes are reported to exist in the prostate metabolizing from androgen precursors to testosterone and DHT. [25] The plasma concentration of DHEA-S is 100-500 times higher than that of testosterone. [26] High circulating levels of DHEA-S provide large amounts of the precursors required for conversion into active androgens in the prostate. The active androgens made locally in the prostate act in the prostate. In our data, the level of DHT in the prostate before ADT was not correlated with the serum level of testosterone, but was correlated with the serum level of DHEA and DHEA-S.[26] These results suggested that DHT in the prostate comes not only from testosterone produced in the testes, but also from adrenal androgens. There are still many questions about the androgen environment in the prostate in patients with prostate cancer. There have been few reports about the relations between histological aggressiveness and the DHT levels in the prostate in patients with prostate cancer. We revealed that the DHT levels in the prostate in patients with Gleason scores of 7 to 10 were significantly lower than those with Gleason scores of 6 and under, although there were no significant differences between the patients with Gleason scores of 7 to 10 and the patients with Gleason scores of 6 and under prostate cancer with respect to serum levels of androgens. [27] The result of the association between the DHT level in the prostate and the Gleason score gives useful information to predict the biological aggressiveness of prostate cancer and consider the treatment of the patients with such cancers. One hypothesis as to the correlation between clinical aggressiveness and low androgen levels in the prostate is that the hormonal milieu with low androgen levels might be varied enough to disrupt the normal growth and maintenance of the prostate tissue, and may cause the resultant compensatory hyperplasia that increases the risk of a consequent selection of androgen independent, aggressive prostate cancer formation due to low androgen levels. [28] Several studies suggested that men with smaller prostates had more high-grade cancers and more advanced diseases. [29-31] Prostate size was inversely associated with the risk of high grade cancer. The Prostate Cancer Prevention Trial (PCPT), a Phase III, randomized, double-blind, placebo-controlled trial of finasteride, a 5-α-reductase inhibitor, for the prevention of carcinoma of the prostate was held. [32] A total of 18,882 essentially healthy men, aged 55 and older, had been randomized to receive finasteride (5 mg daily) or placebo for seven years. PCPT results suggested that finasteride could reduce the frequency of prostate cancer by 25% compared with placebo. However, the patients with Gleason scores of 7 to 10 were detected significantly more frequently in the finasteride group than in the placebo group. Several questions were raised by the results of the trial that finasteride could induce the development of high grade disease. They did not find evidence that the drug caused changes in tumor composition that might contribute to aggressive cancer, though they don't entirely rule out the possibility that finasteride may have led to high-grade prostate cancer in some men in the study. One possible explanation was the occurrence of over-grading due to histological alterations. Several reports, however, showed that although finasteride use might cause some alterations in the assignment of the Gleason grade, a consistent hormonal therapy effect with finasteride treatment has not been observed. [33] Lucia et al. revealed that finasteride may have contributed to the increased rate of high-grade cancers detected in the PCPT by making the prostate smaller, helping the biopsy find the cancer. [34] Moreover, the results of the Reduction by Dutasteride of

Prostate Cancer Events (REDUCE) trial using the dual 5-α-reductase isoenzyme inhibitor dutasteride, has recently been reported.[35] The REDUCE trial, contrary to the Prostate Cancer Prevention Trial (PCPT), is performed in 8,231 men ages 50-75, who would have been candidates for biopsy anyway because of PSA values of 2.5 - 10 ng/ml. Although over the course of 4 years, significantly fewer prostate cancers were detected in men taking dutasteride than in those taking placebo, representing a relative risk reduction of 22.8% (P <0.001), there were 12 tumors with a Gleason score of 8 to 10 in the dutasteride group, as compared with only 1 in the placebo group (P=0.003). These findings and our results suggest that biologically aggressive prostate cancer can exist under a low DHT environment, and may proliferate under the low DHT environment with finasteride or dutasteride medication where the prostate cancer of a low malignancy with high DHT dependency cannot easily exist. High levels of androgen receptor (AR) are said to be associated with the increased proliferation, markers of aggressive disease, and to be predictive of decreased biochemical recurrence-free survival independently. [36] This confirms the role of AR in tumor growth and progression in hormonally naive prostate cancer. Several reports and our results revealed that 17β-HSD5 (known as AKR1C3) positive cases were significantly associated with clinical stage. [37, 38] Fung et al. revealed that elevated expression of AKR1C3 is highly associated with prostate cancer. [37] We also revealed that both AR and androgen-converting enzymes were up-regulated in the high-grade or advanced prostate cancer. [38] AKR1C3 (17β-HSD5) may be involved in increasing the local concentration of testosterone in prostate cancer tissues, resulting in the progression, invasion and further development of prostate cancer following ADT.

5. Intraprostatic androgen milieu during androgen deprivation therapy

The castration level of serum testosterone is disputed; however, historically, circulating testosterone levels have been used to assess the efficacy of androgen depletion with a target total testosterone level below 50 ng/dl (<1.74 nmol/l). [39-42] In men with prostate cancer, orchiectomy reduces serum testosterone to anorchid levels within 12 hours. The clinical significance of different serum levels of testosterone yielded during ADT has not yet been well elucidated. The serum testosterone level in men being treated with ADT has never been categorically established. [43] The typical serum testosterone level in men after an orchiectomy is 14 ng/dl, which is equivalent to 0.5 nmol/l. Over the years, there have been many specialists who have argued that the appropriate serum testosterone level for a man who is being well-controlled on ADT should, in fact, be < 20 ng/dl (0.7 nmol/l). Morote et al. have shown that 25% of men receiving continuous ADT with a GnRH agonist have a serum testosterone level > 50 ng/dl. [44] Forty-four percent of the same group of men studied had a serum testosterone level that was consistently < 20 ng/dl. Also, in the same group of men, they demonstrated a direct correlation between serum testosterone levels and time to development of CRPC. Perachino et al. have also reported a significant association between serum testosterone levels 6 months after initiation of ADT and overall survival. [45] Several reports showed that DHT in the prostate after ADT is supplied by the precursors of androgens from the adrenal origin. We showed that after ADT with castration and flutamide, the DHT level in the prostatic tissue remained at approximately 25% of the amount measured before ADT in the same patients. [26] Previous reports revealed that the mean DHT levels in the prostate tissue treated with ADT were between 10% and 40% of those of untreated. [26, 46-50] Testosterone is converted to DHT by 5-α reductase in the prostate. Labrie et al. showed that even if testosterone levels in blood drop to low levels by castration, DHT levels in the prostate were maintained about 40% before the treatment. [47] These results showed that the considerable levels of DHT exist in the prostate after castration. We also revealed that the levels of DHT in the prostate before ADT were correlated with the serum levels of adrenal androgens. [26] We could not recognize the correlation between testosterone levels in blood and DHT levels in the prostate before the treatment; however, we recognized the correlation between DHT levels in the prostate and DHEA levels (or DHEA-S levels) in blood. The levels of DHT in the prostate after ADT using a GnRH agonist and flutamide were also correlated with the serum level of testosterone. The serum DHT levels after ADT were correlated with serum levels of adrenal androgen. The testosterone levels in blood after ADT are supplied from the adrenal androgen precursors converted in the prostate, and the adrenal androgen precursors are converted into DHT in the peripheral organs including the prostate. These results showed that DHT in the prostate can be made not only from testosterone derived from the testis but also from the adrenal precursors. These findings suggest that serum testosterone after ADT mostly comes from adrenal androgens converted in the prostatic cells. These results revealed that the prostate is the main DHT producing organ and DHT levels in the prostate are correlated with the adrenal androgen precursor levels and testosterone levels in the prostate.

Substantial levels of DHT remain in the prostate after castration; however, the influence on the change in the DHT levels in the prostate before and after ADT in connection with prostate cancer aggressiveness has not yet been elucidated. We revealed that the change in the DHT levels before and after ADT in the prostate with the prostate cancer of Gleason scores of 7 to 10 was significantly smaller than that in the prostate with the prostate cancer of Gleason scores of 6 or less.[51] Recently, 5-α-reductase type 1(SRD5A1) is reported to express in aggressive and recurrent prostate cancer. [38,52, 53] Arai et al. showed that the levels of adrenal androgens in prostate cancer tissues after ADT were similar to those in untreated prostate cancer. [54] Especially, DHEA was the most existing androgen precursor in prostate cancer tissues after ADT. The levels of DHEA were high in prostate cancer tissues, irrespective of ADT. They assumed that DHEA played a significant role in the synthesis of testosterone and DHT in prostate cancer tissues after ADT. Several reports revealed that AR signaling pathway is an important mechanism in proliferation of aggressive prostate cancer during ADT.[55] Stanbrough et al. revealed that AR transcriptional activity is reactivated in androgen-independent prostate cancer and identifies the intracellular conversion of adrenal androgens to testosterone as a mechanism mediating this reactivation. [56] These findings and our results suggest that the low DHT levels in the prostate with aggressive prostate cancers are probably sufficient to propagate the growth of the tumor, and the prostate with aggressive prostate cancer can produce androgens from the adrenal precursors more autonomously than that with non-aggressive prostate cancer does under the low testosterone environment with testicular suppression. Mostaghel et al. showed that the reduction of circulating androgens to castrate levels and interruption of AR signaling by androgen deprivation are neither reliably effective nor uniform in suppressing prostatic androgen-regulated gene and protein expression.[57] Their findings suggest that medical castration based on serum testosterone levels cannot be equated with ablation of androgen levels or androgen-mediated activity in the prostate tissue microenvironment. These findings underscore the need for demonstrating suppression at the target tissue and molecular level before drawing conclusions regarding the clinical efficacy of hormonal treatment strategies. We showed that the serum PSA levels well reflect the androgen milieu in localized prostate cancer patients receiving ADT, which can be explained by the Saturation Model and disease control. [58] The androgen milieu in men with high Gleason score prostate cancer is probably less affected by conventional ADT than that in men with low score cancer, which was suggested to be associated with adrenal androgen levels. We also showed that in patients treated with ADT the pituitary-adrenal axis mediated by adrenocorticotropic hormone has a central role in the regulation of androgen synthesis. [59] Serum adrenocorticotropic hormone and adrenal androgen concentrations were correlated with the post-treatment PSA. Adrenocorticotropic hormone mediated androgen synthesis is a potential target for advanced androgen deprivation therapy.

6. Androgen milieu in the castration-resistant prostate cancer

The pathogenesis of CRPC involves a mixture of multiple pathways that increase and broaden the function of the AR, and others that bypass the AR.[60] Analysis of tumor samples from patients with CRPC has revealed several mechanisms utilized by tumor cells to reactivate the AR signaling at sub-physiological serum concentration of androgens or even in the presence of AR antagonists.[61] CRPC has been used synonymously with androgen-independent prostate cancer and hormone-refractory prostate cancer but is the preferred term, as we now know that many men with CRPC respond to additional manipulations that ablate or block prostate cancer growth stimulation by androgens. CRPC is clinically detected by a rise in PSA, typically defined as three consecutive rises over nadir in the context of castrate levels of serum testosterone and after anti-androgen withdrawal for at least 4 weeks and despite secondary hormonal manipulations and/or radiologic progression. In the face of testicular androgen suppression the adrenal androgens DHEA, DHEA-S and androstenedione retain the potential to stimulate prostate cancer growth since these steroids are converted to testosterone and DHT in the prostate, which are active androgens even after prostate cancer acquires the ability to activate during ADT. Chen et al. showed that a modest increase in AR mRNA was the only change consistently associated with the development of resistance to anti-androgen therapy.[62] This increase in AR mRNA and protein was both necessary and sufficient to convert prostate cancer growth from a hormone-sensitive to a hormone-refractory stage, and was dependent on a functional ligand-binding domain. Conventional AR antagonists showed agonistic activity in cells with increased AR levels; this antagonist-agonist conversion was associated with alterations in the recruitment of coactivators and corepressors to the promoters of AR target genes. Increased levels of AR confer resistance to anti-androgens by amplifying signal output from low levels of residual ligands, and by altering the normal response to antagonists. Mohler et al. revealed that recurrent prostate cancer may develop the capacity to biosynthesize testicular androgens from adrenal androgens or cholesterol. [63, 64] They showed that tissue levels of testosterone were similar in recurrent prostate cancer and benign prostate. They also showed that the DHT level in recurrent prostate cancer tissue was decreased to 18% of the level in benign prostate tissue. Testosterone and dihydrotestosterone occur in recurrent prostate cancer tissue at levels sufficient to activate AR. Montgomery et al. showed that soft tissue metastases in patients with anorchid serum testosterone contain levels of testosterone that are up to three times higher than those in prostate tumors in eugonadal men.[65]

Transcript levels of enzymes involved in androgen synthesis were up-regulated in the same tumors, suggesting that tumoral synthesis of androgens from cholesterol might occur.[66] Androgen-independent prostate cancer cell lines synthesize testosterone from radio-labeled cholesterol in vitro, and human prostate cancer xenografts are capable of synthesizing DHT from acetate and cholesterol, confirming that tumoral androgen synthesis is possible.[67] Thus, experimental and clinical evidence suggests that the enzymes of steroid metabolism are activated in the prostate cancer with CRPC state, and might provide multiple new targets for therapeutic intervention. Moreover, substantial evidences suggest that CRPC may not, in fact, be androgen independent, but occurs in a setting of continued AR-mediated signaling that is driven by the presence of residual tissue androgens. We used androgen independent and androgen sensitive cells, LNCaP cells, and examined androgen metabolism in the cells.[68] We confirmed that DHT converted from the androgen precursors is important in the cellular activity of the cancer cells. This shows that metabolism of the androgen in the prostate cancer cells plays an important role even in the exacerbation with androgen independent and androgen sensitive state after ADT. This conclusion is supported by the evidence that about 30% of recurrent prostate cancers show transient clinical responses to secondary or tertiary hormonal manipulation.[69] As a consequence, strategies to decrease adrenal cortical androgen production in patients with CRPC have been developed and are currently in widespread use. Ryan et al. revealed that higher androstenedione levels predict the likelihood of response to ketoconazole, which is used as an inhibitor of adrenal androgen synthesis, and improved survival compared with patients with lower levels. [70] These data suggest that the therapy with ketoconazole is less effective in patients with low levels of androgens at baseline. Ketoconazole therapy as secondary hormonal therapies may be less effective in the patients with low androgen levels in the prostate.

7. Clinical-translational advances of castration-resistant prostate cancer

Recently, encouraging GnRH antagonists and early phase trial results of promising ADT agents that interfere with AR signaling for patients with hormone-naive prostate cancer or CRPC have been reported.

7.1 Gonadotrophin-releasing hormone (GnRH) antagonists: Degarelix

Medical castration using GnRH agonists currently provides the mainstay of ADT for prostate cancer. Although effective, these agents only reduce testosterone levels after a delay of 14 to 21 days. [71] GnRH antagonists compete with natural GnRH for binding to GnRH receptors, thus decreasing or blocking GnRH action in the body. GnRH antagonists induce fast and profound LH and follicle-stimulating hormone (FSH) suppressions from the pituitary. In men, the reduction in LH subsequently leads to rapid suppression of testosterone release from the testes. Unlike the GnRH agonists, which cause an initial stimulation of the hypothalamic-pituitary-gonadal axis, leading to a surge in testosterone levels, and under certain circumstances, a flare-up of the tumor, GnRH antagonists do not cause a surge in testosterone or clinical flare. [72] Clinical flare is a phenomenon that occurs in patients with advanced disease, which can precipitate a range of clinical symptoms such as bone pain, ureteral obstruction, and spinal cord compression. As testosterone surge does not occur with GnRH antagonists, there is no need for patients to receive an antiandrogen as flare protection during prostate cancer treatment. GnRH agonists also induce an increase in testosterone levels after each reinjection of the drug a phenomenon that does not occur with GnRH antagonists. GnRH antagonists have an immediate onset of action leading to a fast and profound suppression of testosterone and are therefore especially valuable in the treatment of patients with prostate cancer, where fast control of disease is needed. Abarelix, initial GnRH antagonist for prostate cancer, has been linked with immediate-onset systemic allergic reactions.[73] Degarelix is a new type of hormonal therapy for prostate cancer without stimulation of the release of histamine. [74] The reduction in LH subsequently leads to a rapid and sustained suppression of testosterone release from the testes and subsequently reduces the size and growth of the prostate cancer. This in turn results in a reduction in PSA levels in the patient's blood. Degarelix has an immediate onset of action, binding to GnRH receptors in the pituitary gland and blocking their interaction with GnRH. [75] The effectiveness of degarelix was recently evaluated in a Phase III, randomised, 12 month clinical trial (CS21) in 610 patients with prostate cancer, for whom ADT was indicated.[76] Patients were randomised to receive treatment with one of two doses of degarelix or the GnRH agonist, leuprolide. Both degarelix doses were at least as effective as leuprolide at suppressing testosterone to castration levels (<or=0.5 ng/mL) from Day 28 to study end (Day 364). Testosterone levels were suppressed significantly faster with degarelix than with leuprolide, with nearly all of the degarelix patients achieving castration levels by Day 3 of treatment compared with none in the leuprolide group. No patients receiving degarelix experienced a testosterone surge compared with 81% of those patients receiving leuprolide. Furthermore, degarelix resulted in a significantly faster reduction in PSA levels compared with leuprolide indicating faster control of the prostate cancer. Recent results also suggest that degarelix therapy may result in longer control of prostate cancer compared with leuprolide. [77] As with all hormonal therapies, degarelix is commonly associated with hormonal side effects such as hot flushes and weight gain. [76] Due to its mode of administration (subcutaneous injection), degarelix is also associated with injection-site reactions such as injection-site pain, erythema or swelling. Injection-site reactions are usually mild or moderate in intensity and occur predominantly after the first dose, decreasing in frequency thereafter.

7.2 Cytochrome P450, family 17, subfamily A, polypeptide 1 (CYP17A1) inhibitors

The multifunctional 17α-hydroxylase/17,20-lyase encoded by Cytochrome P450, family 17, subfamily A, polypeptide 1 (CYP17A1) is a cytochrome P450 enzyme localized to the endoplasmic reticulum in the adrenals, testes, placenta and ovaries, and lies at the crossroads of sex steroid and glucocorticoid synthesis. It is encoded by a single gene found on chromosome 10 in humans. The enzyme possesses both 17α-hydroxylase activity and C17,20-lyase activity, and requires P450 reductase, cytochrome-b5 reductase (b5), to transfer electrons in the presence of nicotinamide adenine dinucleotide phosphate (NADPH) for both catalytic activities. The degree of C17,20-lyase activity, modulated by cytochrome-b5, determines which metabolic pathway the substrate will follow in terms of sex steroid or glucocorticoid formation.[78, 79] Cytochrome-b5 is required for the C17,20 lyase activity, and high b5/CYP17A1 ratios are associated with the nearly exclusive production of androgens in the testes as opposed to the low ratios observed in the adrenals where glucocorticoids are produced.[80, 81] As the critical catalytic step in all androgen biosynthesis, therapeutic CYP17A1 inhibition to treat prostate cancer and other androgen dependent diseases has been envisioned for over 50 years, with recent discoveries in prostate cancer pathology driving much of the current refocus on CYP17A1 as a therapeutic target.[82, 83] Additionally, some evidence suggests that CYP17A1 mRNA and protein expression correlate with disease stage and relapse.[84, 85] Despite the strong rational for targeting CYP17A1, this target has been largely unexploited with relatively few inhibitors progressing to clinical trials and only ketoconazole, an unspecific inhibitor of CYP17A1, in widespread clinical use.

7.3 Abiraterone acetate

One of CYP17A1 inhibitors, abiraterone acetate, the irreversible inhibitor of 17α-hydroxylase/C17,20-lyase (CYP17A1), is well tolerated and has significant and durable anti-tumor activity both in patients with chemotherapy-naive prostate cancer and in docetaxel-treated patients with CRPC. [86] In patients with CRPC, despite ADT, intra-tumoral androgen levels remain high, with continued AR signaling. The source of these androgens could be adrenal or de novo intra-tumoral synthesis. Researchers tried to inhibit CYP17A1, the key enzyme responsible for androgen synthesis, using abiraterone acetate, which is 10-fold or more potent of inhibition of CYP17A1 than ketoconazole, another inhibitor of CYP17A1. The phase II (open-label, single-arm) portion of the trial was an expansion of a promising phase I trial reported in 2008. [87] All 42 participants were castrated, and 38 had metastases, primarily in bone and/or lymph nodes. Their median age was 70. All received oral abiraterone acetate 1,000 mg daily in 28-day cycles. PSA declined at least 50% in 28 of the 42 patients (67%); eight patients (19%) had PSA decreases of at least 90%. Of the 24 patients who had measurable disease on CT scan, 9 (37.5%) had tumor regression that constituted a partial response. Further, 16 of these 24 patients (67%) showed no evidence of progression at 6 months. Baseline levels of DHEA, DHEA-S, androstenedione and estradiol were associated with the increased likelihood of a PSA decline of at least 50%. Adding dexamethasone 0.5 mg daily at the time of PSA progression reversed abiraterone acetate resistance in 33% of patients. This study and other phase II study revealed that abiraterone acetate has significant antitumor activity in post-docetaxel patients with CRPC. [88-90] Recent results of the phase III trial of abiraterone acetate in post-docetaxel patients has shown an overall survival benefit in advanced CRPC (COU-AA-301). [91] Abiraterone acetate is designed to treat these tumors by inhibiting the production of androgen in the testes, the adrenal glands and prostate cancer tumors themselves. The Phase III trial included 1195 patients from 13 countries whose metastatic, castration-resistant prostate cancer had previously been treated with one of two chemotherapeutic agents that included docetaxel. Among the 398 patients randomly assigned to receive the corticosteroid prednisone plus placebo, median overall survival was 10.9 months. Among the 797 who received abiraterone acetate plus prednisone, median survival was 14.8 months. Significant differences also emerged between the placebo and treatment groups for all of the trial's secondary endpoints, including time to PSA progression, radiographic progression-free survival and PSA response rate. The benefits of abiraterone were determined during a pre-specified interim analysis of the study, prompting the trial's Independent Data Monitoring Committee to recommend unblinding the trial, and allowing anyone on the placebo arm to be offered abiraterone acetate. Several ongoing trials are examining the agent in earlier settings (i.e., a phase III in metastatic CRPC pre-docetaxel, and smaller studies in combination with radiation therapy or as neoadjuvant pre-surgery for localized disease).

The US Food and Drug Administration (FDA) has approved abiraterone acetate (Zytiga, Cougar Biotechnology) in combination with prednisone for the treatment of metastatic CRPC in men who have received prior docetaxel chemotherapy. Herein, several potential strategies for abiraterone are presented to clarify the clinical utilization of this agent in the future. These evidences such as not only decline of PSA levels and the reduction of the tumor size but also the evidences such as the symptom improvement and improved survival duration are expected in future.

7.4 Orteronel (TAK-700) [(1S)-1-(6,7-dimethoxy-2-naphthyl)-1-(1H-imidazol-4-yl)-2-methylpropan-1-ol]

Orteronel is a non-steroidal imidazole CYP17A1 inhibitor (IC50 = 28nM) currently in clinical trials in prostate cancer patients. The compound was found to be selective for CYP17A1 over 11β-hydroxylase by an impressive 260-fold, and exhibited suppressive effects on testosterone biosynthesis in rats and reduction in the weight of prostate and seminal vesicles in the rat. [92, 93] Orteronel was also capable of reducing serum testosterone levels down to castration level after 8 hours following a single oral administration of 1mg/kg to monkeys. A practical asymmetric synthesis of Orteronel has been established in eight steps from 2,3-dihydroxy naphthalene. This phase I/II, open-label, dose-escalation study assesses the safety and tolerability of oral, twice-daily (BID) Orteronel in patients with metastatic CRPC. Secondary objectives include assessment of Orteronel efficacy, as shown by PSA response, and Orteronel pharmacokinetics. Orteronel >= 300 mg BID appears active and well tolerated in patients with metastatic CRPC. The recommended phase II dose is 400 mg BID. [ASCO 2010 Genitourinary Cancers Symposium] Orteronel is performed on two phase 3 clinical trials: one is a randomized, double-blind, multicenter, phase 3 study evaluating orteronel plus prednisone compared with placebo plus prednisone in the treatment of men with progressive, chemotherapy-naive, metastatic CRPC, the other is in men with metastatic CRPC that has progressed following taxane-based therapy.

7.5 TOK-001 (VN/124-1) [3β-hydroxy-17-(1H-benzimidazole-1-yl)androsta-5,16-diene]

The increased efficacy of TOK-001 in several prostate cancer models both in vitro and in vivo is believed to arise from its ability to down regulate the AR as well as competitively block androgen binding. [94, 95]. TOK-001 can act by several mechanisms (CYP17A1 inhibition, competitive inhibition and down-regulation of the AR). In prostate cancer cell lines, TOK-001 inhibited the growth of CRPCs, which had increased AR and were no longer sensitive to bicalutamide. Indeed, ARMOR1(Androgen Receptor Modulation Optimized for Response1) phase1/2 trials with TOK-001 was recently initiated in CRPC patients.

7.6 3β-Hydroxysteroid dehydrogenase inhibitors

Prostate cancer exhibits robust 3β-HSD enzymatic activity, which is required for the AR-mediated response to Δ-5 adrenal androgens and that 3β-HSD may serve as a pharmacologic target for the treatment of CRPC. [96] Pharmacologic inhibition of 3β-HSD might have therapeutic value regardless of the relative contribution of adrenal androgens as opposed to de novo steroidogenesis in the reconstitution of intratumoral testosterone and DHT. We showed that trilostane , a 3β-HSD inhibitor, actually inhibits the in situ conversion of DHEA to androstenedione in prostate cancer cells, suggesting a new therapeutic target to more efficiently suppress intracellular androgen levels.[97] However, trilostane has a direct androgenic ability in cancer cells with mutated or wild-type AR. Trilostane should be used with particular concern when treating prostate cancer, possibly suggesting the combination of trilostane and an AR antagonist such as bicalutamide or designing an inhibitor of 3β-HSD free of AR agonist activity.

7.7 Apoptone (HE3235) (17α-ethynyl-5α-androstan-3α, 17β-diol)

A novel androstane steroid, Apoptone (HE3235), an orally bioavailable synthetic analogue of 3β-androstanediol, has a significant inhibitory activity for 5'-androstenediol-stimulated LNCaP proliferation. [98, 99] Apoptone exhibits a wide range of effects, including alteration of androgen receptor signaling and reductions in levels of intratumoral androgens. This inhibitory activity is accompanied by an increase in the number of apoptotic cells. Animal studies have confirmed the cytoreductive activity of apoptone on LNCaP tumours. The results suggest that this compound may be of clinical use in CRPC. From the results of phase I/II clinical trial, apoptone is a novel, orally delivered agent with clinical activity in advanced CRPC patients. It is well tolerated and has an AUC linear to dose. Based on the safety and activity observed, the trial continues to accrue an expansion cohort at 100 mg/day of patients with chemotherapy-naive CRPC. [100]

7.8 Inhibitors targeting androgen receptor
7.8.1 A new androgen receptor antagonist, MDV3100 (Fig. 2)

As for the conventional anti-androgen, affinity for AR and agonistic activity for AR are matters of concern. Because AR signaling appears to drive this cancer, blocking this signaling should stop its growth, the researchers theorized, and they went on to develop a drug that would do just that. Another novel ADT drug, AR antagonist MDV3100 (a diarylthiohydantoins) is a small-molecule, pure AR antagonist that inhibits AR nuclear translocation and DNA binding. [101, 102] MDV3100 is generally well tolerated, and shows encouraging anti-tumor activity in patients with CRPC. The drug was selected as a result of its activity in models of AR over-expression, in which conventional anti-androgens develop agonist properties. Currently available agents in the setting of AR over-expression actually act as agonists, rather than antagonists, so they actually make the disease worse, while MDV3100 has no known agonist activity. MDV3100 has demonstrated activity in models of bicalutamide-resistant prostate cancer. The results come from a phase 1/2 trial (NCT00510718) of 140 men, 65 of whom were chemotherapy-naive. Patients with progressive, metastatic CRPC were enrolled in dose-escalation cohorts of three to six patients and given an oral daily dose of MDV3100 from 30 mg to 600mg. The primary objective was to identify the safety and tolerability profile of MDV3100 and to establish the maximum tolerated dose. They noted antitumor effects at all doses, including decreases in serum prostate-specific antigen of 50% or more in 78 (56%) patients, responses in soft tissue in 13 (22%) of 59 patients, stabilized bone disease in 61 (56%) of 109 patients, and conversion from unfavorable to favorable circulating tumor cell counts in 25 (49%) of the 51 patients. PET imaging of 22 patients to assess androgen-receptor blockade showed decreased (18)F-fluoro-5α-dihydrotestosterone binding at doses from 60 mg to 480 mg per day (range 20-100%). The median time to progression was 47 weeks (95% CI 34-not reached) for radiological progression. The maximum tolerated dose for sustained treatment (>28 days) was 240 mg. The most common grade 3-4 adverse event was dose-dependent fatigue (16 [11%] patients), which generally resolved after dose reduction. The encouraging antitumor

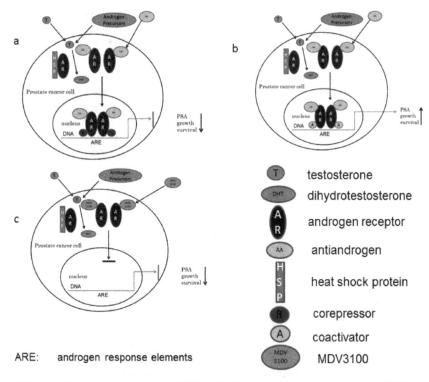

ARE: androgen response elements

T	testosterone
DHT	dihydrotestosterone
AR	androgen receptor
AA	antiandrogen
HSP	heat shock protein
R	corepressor
A	coactivator
MDV 3100	MDV3100

Fig. 2. The nuclear translocation and DNA binding on androgen receptors (AR) of androgens in the prostate cancer cells and action mechanisms of conventional AR antagonists and a new AR antagonist, MDV3100. (a) Conventional AR antagonists block AR with antagonistic action competitively in the prostate cancer cells. (b) Conventional AR antagonists showed agonistic activity in cells with increased AR levels; this antagonist-agonist conversion was associated with alterations in the recruitment of coactivators and corepressors to the promoters of AR target genes. Increased levels of AR confer resistance to anti-androgens by amplifying signal output from low levels of residual ligands, and by altering the normal response to antagonists. (c) MDV3100 is a pure AR antagonist that inhibits AR nuclear translocation and DNA binding. The affinity with AR of MVD3100 is stronger than that of conventional anti-androgens. MDV3100 has no known agonist activity for AR.

activity with MDV3100 in CRPC validates preclinical studies that have implicated AR signaling as a driver of this disease. MDV3100 is performed on two phase 3 clinical trials: one is a randomized, double-blind, multicenter, phase 3 study evaluating MDV3100 compared with placebo in the treatment of men with progressive, chemotherapy-naive, metastatic CRPC (PREVAIL), the other is in men with metastatic CRPC that has progressed following taxane-based therapy (AFFIRM).

ARN-509 is also an AR antagonist that inhibits nuclear translocation and DNA binding of the receptor, thereby modulating expression of genes that drive prostate cancer growth. Phase 1/2 clinical trial of ARN-509 in patients with CRPC was announced. (NCT01171898)

7.8.2 An inhibitor of the amino terminal domain (NTD) of the AR: EPI-001

AR is activated by androgen or by other factors when androgen is removed, resulting in the transactivation of the amino terminal domain (NTD) of AR and AR binding to androgen response elements (AREs) in the promoters of androgen-regulated genes. All current therapies that target the AR are dependent on the presence of its C-terminal ligand-binding domain (LBD). A library of extracts from marine sponges for an inhibitor of AR NTD transactivation were screened and the small molecule EPI-001 was identified, which inhibited transcriptional regulation of androgen-regulated genes, but not those regulated by the related progesterone and glucocorticoid steroid receptors. [103] Importantly, EPI-001 was effective at inhibiting both ligand-dependent and ligand-independent transactivation of AR, as well as inhibiting constitutively active AR splice variants that are devoid of LBD. EPI-001 has a new mode of action, as it targets the transactivation of AR regardless of the presence of androgen, and is a promising therapy to delay the progression of CRPC.

8. The prospects of the androgen deprivation therapy on the ground of androgen milieu in the prostate

Conventional ADTs that we have used cannot decrease DHT levels in the prostate sufficiently to restrain the growth of the cancer in patient with aggressive prostate cancer, as we mentioned above. The androgen levels in blood were low; however, it became clear that the AR signals play important roles for progress of the cancers from the studies of the prostate cancer that became exacerbation after ADT. The androgen milieu in men with high Gleason score prostate cancer is probably less affected by conventional ADT than that in men with low score cancer, which was suggested to be associated with adrenal androgen levels. In patients treated with ADT the pituitary-adrenal axis mediated by adrenocorticotropic hormone has a central role in the regulation of androgen synthesis. Adrenocorticotropic hormone mediated androgen synthesis is a potential target for advanced ADT. Importantly, the suboptimal suppression of androgen activity in the prostate cancer may account for the heterogeneity in treatment effect observed across individual patients, and, moreover, may contribute to the outgrowth of resistant prostate cancer clones adapted to survive in a low androgen environment, suggesting that more effective methods for suppressing the androgen axis in the tumoral microenvironment are required. From the results of the high reactivity of a CYP17A1 inhibitor and a new AR antagonist for patients with CRPC, the androgen syntheses and the maintenances of the AR signal system in the prostate cancer play important roles in etiological mechanisms of CRPC. As for the ADT for the patients with aggressive prostate cancer, it is important to restrain productions of testosterone and DHT and to restrain AR activity together with castration from early period of treatment. The results with new ADT agents, such as MDV3100 and abiraterone acetate seem to validate the hypothesis that androgens and the AR are vital to progression of metastatic CRPC.

9. Conclusions

The patients with prostate cancer of high Gleason score have low DHT levels in the prostatic tissue. Biologically aggressive prostate cancer can occur under a low DHT level environment where the prostate cancer of a low malignancy with high DHT dependency cannot easily occur. Conventional ADTs that we have used cannot decrease DHT levels in the prostate sufficiently to restrain the growth of the cancer in patients with aggressive prostate cancer. Persistent levels of DHT in the prostate after castration are derived from adrenal androgens in the prostate. The androgen milieu in men with high Gleason score prostate cancer is probably less affected by conventional ADT than that in men with low score cancer, which was suggested to be associated with adrenal androgen levels. In patients treated with ADT the pituitary-adrenal axis mediated by adrenocorticotropic hormone has a central role in the regulation of androgen synthesis. These locally produced androgens can play important roles in the pathogenesis and development of prostate cancer. AR signaling pathway is an important mechanism in proliferation of aggressive prostate cancer during ADT. AR transcriptional activity is reactivated in CRPC and identifies the intracellular conversion of adrenal androgens to DHT as a mechanism mediating this reactivation. New ADTs using CYP17A1 inhibitors such as abiraterone acetate and AR antagonists such as MDV3100 for patients with CRPC, which will break through the limitation of the efficacy of conventional ADTs that have been used for nearly 70 years, have been developing. Therefore, it is important to examine the status of in situ androgen metabolism and/or the AR signal system in detail in order to improve the clinical response to ADT in patients diagnosed with biologically aggressive prostate cancer from now on.

10. Acknowledgments

The author is supported by Grants-in-Aid for Scientific Research C 2009 (No. 21592035) and Suzuki Foundation for Urological Medicine.

11. References

[1] Heinlein CA, Chang C., Androgen receptor in prostate cancer., Endocr Rev. 2004;25(2):276-308.
[2] Huggins C, Hodges CV. Studies on prostate cancer. Effect of castration, estrogen and androgen injection on serum phosphatases in metastatic carcinoma of the prostate. Cancer Res 1941; 1:293-7.
[3] McLeod DG, Crawford ED, DeAntoni EP. Combined androgen blockade: the gold standard for metastatic prostate cancer. Eur Urol. 1997;32 Suppl 3:70-7.
[4] Pienta KJ, Bradley D. Mechanisms underlying the development of androgen-independent prostate cancer. Clin Cancer Res. 2006; 12: 1665-71.
[5] Di Lorenzo G, Buonerba C, Autorino R, De Placido S, Sternberg CN. Castration-resistant prostate cancer: current and emerging treatment strategies. Drugs. 2010;70(8):983-1000.
[6] Winters SJ, Clark BJ. Testosterone Synthesis, Transport, and Metabolism. In Bagatell CJ, Bremner WJ (eds), Androgens in Health and Disease. pp3-22. Humana Press, 2003.
[7] Rommerts FFG. Testosterone: overview of biosynthesis, transport, metabolism and non-genomic actions. In Nieschlag E, Behre HM, Niechlag S (eds) Testosterone. 3rd edn, pp1-38. Cambridge, 2004.
[8] Haider SG., Cell biology of Leydig cells in the testis., Int Rev Cytol. 2004;233:181-241.
[9] Midzak AS, Chen H, Papadopoulos V, Zirkin BR. Leydig cell aging and the mechanisms of reduced testosterone synthesis. Mol Cell Endocrinol. 2009;299(1):23-31.

[10] Endogenous Hormones and Prostate Cancer Collaborative Group, Roddam AW, Allen NE, Appleby P, Key TJ., Endogenous sex hormones and prostate cancer: a collaborative analysis of 18 prospective studies., J Natl Cancer Inst. 2008;100(3):170-83.

[11] Morote J, Ramirez C, Gomez E, Planas J, Raventos CX, de Torres IM, Catalan R., The relationship between total and free serum testosterone and the risk of prostate cancer and tumour aggressiveness., BJU Int. 2009;104(4):486-9.

[12] Luu-The V, Belanger A, Labrie F., Androgen biosynthetic pathways in the human prostate., Best Pract Res Clin Endocrinol Metab. 2008;22(2):207-21.

[13] Penning TM, Byrns MC., Steroid hormone transforming aldo-keto reductases and cancer., Ann N Y Acad Sci. 2009;1155:33-42.

[14] Ghayee HK, Auchus RJ., Clinical implications of androgen synthesis via 5α-reduced precursors., Endocr Dev. 2008;13:55-66.

[15] Zhu YS, Imperato-McGinley JL., 5α-reductase isozymes and androgen actions in the prostate., Ann N Y Acad Sci. 2009;1155:43-56.

[16] Uemura M, Tamura K, Chung S, Honma S, Okuyama A, Nakamura Y, Nakagawa H. Novel 5 α-steroid reductase (SRD5A3, type-3) is overexpressed in hormone-refractory prostate cancer. Cancer Sci. 2008;99(1):81-6.

[17] Godoy A, Kawinski E, Li Y, Oka D, Alexiev B, Azzouni F, Titus MA, Mohler JL. 5α-reductase type 3 expression in human benign and malignant tissues: A comparative analysis during prostate cancer progression. Prostate. 2010 Dec 28. [Epub ahead of print]

[18] Auchus RJ., The backdoor pathway to dihydrotestosterone., Trends Endocrinol Metab. 2004;15(9):432-8.

[19] Ghayee HK, Auchus RJ., Basic concepts and recent developments in human steroid hormone biosynthesis., Rev Endocr Metab Disord. 2007;8(4):289-300.

[20] Sharifi N, McPhaul MJ, Auchus RJ. "Getting from here to there"--mechanisms and limitations to the activation of the androgen receptor in castration-resistant prostate cancer. J Investig Med. 2010;58(8):938-44.

[21] Morgentaler A., Testosterone and prostate cancer: an historical perspective on a modern myth., Eur Urol. 2006;50(5):935-9.

[22] Isbarn H, Pinthus JH, Marks LS, Montorsi F, Morales A, Morgentaler A, Schulman C., Testosterone and prostate cancer: revisiting old paradigms., Eur Urol. 2009;56(1):48-56.

[23] Morgentaler A, Traish AM., Shifting the paradigm of testosterone and prostate cancer: the saturation model and the limits of androgen-dependent growth., Eur Urol. 2009;55(2):310-20.

[24] Weiss JM, Huang WY, Rinaldi S, Fears TR, Chatterjee N, Hsing AW, Crawford ED, Andriole GL, Kaaks R, Hayes RB. Endogenous sex hormones and the risk of prostate cancer: a prospective study. Int J Cancer. 2008;122(10):2345-50.

[25] Bartsch W, Klein H, Schiemann U, Bauer HW, Voigt KD. Enzymes of androgen formation and degradation in the human prostate. Ann N Y Acad Sci. 1990;595:53-66.

[26] Nishiyama T, Hashimoto Y, Takahashi K. The influence of androgen deprivation therapy on dihydrotestosterone levels in the prostatic tissue of patients with prostate cancer. Clin Cancer Res. 2004;10(21):7121-6.

[27] Nishiyama T, Ikarashi T, Hashimoto Y, Suzuki K, Takahashi K. Association between the dihydrotestosterone level in the prostate and prostate cancer aggressiveness using the Gleason score. J Urol. 2006;176(4 Pt 1):1387-91.

[28] Prehn RT. On the prevention and therapy of prostate cancer by androgen administration. Cancer Res. 1999;59(17):4161-4.

[29] Freedland SJ, Isaacs WB, Platz EA, Terris MK, Aronson WJ, Amling CL, Presti JC Jr, Kane CJ. Prostate size and risk of high-grade, advanced prostate cancer and biochemical progression after radical prostatectomy: a search database study. J Clin Oncol. 2005;23(30):7546-54.

[30] Kwon T, Jeong IG, You D, Park MC, Hong JH, Ahn H, Kim CS. Effect of prostate size on pathological outcome and biochemical recurrence after radical prostatectomy for prostate cancer: is it correlated with serum testosterone level? BJU Int. 2010;106(5):633-8.

[31] Newton MR, Phillips S, Chang SS, Clark PE, Cookson MS, Davis R, Fowke JH, Herrell SD, Baumgartner R, Chan R, Mishra V, Blume JD, Smith JA Jr, Barocas DA. Smaller prostate size predicts high grade prostate cancer at final pathology. J Urol. 2010;184(3):930-7.

[32] Thompson IM, Goodman PJ, Tangen CM, Lucia MS, Miller GJ, Ford LG, Lieber MM, Cespedes RD, Atkins JN, Lippman SM, Carlin SM, Ryan A, Szczepanek CM, Crowley JJ, Coltman CA Jr. The influence of finasteride on the development of prostate cancer. N Engl J Med. 2003;349(3):215-24.

[33] Rubin MA, Allory Y, Molinie V, Leroy X, Faucon H, Vacherot F, Huang W, Kuten A, Salomon L, Rebillard X, Cussenot O, Abbou C, de la Taille A. Effects of long-term finasteride treatment on prostate cancer morphology and clinical outcome. Urology. 2005;66(5):930-4.

[34] Lucia MS, Epstein JI, Goodman PJ, Darke AK, Reuter VE, Civantos F, Tangen CM, Parnes HL, Lippman SM, La Rosa FG, Kattan MW, Crawford ED, Ford LG, Coltman CA Jr, Thompson IM. Finasteride and high-grade prostate cancer in the Prostate Cancer Prevention Trial. J Natl Cancer Inst. 2007;99(18):1375-83.

[35] Andriole GL, Bostwick DG, Brawley OW, Gomella LG, Marberger M, Montorsi F, Pettaway CA, Tammela TL, Teloken C, Tindall DJ, Somerville MC, Wilson TH, Fowler IL, Rittmaster RS; REDUCE Study Group. Effect of dutasteride on the risk of prostate cancer. N Engl J Med. 2010 Apr 1;362(13):1192-202.

[36] Li R, Wheeler T, Dai H, Frolov A, Thompson T, Ayala G. High level of androgen receptor is associated with aggressive clinicopathologic features and decreased biochemical recurrence-free survival in prostate: cancer patients treated with radical prostatectomy. Am J Surg Pathol. 2004;28(7):928-34.

[37] Fung KM, Samara EN, Wong C, Metwalli A, Krlin R, Bane B, Liu CZ, Yang JT, Pitha JV, Culkin DJ, Kropp BP, Penning TM, Lin HK. Increased expression of type 2 3α-hydroxysteroid dehydrogenase/type 5 17β-hydroxysteroid dehydrogenase (AKR1C3) and its relationship with androgen receptor in prostate carcinoma. Endocr Relat Cancer. 2006;13(1):169-80.

[38] Wako K, Kawasaki T, Yamana K, Suzuki K, Jiang S, Umezu H, Nishiyama T, Takahashi K, Hamakubo T, Kodama T, Naito M. Expression of androgen receptor through androgen-converting enzymes is associated with biological aggressiveness in prostate cancer. J Clin Pathol. 2008;61(4):448-54.

[39] Maatman TJ, Gupta MK, Montie JE. Effectiveness of castration versus intravenous estrogen therapy in producing rapid endocrine control of metastatic cancer of the prostate. J Urol. 1985;133:620-1.

[40] Oefelein MG, Feng A, Scolieri MJ, Ricchiutti D and Resnick MI Reassessment of the definition of castrate levels of testosterone: implications for clinical decision making. Urology 2000; 56: 1021-1024.

[41] Tammela T. Endocrine treatment of prostate cancer. J Steroid Biochem Mol Biol. 2004;92:287-95.

[42] Tombal B. Appropriate Castration with Luteinising Hormone Releasing Hormone (LHRH) Agonists: What is the Optimal Level of Testosterone? Eur Urol Suppl 2005; 4:14-9.

[43] Crawford ED, Rove KO. Incomplete testosterone suppression in prostate cancer. N Engl J Med. 2010;363(20):1976.

[44] Morote J, Orsola A, Planas J, Trilla E, Raventos CX, Cecchini L, Catalan R. Redefining clinically significant castration levels in patients with prostate cancer receiving continuous androgen deprivation therapy. J Urol. 2007 ;178(4 Pt 1) :1290-5.

[45] Perachino M, Cavalli V, Bravi F. Testosterone levels in patients with metastatic prostate cancer treated with luteinizing hormone-releasing hormone therapy: prognostic significance? BJU Int. 2010 Mar;105(5):648-51.

[46] Labrie F, Belanger A, Luu-The V, Labrie C, Simard J, Cusan L, Gomez J, Candas B. Gonadotropin-releasing hormone agonists in the treatment of prostate cancer. Endocr Rev. 2005; 26: 361-79.

[47] Labrie F, Belanger A, Dupont A, Luu-The V, Simard J, Labrie C. Science behind total androgen blockade: from gene to combination therapy. Clin Invest Med. 1993; 16: 475-92.

[48] Hammond GL. Endogenous steroid levels in the human prostate from birth to old age: a comparison of normal and diseased tissues. J Endocrinol. 1978; 78: 7-19.

[49] Belanger B, Belanger A, Labrie F, Dupont A, Cusan L, Monfette G. Comparison of residual C-19 steroids in plasma and prostatic tissue of human, rat and guinea pig after castration: unique importance of extratesticular androgens in men. J Steroid Biochem. 1989; 32: 695-8.

[50] Geller J, Albert JD. Effects of castration compared with total androgen blockade on tissue dihydrotestosterone (DHT) concentration in benign prostatic hyperplasia (BPH). Urol Res. 1987; 15: 151-3.

[51] Nishiyama T, Ikarashi T, Hashimoto Y, Wako K, Takahashi K. The change in the dihydrotestosterone level in the prostate before and after androgen deprivation therapy in connection with prostate cancer aggressiveness using the Gleason score. J Urol. 2007;178(4 Pt 1):1282-8.

[52] Titus MA, Gregory CW, Ford OH 3rd, Schell MJ, Maygarden SJ, Mohler JL. Steroid 5α-reductase isozymes I and II in recurrent prostate cancer. Clin Cancer Res. 2005;11(12):4365-71.

[53] Thomas LN, Lazier CB, Gupta R, Norman RW, Troyer DA, O'Brien SP, Rittmaster RS. Differential alterations in 5α-reductase type 1 and type 2 levels during development and progression of prostate cancer. Prostate. 2005;63:231-9.

[54] Arai S, Miyashiro Y, Shibata Y, Tomaru Y, Kobayashi M, Honma S, Suzuki K. Effect of castration monotherapy on the levels of adrenal androgens in cancerous prostatic tissues. Steroids. 2011 Feb;76(3):301-8.

[55] Grossmann ME, Huang H, Tindall DJ. Androgen receptor signaling in androgen-refractory prostate cancer. J Natl Cancer Inst. 2001 ;93 :1687-97.

[56] Stanbrough M, Bubley GJ, Ross K, Golub TR, Rubin MA, Penning TM, Febbo PG, Balk SP. Increased expression of genes converting adrenal androgens to testosterone in androgen-independent prostate cancer. Cancer Res. 2006;66(5):2815-25.

[57] Mostaghel EA, Page ST, Lin DW, Fazli L, Coleman IM, True LD, Knudsen B, Hess DL, Nelson CC, Matsumoto AM, Bremner WJ, Gleave ME, Nelson PS. Intraprostatic androgens and androgen-regulated gene expression persist after testosterone suppression: therapeutic implications for castration-resistant prostate cancer. Cancer Res. 2007;67:5033-41.

[58] Takizawa I, Nishiyama T, Hara N, Isahaya E, Hoshii T, Takahashi K. Serum prostate-specific antigen levels reflect the androgen milieu in patients with localized prostate cancer receiving androgen deprivation therapy: Tumor malignant potential and androgen milieu., Prostate. 2010;70(13):1395-401.

[59] Takizawa I, Hara N, Nishiyama T, Isahaya E, Hoshii T, Takahashi K. Adrenocorticotropic hormone is involved in regulation of androgen synthesis in men receiving androgen deprivation therapy for localized prostate cancer. J Urol. 2010;184(5):1971-6.

[60] Attar RM, Takimoto CH, Gottardis MM. Castration-resistant prostate cancer: locking up the molecular escape routes. Clin Cancer Res. 2009;15(10):3251-5.

[61] Yuan X, Balk SP. Mechanisms mediating androgen receptor reactivation after castration. Urol Oncol. 2009;27(1):36-41.

[62] Chen CD, Welsbie DS, Tran C, Baek SH, Chen R, Vessella R, Rosenfeld MG, Sawyers CL. Molecular determinants of resistance to antiandrogen therapy. Nat Med. 2004;10(1):33-9.

[63] Mohler JL, Gregory CW, Ford OH 3rd, Kim D, Weaver CM, Petrusz P, Wilson EM, French FS. The androgen axis in recurrent prostate cancer. Clin Cancer Res. 2004;10(2):440-8.

[64] Titus MA, Schell MJ, Lih FB, Tomer KB, Mohler JL. Testosterone and dihydrotestosterone tissue levels in recurrent prostate cancer. Clin Cancer Res. 2005;11(13):4653-7.

[65] Montgomery RB, Mostaghel EA, Vessella R, Hess DL, Kalhorn TF, Higano CS, True LD, Nelson PS. Maintenance of intratumoral androgens in metastatic prostate cancer: a mechanism for castration-resistant tumor growth. Cancer Res. 2008;68(11):4447-54.

[66] Locke JA, Guns ES, Lubik AA, Adomat HH, Hendy SC, Wood CA, Ettinger SL, Gleave ME, Nelson CC. Androgen levels increase by intratumoral de novo steroidogenesis during progression of castration-resistant prostate cancer. Cancer Res. 2008;68(15):6407-15.

[67] Dillard PR, Lin MF, Khan SA. Androgen-independent prostate cancer cells acquire the complete steroidogenic potential of synthesizing testosterone from cholesterol. Mol Cell Endocrinol. 2008;295(1-2):115-20.

[68] Suzuki K, Nishiyama T, Hara N, Yamana K, Takahashi K, Labrie F. Importance of the intracrine metabolism of adrenal androgens in androgen-dependent prostate cancer. Prostate Cancer Prostatic Dis. 2007;10(3):301-6.

[69] Lam JS, Leppert JT, Vemulapalli SN, Shvarts O, Belldegrun AS. Secondary hormonal therapy for advanced prostate cancer. J Urol. 2006;175(1):27-34.

[70] Ryan CJ, Halabi S, Ou SS, Vogelzang NJ, Kantoff P, Small EJ. Adrenal androgen levels as predictors of outcome in prostate cancer patients treated with ketoconazole plus antiandrogen withdrawal: results from a cancer and leukemia group B study. Clin Cancer Res. 2007;13(7):2030-7.

[71] Van Poppel H. Evaluation of degarelix in the management of prostate cancer. Cancer Manag Res. 2010 Jan 25;2:39-52.

[72] van Poppel H, Nilsson S. Testosterone surge: rationale for gonadotropin-releasing hormone blockers? Urology. 2008 Jun;71(6):1001-6.

[73] Debruyne F, Bhat G, Garnick MB. Abarelix for injectable suspension: first-in-class gonadotropin-releasing hormone antagonist for prostate cancer. Future Oncol. 2006 Dec;2(6):677-96.

[74] Koechling W, Hjortkjaer R, Tanko LB. Degarelix, a novel GnRH antagonist, causes minimal histamine release compared with cetrorelix, abarelix and ganirelix in an ex vivo model of human skin samples. Br J Clin Pharmacol. 2010 Oct;70(4):580-7.

[75] Princivalle M, Broqua P, White R, Meyer J, Mayer G, Elliott L, Bjarnason K, Haigh R, Yea C. Rapid suppression of plasma testosterone levels and tumor growth in the dunning rat model treated with degarelix, a new gonadotropin-releasing hormone antagonist. J Pharmacol Exp Ther. 2007 Mar;320(3):1113-8.

[76] Klotz L, Boccon-Gibod L, Shore ND, Andreou C, Persson BE, Cantor P, Jensen JK, Olesen TK, Schroder FH. The efficacy and safety of degarelix: a 12-month, comparative, randomized, open-label, parallel-group phase III study in patients with prostate cancer. BJU Int. 2008 Dec;102(11):1531-8.

[77] Tombal B, Miller K, Boccon-Gibod L, Schroder F, Shore N, Crawford ED, Moul J, Jensen JK, Kold Olesen T, Persson BE. Additional Analysis of the Secondary End Point of Biochemical Recurrence Rate in a Phase 3 Trial (CS21) Comparing Degarelix 80mg Versus Leuprolide in Prostate Cancer Patients Segmented by Baseline Characteristics. Eur Urol. 2010 May;57(5):836-42.

[78] Lee-Robichaud P, Shyadehi AZ, Wright JN, Akhtar ME, Akhtar M. Mechanistic kinship between hydroxylation and desaturation reactions: acyl-carbon bond cleavage promoted by pig and human CYP17 (P-450(17)α; 17 α-hydroxylase-17,20-lyase). Biochemistry. 1995;34(43):14104-13.

[79] Akhtar MK, Kelly SL, Kaderbhai MA. Cytochrome b(5) modulation of 17α-hydroxylase and 17-20 lyase (CYP17) activities in steroidogenesis. J Endocrinol. 2005;187(2):267-74.

[80] Katagiri M, Kagawa N, Waterman MR. The role of cytochrome b5 in the biosynthesis of androgens by human P450c17. Arch Biochem Biophys. 1995;317(2):343-7.

[81] Dharia S, Slane A, Jian M, Conner M, Conley AJ, Parker CR Jr. Colocalization of P450c17 and cytochrome b5 in androgen-synthesizing tissues of the human. Biol Reprod. 2004;71(1):83-8.

[82] Gaunt R, Steinetz BG, Chart JJ. Pharmacologic alteration of steroid hormone functions. Clin Pharmacol Ther. 1968;9(5):657-81.

[83] Arth GE, Patchett AA, Jefopoulus T, Bugianesi RL, Peterson LH, Ham EA, Kuehl FA Jr, Brink NG. Steroidal androgen biosynthesis inhibitors. J Med Chem. 1971;14(8):675-9.

[84] Montgomery RB, Mostaghel EA, Vessella R, Hess DL, Kalhorn TF, Higano CS, True LD, Nelson PS. Maintenance of intratumoral androgens in metastatic prostate cancer: a mechanism for castration-resistant tumor growth. Cancer Res. 2008;68(11):4447-54.

[85] Stigliano A, Gandini O, Cerquetti L, Gazzaniga P, Misiti S, Monti S, Gradilone A, Falasca P, Poggi M, Brunetti E, Agliano AM, Toscano V. Increased metastatic lymph node 64 and CYP17A1 expression are associated with high stage prostate cancer. J Endocrinol. 2007;194(1):55-61.

[86] Attard G, Reid AH, Yap TA, Raynaud F, Dowsett M, Settatree S, Barrett M, Parker C, Martins V, Folkerd E, Clark J, Cooper CS, Kaye SB, Dearnaley D, Lee G, de Bono JS. Phase I clinical trial of a selective inhibitor of CYP17, abiraterone acetate, confirms that castration-resistant prostate cancer commonly remains hormone driven. J Clin Oncol. 2008;26(28):4563-71.

[87] Attard G, Reid AH, A'Hern R, Parker C, Oommen NB, Folkerd E, Messiou C, Molife LR, Maier G, Thompson E, Olmos D, Sinha R, Lee G, Dowsett M, Kaye SB, Dearnaley D, Kheoh T, Molina A, de Bono JS. Selective inhibition of CYP17 with abiraterone acetate is highly active in the treatment of castration-resistant prostate cancer. J Clin Oncol. 2009;27(23):3742-8.

[88] Danila DC, Morris MJ, de Bono JS, Ryan CJ, Denmeade SR, Smith MR, Taplin ME, Bubley GJ, Kheoh T, Haqq C, Molina A, Anand A, Koscuiszka M, Larson SM, Schwartz LH, Fleisher M, Scher HI. Phase II multicenter study of abiraterone acetate plus prednisone therapy in patients with docetaxel-treated castration-resistant prostate cancer. J Clin Oncol. 2010;28(9):1496-501.

[89] Reid AH, Attard G, Danila DC, Oommen NB, Olmos D, Fong PC, Molife LR, Hunt J, Messiou C, Parker C, Dearnaley D, Swennenhuis JF, Terstappen LW, Lee G, Kheoh T, Molina A, Ryan CJ, Small E, Scher HI, de Bono JS. Significant and sustained antitumor activity in post-docetaxel, castration-resistant prostate cancer with the CYP17 inhibitor abiraterone acetate. J Clin Oncol. 2010;28(9):1489-95.

[90] Ryan CJ, Smith MR, Fong L, Rosenberg JE, Kantoff P, Raynaud F, Martins V, Lee G, Kheoh T, Kim J, Molina A, Small EJ. Phase I clinical trial of the CYP17 inhibitor abiraterone acetate demonstrating clinical activity in patients with castration-resistant prostate cancer who received prior ketoconazole therapy. J Clin Oncol. 2010;28(9):1481-8.

[91] de Bono JS, Logothetis CJ, Molina A, Fizazi K, North S, Chu L, Chi KN, Jones RJ, Goodman OB Jr, Saad F, Staffurth JN, Mainwaring P, Harland S, Flaig TW, Hutson TE, Cheng T, Patterson H, Hainsworth JD, Ryan CJ, Sternberg CN, Ellard SL, Fléchon A, Saleh M, Scholz M, Efstathiou E, Zivi A, Bianchini D, Loriot Y, Chieffo N, Kheoh T, Haqq CM, Scher HI; COU-AA-301 Investigators. Abiraterone and increased survival in metastatic prostate cancer. N Engl J Med. 2011;364(21):1995-2005.

[92] Matsunaga N, Kaku T, Itoh F, Tanaka T, Hara T, Miki H, Iwasaki M, Aono T, Yamaoka M, Kusaka M, Tasaka A. C17,20-lyase inhibitors I. Structure-based de novo design and SAR study of C17,20-lyase inhibitors. Bioorg Med Chem. 2004;12(9):2251-73.

[93] Matsunaga N, Kaku T, Ojida A, Tanaka T, Hara T, Yamaoka M, Kusaka M, Tasaka A. C(17,20)-lyase inhibitors. Part 2: design, synthesis and structure-activity

relationships of (2-naphthylmethyl)-1H-imidazoles as novel C(17,20)-lyase inhibitors. Bioorg Med Chem. 2004;12(16):4313-36.

[94] Handratta VD, Vasaitis TS, Njar VC, Gediya LK, Kataria R, Chopra P, Newman D Jr, Farquhar R, Guo Z, Qiu Y, Brodie AM. Novel C-17-heteroaryl steroidal CYP17 inhibitors/antiandrogens: synthesis, in vitro biological activity, pharmacokinetics, and antitumor activity in the LAPC4 human prostate cancer xenograft model. J Med Chem. 2005;48(8):2972-84.

[95] Vasaitis T, Belosay A, Schayowitz A, Khandelwal A, Chopra P, Gediya LK, Guo Z, Fang HB, Njar VC, Brodie AM. Androgen receptor inactivation contributes to antitumor efficacy of 17α-hydroxylase/17,20-lyase inhibitor 3β-hydroxy-17-(1H-benzimidazole-1-yl)androsta-5,16-diene in prostate cancer. Mol Cancer Ther. 2008;7(8):2348-57.

[96] Evaul K, Li R, Papari-Zareei M, Auchus RJ, Sharifi N. 3β-hydroxysteroid dehydrogenase is a possible pharmacological target in the treatment of castration-resistant prostate cancer. Endocrinology. 2010;151(8):3514-20.

[97] Takizawa I, Nishiyama T, Hara N, Hoshii T, Ishizaki F, Miyashiro Y, Takahashi K. Trilostane, an inhibitor of 3β-hydroxysteroid dehydrogenase, has an agonistic activity on androgen receptor in human prostate cancer cells. Cancer Lett. 2010;297(2):226-30.

[98] Trauger R, Corey E, Bell D, White S, Garsd A, Stickney D, Reading C, Frincke J. Inhibition of androstenediol-dependent LNCaP tumour growth by 17α-ethynyl-5α-androstane-3α, 17β-diol (HE3235). Br J Cancer. 2009;100(7):1068-72.

[99] Koreckij TD, Trauger RJ, Montgomery RB, Pitts TE, Coleman I, Nguyen H, Reading CL, Nelson PS, Vessella RL, Corey E. HE3235 inhibits growth of castration-resistant prostate cancer. Neoplasia. 2009;11(11):1216-25.

[100] Ahlem C, Kennedy M, Page T, Bell D, Delorme E, Villegas S, Reading C, White S, Stickney D, Frincke J. 17α-Alkynyl 3α, 17β-androstanediol non-clinical and clinical pharmacology, pharmacokinetics and metabolism. Invest New Drugs. 2010 Sep 3. [Epub ahead of print]

[101] Tran C, Ouk S, Clegg NJ, Chen Y, Watson PA, Arora V, Wongvipat J, Smith-Jones PM, Yoo D, Kwon A, Wasielewska T, Welsbie D, Chen CD, Higano CS, Beer TM, Hung DT, Scher HI, Jung ME, Sawyers CL. Development of a second-generation antiandrogen for treatment of advanced prostate cancer. Science. 2009;324(5928):787-90.

[102] Scher HI, Beer TM, Higano CS, Anand A, Taplin ME, Efstathiou E, Rathkopf D, Shelkey J, Yu EY, Alumkal J, Hung D, Hirmand M, Seely L, Morris MJ, Danila DC, Humm J, Larson S, Fleisher M, Sawyers CL; Prostate Cancer Foundation/Department of Defense Prostate Cancer Clinical Trials Consortium. Antitumour activity of MDV3100 in castration-resistant prostate cancer: a phase 1-2 study. Lancet. 2010;375(9724):1437-46.

[103] Andersen, R. J. et al. Regression of castrate-recurrent prostate cancer by a small-molecule inhibitor of the amino-terminus domain of the androgen receptor. Cancer Cell 2010;17: 535-546.

5

The Role of Cancer Stem Cells and MicroRNAs in Human Prostate Cancer

Mustafa Ozen[1,2,3] and Serhat Sevli[1]
[1]Department of Medical Genetics Istanbul University Cerrahpasa Medical School, Istanbul
[2]Bezmialem Vakif University, Istanbul
[3]Department of Pathology & Immunology Baylor College of Medicine, Houston, TX
[1,2]Turkey
[3]USA

1. Introduction

The Cancer Stem Cell (CSC) s are potentially tumorigenic cells supporting initiation, survival and spread of the tumor. Several researches have been reported that CSCs are present and active in a variety of tumors including lung, brain, and breast, prostate and ovarian cancers. Inspite of the debate between basal or luminal origin of prostate cancer, the accepted idea is that progenitor cells of both cell types give rise to the disease. The other names given to the prostate cancer originating cells are stromal-like or stem-like, tumor progenitor and tumor initiating cells. The idea of CSCs is generated by their differentiation potential and slow growing and also tumors' clonality and possessing minor amounts of stem cell like cells.

CSCs are identified by their tissue specific stem cell-like properties. The most common surface markers for isolation of prostate cancer stem cells are CD44, integrin-alpha(2) beta(1) and CD133. Other methods are Hoechst 33342 dye exclusion, and holoclone formation for showing stemness of CSCs.

True identification and characterization of CSCs is promising for development of novel treatment options by targeting specifically CSCs. Classic therapies target the fast-dividing and differentiated cancer cells. However, CSCs grow and divide slowly and are mostly resistant against most cancer therapies. After the therapy, some cells responsible from tumor relapse and metastasis remain intact.

MicroRNAs are the most popular small RNAs regulating mRNA expression. MiRNAs are transcribed from the DNA as primary-miRNA form and are cut by special nucleases and obtain hairpin precursor-miRNA structure. The adult single stranded 20-25 nucleotides miRNA in cytoplasm inhibit protein synthesis by targeting semi-complementary sequences on 3'-untranslated regions of mRNA. MiRNAs have specific mRNA targets and approximately 30% of transcripts are controlled by miRNAs. The alterations of miRNA expression in different tumor types and widespread deregulation in Prostate Tumors have been identified in recent years. The miRNAs are determined as potential therapeutic targets and diagnostic tumor markers from both tissue and blood, due to their specifically over-expressed or down-regulated expression in variable tumor types. miRNAs, commonly upregulated in tumor cells and inhibit tumor suppressor genes and promote cell proliferation in tumor cells are termed as oncogenic miRNAs or oncomirs. On the other hand, the miRNAs which are commonly down-regulated in tumor cells and inhibit tumor development are called tumor suppressor miRNAs.

Additionally, differential expression of miRNAs in Cancer Stem Cells of prostate tumors has been under investigation in recent years. Those two popular topics are seemed to provide novel information on the way of understanding the prostate cancer molecularly and providing new insights for prostate cancer diagnosis and therapy.

2. Prostate cancer stem cells (CSCs)

Prostate Cancer is one of the most frequent tumors among men in the developed countries. The locally advanced or metastatic types of prostate tumors mostly do not respond to current treatment options. Androgen independent prostate tumors are mostly lethal after androgen-ablation therapy and so the chemotherapy and radiotherapy resistant tumors are (Collins & Maitland, 2006).

The epithelial cell layer of prostate tissue is divided into two layers of basal and luminal that contain three subpopulation of cells; Basal cells, neuroendocrine cells and luminal cells. These cells are distinguished by their localization, morphology and phenotypes. The basal and neuroendocrine cells are along the basement membrane of prostate and the latter secretes neuroendocrine peptides to promote epithelial viability and growth of the gland. The luminal cells stay above basal cell layer and function to secrete prostate specific molecules through luminal space. The prostatic stem cells are commonly present in these epithelial cell populations, especially in basal cell subpopulation (Lawson & Witte, 2007; Miki & Rhim, 2008). The molecular markers of prostatic epithelial cells are characterized to identify the origin of normal and CSCs (Lawson & Witte, 2007). The androgen dependent luminal secretory cells express AR, prostate specific antigen, prostatic acid phosphatase, CD57, and low molecular weight cytokeratin (Miki & Rhim, 2008). The androgen independent non-secretory basal cells do not express androgen receptor (or low levels of AR), prostate specific antigen or prostatic acid phosphatase but present CD44, p63, and high molecular weight cytokeratin. The normal stem cells among basal cells amplify to differentiate into androgen independent transit amplifying cells (TACs) and these cells further differentiate to form androgen dependent luminal cells (Miki & Rhim, 2008; Wang & Shen, 2011).

2.1 The cancer stem cell theory

The cancer stem cell theory proposed more than a century ago. However, its molecular details have been understood in recent years. In 1950s, the first reliable studies about CSCs were conducted by Ernest McCulloch and James Till in Toronto. In recent years by the development of flow cytometry and xenotransplantation techniques, researchers know more about their molecular roles and pathogenic properties. The CSCs are also called cancer progenitor cells or tumor initiating cells, meaning that they have intrinsic and/or acquired capacity to initiate tumor and these cells are resistant against current clinical treatment strategies (Masters et al., 2008).

There are epithelial somatic stem cells and progenitor cells in basal and neuroendocrine cell layers of prostate tissue. When investigators retrieve androgen from the tissue, the epithelial cells die. Arise of epithelial layer after providing the androgen back, supports the idea of

presence of stem-like cells in prostate tissue. Additionally, prostate stem cells should be androgen-independent cells surviving without of it (Lawson & Witte, 2007).
Early evidences about cancer provided the idea that prostate cancer is formed by a one mutated cell that the entire tumor is homogenous clone of that originating cell. Cancer stem cell theory fits the clonality part today. It is well-known that tumor consists of heterogeneous cells with different tumorigenic capacity and possibly more than one initiator cells.
There are two important ideas about CSCs and prostate cancer connection: CSCs can potentially contribute to tumor development and they cause initiation and advancement of prostate tumors themselves (Collins & Maitland, 2006).
Both somatic stem cells and CSCs are capable of organogenesis. Somatic adult stem cells have potential to form multilineage of cells in a tissue. The CSCs are also able to repopulate tumor cells in distinct locations (Miki & Rhim, 2008). The cancer stem cell model suggests that tumor arises from tumor-initiating, self-renewing and differentiating stem-like cell. The differentiated cancer cells lack tumorigenesis capacity (Wang & Shen, 2011).
Prostate cancer as well as other solid tumor types comprise of heterogeneous cell types. The current cancer stem cell theory suggest that the prostate tumor contain minor amount of self-renewing cells possessing stem cell phenotypes and they are possibly responsible from proliferation, recurrence, and resistance to apoptosis of tumors (Lam & Reiter, 2006). According to recent experimental evidences, tumors also arise from stem-cell derived progenitor cells or differentiated cells (Lam and Reiter, 2006; Miki and Rhim, 2008; Wang and Shen, 2011). Thus the tumor-initiating cells might not always mean that they have CSC properties but by the oncogenic transformations differentiated cells or progenitor cells may have in vivo tumorigenic capacity and this is compatible with clonal evolution model.

Cancer Stem Cells			
Clinical Implications	Properties	Origin	Specific Pathways
Current treatments often fail to eliminate CSCs	Aberration in mitosis rate due to genomic mutations	Present in the tissue where tumor arise	Sonic hedgehog
	Differentiation and self renewal capability	Originated from stem, progenitor, or differentiated cells	Wnt/B-catenin
	Small population of cells with similar marker proteins		Notch signaling system

Table 1. Important features of cancer stem cells. Derived from the article of (Lobo et al., 2007)

The stem cell specific pathways, Wnt/β-catenin, Notch, and Hedgehog signaling pathways are frequently activated and implicated in self-renewal and cell fate of CSCs. The TGFβ signaling aims to keep the stem cells in quiescent state. The Epithelial growth factor receptor, EGFR, Platelet derived growth factor receptor, PDGFR, Stem cell factor, SCF, PTEN, and TP53 genes are also functioning in regulation of CSCs (Kelly & Yin, 2008; Korkaya & Wicha, 2007; Mimeault et al., 2007).

Another cancer organization model is the clonal evolution of tumor. According to this model of carcinogenesis, the tumors have a distinct type of and several tumor-initiating cells; thus the tumor may consist of more than one clone of cells. The cancer stem cell and clonal evolution theories support each other when the tumor may contain different clones originated from different stem or progenitor cells as schematized in Figure 1. Thus the cancer therapy should target all these clones specifically or commonly (Wang & Shen, 2011).

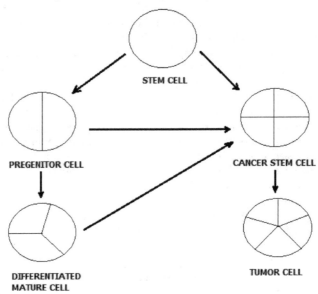

Fig. 1. Cancer stem cell formation

2.2 Identification of prostate cancer stem cell (PCSC) s

The cells being potentially prostate CSCs are identified generally by three experimental methods: clonal assay, separation by cell surface markers, and side population analysis. The studies show the existence of prostate CSCs using the primary prostate tumor samples, prostate cancer cell lines and animal models (Miki & Rhim, 2008).

We can separate the CSCs in prostate tumors by specific molecular markers. The surface markers for stem cells of one tissue or tumor do not always match to another tissue or tumor.

AR expression is the most common phenotype. The CSCs possess high *in vitro* proliferation potential. The cells of primary prostate cancer that show higher proliferation capacity do not express AR (Lawson & Witte, 2007). The normal prostate stem cells are also lack AR expression, thus both prostate CSCs and normal SCs do not need androgen for growth (Miki & Rhim, 2008).

Commonly accepted antigen profile for prostate specific CSCs is CD44+α2β1hiCD133+. This profile is in accordance with the normal prostate SCs (Lawson & Witte, 2007). The cells separated only by CD44 presence have enhanced proliferative activity in vitro. The CD44+ prostate cancer cells also lack of AR and they have tumor initiating and metastasis functions. The CSCs are known with their similar stemness genes' expression. Other than CD44 and CD133, prostate cancer cells also express higher levels of OCT3, OCT4, Nanog, Sox2, CD117, β-catenin, and BMI1 (Lawson & Witte, 2007).

The prostate cancer cells that express high levels of α2β1integrin have high colony-forming efficiency in vitro. The cells with CD133+/α2β1hi AND CD44+/CD133+ phenotype possess increased colony forming efficiency and tumor initiation after in vivo injection (Wang & Shen, 2011).

Stem Cell Surface Markers	Human	Mice
CD34	+	+
CD133	+	+
CD117	+	+
SCA1	+	+
CD44	+	-
CD24	+	-
CD20	+	-
CD105	+	-
CD326 (EpCAM)	+	-

Table 2. List of common cancer stem cell markers identified in human and mice

Xenotransplantation is a widely used functional assay in order to study tumor initiating properties of the CSCs. The CSCs from prostate cancer cell lines or primary prostate tumors have potential to generate prostate tumors in vivo. The observation of tumor generation in basal, luminal or neuroendocrinal layers shows the multilineage differentiation capacity of prostate CSCs (Lawson & Witte, 2007; Wang & Shen, 2011). The transplantation is performed on immune-deficient mice and every time at least 100 separated CSCs are required to produce tumors. The aim in CSCs theory is to find right cell, which is able to produce tumor itself in vivo. In other words, today our knowledge about the CSC characteristics is limited (Masters et al., 2008).

Side population analysis is the third method in order to identify and separate CSCs. During flow cytometer analysis, some cells are defined by pumping out the DNA-binding dye Hoechst 33342 and form a minor side population. For prostate cancer cells, these side population cells show stem cell like properties (Miki & Rhim, 2008).

Prostate cancer research uses mainly three types of samples as primary tumor cells, prostate cancer cell lines and animal models that present prostate tumor. The primary prostate cancer cells display the original characteristics of the tumor but we have limited access to biopsy samples and they possess limited lifespan even with specific culture techniques. Additionally, the cancer stem or progenitor cell amount is minor than other tumor or possibly contaminated normal epithelial cells (Miki & Rhim, 2008).

The permanent prostate cancer cell lines have unlimited proliferation ability, and have more cells with cancer stem cell profile, but they reflect the tumor characteristics more generally.

The mouse models are also useful tools in order to understand the tumorigenic capacity of CSCs with different surface markers. In mouse the prostate CSCs express the Sca-1 (stem cell antigen-1) and the cells possessing that marker can regenerate tumors in vivo. The most important issue about mouse models is that they have unknown phenotypes different from human tumors which are not fully characterized (Miki & Rhim, 2008).

2.3 PCSCs in prostate cancer diagnosis and development

The revealing of the signaling pathways and functional genes in cancer stem cells' self-renewal and survival is important for the identification of novel therapeutic targets.

Androgen-independent prostate cancers arise after androgen-ablation therapy for some patients. The initial idea is that minor amount of androgen-independent prostate cancer stem cells with basal cell characteristics is responsible for this transition (Kelly & Yin, 2008). Although there are cases consisting of AR mutations or alterations in AR-signaling pathways causing the androgen-refractory prostate cancer. AR mutations may also exist in metastatic and tumorigenic cells. The selection of cells with AR mutation must include self-renewing cells, which are metastatic cell of origin and androgen-independent but AR expressing cells. The metastatic prostate cancer should contain self-renewing cells in order to colonize in target tissue. Another alternative is that an AR expressing prostate cancer cell of origin acquires mutations causing the cell to have stem-cell properties. The progenitor cells are most likely candidates. Translocations are also common in prostate cancer originating cells and PIN (prostatic intraepithelial neoplasia). The TMPRSS2-ETS fusion gene formation after translocation cause over expression of ETS family transcription factors which are regulated by androgens (Kelly & Yin, 2008).

2.4 Impact of PCSCs in the treatment of prostate cancer and potential applications

Throughout the years, the only experience obtained about prostate cancer therapy is that the prostate cancer recurs. Androgen-ablation therapy, chemotherapy, radiotherapy and even radical prostatectomy may not help to eliminate the tumor-initiating or metastatic cells. The cancer stem cell theory is a promising finding to overcome the therapy resistant tumors. The CSCs are androgen independent, replication quiescent, and therapy resistant cells and novel therapies targeting specifically to these cells is logical than targeting differentiated prostate cancer cells.

Initially the cancer was thought as a homogeneous mass of aggressively proliferative tumor cells that were targeted by cancer therapy. The cancer stem cell theory provided a novel approach to therapy since the CSCs subpopulation are distinct from other tumor cells.

Drug testing clinical trials should quantify the cancer stem cell eradication rather than total tumor decay. However, it is hard for those studies to target specifically CSCs from normal tissue specific stem cells, since both have similar expressional and antigenic profiles (Lawson & Witte, 2007). Therefore, new markers needed to differentiate CSCs from tissue specific stem cells. MicroRNAs might be considered as novel molecules in this respect.

3. MicroRNAs and prostate cancer

MicroRNAs (miRNAs) are short (18-25nt) non-coding RNAs regulating gene expression during translation. They specifically target mRNAs and cause inhibition of translation, degradation of transcript or de-adenylation of poly(A) tail. In recent years miRNAs were discovered in viruses, plants and animal cells and total of 16772 miRNA have been identified 1424 of them belonging to homo sapiens (miRBase:Release17.0: April 2011) (Griffiths-Jones, 2004; Griffiths-Jones et al., 2006; Griffiths-Jones et al., 2008).

The microRNAs incompletely hybridize on target mRNAs and attract RNA Induced Silencing Complex (RISC) proteins in order to inhibit the protein synthesis. The miRNAs mostly on 5-Untranslated region of mRNA transcripts but hybridization on coding and 3-UTR sequences were shown. The incomplete hybridization of miRNA occurs by a certain motif as the first 7-8 nts called seed match hybridize totally and a loop with variable hybridization pattern follow. This motif has been analyzed via verified mRNA-miRNA matches and novel target predictions can be performed by computer algorithms (Bartel, 2004).

MicroRNA dysregulation has crucial outcomes on cellular mechanisms. Since one type of miRNA can target tens of different mRNA and all the miRNA-mRNA interactions have not been solved yet, the direct effect of miRNA expressional alteration is not clearly known. In tumors, there are enormous data about alteration of miRNA expression. Those alterations are originating from mutations in miRNA genes, mutation in genes of miRNA bio-processing pathway proteins, and RISC group proteins (Sevli et al., 2010). The miRNA genes are mostly located on fragile sites of chromosomes and in prostate cancer widespread deregulation of miRNAs was shown (Ozen et al., 2008).

The miRNA profiling studies have been performed initially by microarray technology. The identified miRNAs are verified by RT-PCR analysis. The samples most suitable for profiling studies are primary tumors, prostate cell lines, and tumor xenograft models. Further functional studies in order to identify the target mRNA transcripts of miRNAs and possible therapeutic roles, transfection of miRNA genes or pre-miRNA forms are performed several techniques such as lipofection, viral-transfection, electroporation etc. (Sevli et al., 2010). Expressional alterations of the miRNA target transcripts can be observed as changes in transcript of protein level since the miRNA mechanism could inhibit the protein translation keeping the mRNA stable or the RISC complex may cut the mRNA causing it to get into degradation. Whichever pathway would take place depends on the RISC components (Kim & Lee, 2009).

3.1 The miRNA expression profiling in prostate cancer

MicroRNAs are classified as tumor suppressor or oncomiRs depending on their expressional alteration or type of targeted mRNA. Tumor suppressor miRNAs target oncogenes keeping their protein products at normal levels and commonly down-regulated in tumors. OncomiRs target tumor suppressor transcripts and commonly up-regulated in tumors causing dysfunction of tumor-suppressor genes (Sevli et al., 2010).

It is thought that certain miRNAs are specifically deregulated in different cancer types; however, alteration of some miRNAs is observed in most of the tumors. Among them miR-21, miR291, and miR17-5p are significantly up-regulated in most of the solid tumors; therefore, they are called oncomiRs (Lu et al., 2008). Individual studies have shown that their over expression provides tumorigenesis and inhibition induces apoptosis or decreased rate of proliferation. On the other hand, we are not totally sure whether their expressional up-regulation is sufficient for prostate cancer development alone, or not. Tumor suppressor miRNA act in the opposite way of oncomiRs. Tumor suppressor miRNAs are down-regulated in cancers and studies ectopically over-expressing those tumor suppressor miRNAs have shown the inhibition of proliferation, invasion and proliferation capacity (Sevli et al., 2010).

Expression profiling studies on prostate cancer has provided some miRNAs that are significantly up- or down-regulated and functional studies with these miRNAs have revealed the importance of miRNAs in tumor progression and pathogenesis. Hsa-miR-125b is over-expressed in clinical samples and androgen independent cell lines. Its upregulation is related with the androgen-independence and survival of the tumor. miR-125b targets the Her2 and Bak1 transcripts. Her2 protein has role in androgen independence in prostate cancer and Bak1 together with Bax protein have interaction in apoptotic signaling pathway (Sevli et al., 2010).

Hsa-miR-21 is also over expressed in prostate cancer and effects tumorigenesis, invasion and metastasis by inhibiting the synthesis of proteins in those pathways. miR-21 also induces the motility of cancer cells and inhibits apoptosis (Sevli et al., 2010).

MiR-15a/16-1 cluster contains two different mature miRNA, transcribed together in primary microRNA form and processed by Drosha and Dicer RNases to get into mature form. These two miRNAs are down-regulated in some cancer types including prostate cancer. In order to check the direct roles of tumor suppressor miRNA in prostate cancer progression, knock-out animal models were investigated and hyperplasia together with increased cell proliferation and invasion of prostate tumor cells were observed in mice (Aqeilan, 2010). Ectopic turn-over of down-regulated tumor suppressor miRNAs by intra-cell delivery techniques provides the information about the therapeutic capacity of tumor suppressor miRNAs. Over-expression of miR-15a/16-1 has significant tumor regression capacity in vivo (Sevli et al., 2010).

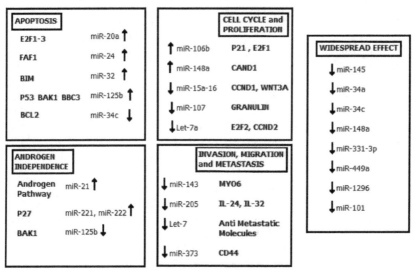

Fig. 2. A list of miRNAs with altered expression, providing their targeted messenger RNAs and pathways. Derived from (Catto et al., 2011; Sevli et al., 2010)

MiR-145 and miR143 are two of the most common deregulated tumor suppressor miRNA in all cancer types. miR-145/miR143 are also transcribed together as cluster and cleaved during maturation process. Down-regulation of miR-145 was observed prostate cancer (but not for miR143) and ectopic over-expression of miR-145 also cause anti-tumorigenic effect (our unpublished data).

Some miRNAs are reported to have functions on the androgen independency of prostate tumors. By comparing the androgen-dependent and androgen-independent prostate samples, miR-146a was revealed as taking role in androgen independency of prostate cancers.

Transcription of microRNAs is regulated by transcription factors since microRNA genes have their own promoters or they are co-regulated by the genes that host the miRNA genes in their intronic sequences. P53, a significant tumor suppressor protein is activated by the DNA-damage and induce expression of genes that carry p53 response elements on promoter sequences for promoting the repair mechanism. miR-34a, described in the last section, and miR145 are regulated by p53 protein. P53 also interacts with Drosha complex to promote the pri-microRNA to pre-microRNA conversion of miR-145's and some other microRNAs maturation (Suzuki et al., 2009).

There are some other microRNAs that are dysregulated in prostate cancer and the research findings are quite similar. The complete list of most significantly altered or mostly observed microRNAs are given in the Table-3. As the reference only one consistent article was chosen, but some other miRNAs that have distinct role in prostate cancer progression may be present and published.

Up-regulated	Reference	Down-regulated	Reference
Let-7	(Ozen et al., 2008; Volinia et al., 2006),	miR-125b	(Ozen et al., 2008; Schaefer et al., 2010)
miR-182	(Schaefer et al., 2010)	miR-15a/16-1	(Schaefer et al., 2010)
miR-96	(Schaefer et al., 2010)	miR-34a	(Lodygin et al., 2008)
miR375	(Schaefer et al., 2010)	miR-205	(Schaefer et al., 2010; Tang et al., 2011)
		miR-145	(Ozen et al., 2008; Schaefer et al., 2010)
		miR-221	(Schaefer et al., 2010; Tong et al., 2009)
		miR-222	(Schaefer et al., 2010; Tong et al., 2009)
		miR-181b	(Schaefer et al., 2010)
		miR-31	(Schaefer et al., 2010)
		miR-200c	(Tang et al., 2011)
Androgen-Independence			
Up-regulated	Reference	Down-regulated	Reference
miR-184	(Lin et al., 2008)	miR-128b	(Lin et al., 2008)
miR-361	(Lin et al., 2008)	miR-221	(Lin et al., 2008)
miR424	(Lin et al., 2008)	miR-222	(Lin et al., 2008)
miR-616	(Ma et al., 2011)	miR-146a/b	(Lin et al., 2008)
		miR-148a	(Lin et al., 2008)
		miR-663	(Lin et al., 2008)
Cancer Stem Cell , Metastases, or Invasion related			
Up-regulated	Reference	Down-regulated	Reference
miR-377	(Brase et al., 2011)	miR-34a	(Liu et al., 2011)
miR141	(Brase et al., 2011)	miR-143	(Peng et al., 2011)
		miR-145	(Peng et al., 2011)
		miR-15	(Musumeci et al., 2011)
		miR-16	(Musumeci et al., 2011)

Table 3. Differentially expressed miRNA implicated in prostate cancer (modified from (Sevli et al., 2010))

3.2 miRNAs as potential targets for development of therapy in prostate cancer

MicroRNAs have great potential as target for anti-cancer oligo-nucleotide therapy. Although their critical role in post-transcriptional gene expression is solved, more should be revealed about the specific deregulated miRNAs in individual tumors and the mRNA targets of them. Therapeutic delivery of down-regulated miRNAs is promising and lots of studies were performed to evaluate the potential miRNAs. The up-regulated miRNAs in prostate tumors can be inhibited by delivery of anti-miR molecules that specifically bind and form non-functional double stranded mature-miRNA molecules.

miRNA can also be used as cancer immunotherapy agents. Their immune regulatory functions were identified for certain miRNAs. miR-222 and miR-339 have role in targeting of tumors by immune cells. Some other miRNAs were identified in T-cells for immune cell regulated cancer therapy (Okada et al., 2010).

4. PCSCs and miRNAs: Future developments of identification of new approaches for prostate cancer progression and therapy

Some miRNAs have direct role in survival of prostate CSCs. CD44 as already known is the significant marker for CSCs in prostate tumors. The differential expression studies on CD44 positive and negative cells revealed that miR-34a is down regulated in tumors with enriched CD44 marker. Ectopic expression of miR-34a in CD44+ cells caused the decreased clonogenicity and recurrence/metastases capacity. The CD44- cells have higher miR-34a expression and down-regulation of miR-34a with antagonist antimiR molecules caused increased rate of metastasis and tumorigenesis. The CD44 transcript was found as direct target of miR-34a (Liu et al., 2011). MiR-34a is also induced by P53 tumor suppressor protein and commonly down-regulated in cancers which have decreased p53 expression. Mir-34a degrades the SIRT1, a sirtuin class III histone deacetylase protein, of which up-regulation was shown in less miR-34a expressing prostate samples.

5. Conclusion

Despite the recent developments on cancer diagnosis and therapy, prostate cancer still remains one of the leading cause of cancer deaths in men. New tools for precise diagnosis, distinguishing those patients who will be recurred early requiring more extensive treatments than those who will live their lifetime without not much getting affected by the disease are needed. Unlike some other types of tumors, prostate cancer is one of the tumor types in which limited treatment options are available; therefore, there is a need for novel therapy tools as well. In this chapter, two highly attracted topics, cancer stem cells and microRNAs are summarized as their role and implications in human prostate cancer arise. We believe this chapter will help to those who are interested in cancer stem cells and microRNAs not only in prostate cancer but in other applicable diseases as well.

6. Acknowledgement

Some of the research presented in this chapter is supported by a grant (108S051) from The Scientific and Technological Research Council of Turkey (TUBITAK).

7. References

Aqeilan, R.I., Calin, G.A., & Groce, C.M. (2010). miR-15a and miR-16-1 in cancer: discovery, function and future perspectives. *Cell Death and Differentiation*, Vol.17, No.2, (February, 2010), pp. 215-220,

Bartel, D.P. (2004). MicroRNAs: genomics, biogenesis, mechanism, and function. *Cell,* Vol.116, No.2, (2007), pp. 281-297,

Brase, J.C., Johannes, M., Schlomm, T., Fälth, M., Haese, A., Steuber, T., Beissbarth, T., Kuner, R., & Sültmann, H. (2011). Circulating miRNAs are correlated with tumor progression in prostate cancer. *International Journal of Cancer,* Vol.128, No.3, (February, 2011), pp. 608-616,

Catto, J.W., Alcaraz, A., Bjartell, A.S., De Vere White, R., Evans, C.P., Fussel, S., Hamdy, F.C., Kallioniemi, O., Mengual, L., Schlomm, T., Visakorpi, T. (2011). MicroRNA in prostate, bladder, and kidney cancer: a systematic review. *European Urology,* Vol.59, No.5, (May, 2011), pp. 671-681

Collins, A.T. & Maitland, N.J. (2006). Prostate Cancer Stem Cells. *European Journal of Cancer,* Vol.42, No.9, (June 2006), pp. 1213-1218,

Griffiths-Jones, S., Saini, H.K., van Dongen, S., & Enright, A.J. (2008). miRBase:tools for microRNA genomics. *Nucleic Acids Research,* Vol.36, No.1, (2008), pp. 154-158,

Griffiths-Jones, S., Grocock, R.J., van Dongen, S., Bateman, A., & Enright, A.J. (2006). miRBase: microRNA sequences, targets and gene nomenclature. *Nucleic Acids Research,* Vol.34, No.1, (2006), pp. 140-144,

Griffiths-Jones, S. (2004). The microRNA registry. *Nucleic Acids Research,* Vol.32, No.1, (2004), pp. 109-111,

Kelly, K. & Yin, J.J. (2008). Prostate Cancer and Metastasis Initiating Stem Cells. *Cell Research,* Vol.18, No.5, (May 2008), pp. 528-537,

Kim, W.C. & Lee, C.H. (2009). The role of mammalian ribonucleases (RNases) in cancer. *Biochimica et Biophysica acta,* Vol.1796, No.2, (December 2009), pp.99-113,

Korkaya, H. & Wicha, M.S. (2007). Selective Targeting of Cancer: A New Concept in Cancer Therapeutics. *Biodrugs: Clinical Immunotherapeutics, Biopharmaceyticals, and Gene Therapy,* Vol.21, No.5, (2007), pp. 299-310,

Lam, J.S. & Reiter, R.E. (2006). Stem Cells in Prostate and Prostate Cancer Development. *Urologic Oncology,* Vol.24, No.2, (March-April 2006), pp. 131-140,

Lawson, D.A. & Witte, O.N. (2007). Stem Cells in Prostate Cancer Initiation and Progression. *The Journal of Clinical Investigation,* Vol.117, No.8, (August, 2007), pp. 2044-2050,

Lin, S.L., Chiang, A., Chang, D., Ying, S.Y. (2008). Loss of mir-146a function in hormone-refractory prostate cancer. *The RNA,* Vol.14, No.3, (March, 2008), pp. 417-424,

Liu, C., Kelnar, K.,Liu, B., Chen, X., Calhoun-Davis, T., Li, H., Patrawala, L., Yan, H., Jeter, C., Honorio, S., Wiggins, J.F., Bader, A.G., Fagin, R., Brown, D., & Tang, D.G. (2011). The MicroRNA miR-34a Inhibits Prostate Cancer Stem Cells and Metastasis by Directly repressing CD44. *Nature Medicine,* Vol.17, No.2, (February, 2011), pp. 211-215,

Lu, Z., Liu, M., Stribinskis, V., Klinge, C.M., Ramos, K.S., Colburn, N.H., & Li, Y. (2008). MicroRNA-21 promotes cell transformation by targeting the programmed cell death 4 gene. *Oncogene,* Vol.27, No.31, (July, 2008), pp. 4373-4379,

Lobo, N.A., Shimono, Y., Qian, D., & Clarke, M.F. (2007). The Biology of the Cancer Stem Cells. *Annual Review of Cell and Developmental Biology,* Vol.23, No.1, (2007), pp. 675-699,

Lodygin, D., Tarasov, V., Epanchintsev, A., Berking, C., Knyazeva, T., Körner, H., Knyazev, P., Diebold, J., & Hermeking, H. (2008). Inactivation of miR-34a by aberrant CpG methylation in multiple types of cancer. *Cell Cycle,* Vol.7, No.16, (August, 2008), pp. 2591-2600,

Ma, S., Chan, Y.P., Kwan, P.S., Lee, T.K., Yan, M., Tang, K.H., Ling, M.T., Vielkind, J.R., Guan, X.Y., & Chan, K.W. (2011). MicroRNA-616 induces androgen-independent growth of prostate cancer cells by suppressing expression of tissue factor pathway inhibitor TFPI-2. *Cancer Research,* Vol.71, No.2, (January, 2011), pp. 583-592,

Masters, J.R., Kane, C., Yamamoto, H., & Ahmed, A. (2008). Prostate Cancer Stem Cell Therapy: Hype or Hope?. *Prostate Cancer and Prostatic Diseases*, Vol.11, No.4, (December 2008), pp. 316-319,

Miki, J. & Rhim, J.S. (2008). Prostate Cell Cultures as in vitro Models for the Study of Normal Stem Cells and Cancer Stem Cells. *Prostate Cancer and Prostatic Diseases*, Vol.11, No.1, (March 2008), pp. 32-39,

Mimeault, M., Hauke, R., Mehta, P.P., & Batra, S.K. (2007). Recent Advances in Cancer Stem/Progenitor Cell Research: Therapeutic Implications for Overcoming Resistance to the Most Aggressive Cancers. *Journal of Cellular and Molecular Medicine*, Vol.11, No.5, (September-October, 2007), pp. 981-1011,

Musumeci, M., Coppola, V., Addario, A., Patrizii, M., Maugeri-Saccà, M., Memeo, L., Colarossi, C., Francescangeli, F., Biffoni, M., Collura, D., Giacobbe, A., D'Urso, L., Falchi, M., Venneri, M.A., Muto, G., De Maria, R., & Bonci, D. (2011). Control of tumor and microenvironment cross-talk by miR-15a and miR-16 in prostate cancer. *Oncogene*, (May, 2011), Epub ahead of print,

Okada, H., Kohanbash, G., & Lotze, M.T. (2010). MicroRNAs in Immune Regulation: Opportunities for Cancer Immunotherapy. *The International Journal of Biochemistry and Cell Biology*, Vol.42, No.8, (August, 2010), pp. 1256-1261,

Ozen, M., Creighton, C.J., Ozdemir, M., Ittmann, M. (2008). Widespread deregulation of microRNA expression in human prostate cancer. *Oncogene*, Vol.27, No.12, (March 2008), pp. 1788-1793,

Peng, X., Guo, W., Liu, T., Wang, X., Tu, X., Xiong, D., Chen, S., Lai, Y., Du, H., Chen, G., Liu, G., Tang, Y., Huang, S., & Zou, X. (2011). Identification of miRs-143 and -145 that Is Associated with Bone Metastasis of Prostate Cancer and Involved in the Regulation of EMT. *PLOS One*, Vol.6, No.5, (May 2011), e20341,

Sevli, S., Uzumcu, A., Solak, M., Ittman, M., & Ozen, M. (2010). The Function of MiRNAs, the Small but Potent Molecules, in Human Prostate Cancer. *The Prostate Cancer and Prostatic Diseases*, Vol.13, No.3, (September 2010), pp. 208-217,

Schaefer, A., Jung, M., Mollenkopf, H.J., Wagner, I., Stephan, C., Jentzmik, F., Miller, K., Lein, M., Kristiansen, G., & Jung, K. (2010). Diagnostic and prognostic implications of microRNA profiling in prostate carcinoma. *International Journal of Cancer*, Vol.126, No.5, (March, 2010), pp. 1166-1176,

Suzuki, H.I., Yamagata, K., Sugimoto, K., Iwamoto, T., Kato, S., & Miyazono, K. (2009). Modulation of microRNA processing by p53. *Nature*, Vol.460, No.7254, (July, 2009), pp. 529-533,

Tang, X., Tang, X., Gal, J., Kyprianou, N., Zhu, H., & Tang, G. (2011). Detection of microRNAs in prostate cancer cells by microRNA array. *Methods in Molecular Biology*, Vol.732, No.1, (2011), pp. 69-88,

Tong, A.W., Fulgham, P., Jay, C., Chen, P., Khalil, I., Liu, S., Senzer, N., Eklund, A.C., Han, J., & Nemunaitis, J. (2009). MicroRNA profile analysis of human prostate cancers. *Cancer Gene Therapy*, Vol.16, No.3, (March, 2009), pp.206-216,

Wang, Z.A. & Shen, M.M. (2011). Revisiting the Concept of Cancer Stem Cells in Prostate Cancer. *Oncogene*, Vol.30, No.11, (March, 2011), pp. 1261-1271,

Volinia, S., Calin, G.A., Liu, C.G., Ambs, S., Cimmino, A., Petrocca, F., Visone, R., Iorio, M., Roldo, C., Ferracin, M., Prueitt, R.L., Yanaihara, N., Lanza, G., Scarpa, A., Vecchione, A., Negrini, M., Harris, C.C., Croce, C.M. (2006). A microRNA expression signature of human solid tumors defines cancer gene targets. *Proceedings of the National Academy of Sciences of the United States of America*, Vol.103, No.7, (February, 2006), pp. 2257-2261,

The Role of Vitamin D in the Prevention and Treatment of Prostate Cancer

Sophia L. Maund and Scott D. Cramer
Wake Forest University School of Medicine
University of Colorado, DenverAnschutz Medical Campus
USA

1. Introduction

Prostate cancer is the most common non-cutaneous cancer in American men and the second most deadly (Jemal et al., 2010). One in six American men will get prostate cancer in his lifetime, and the risk increases with age. Prostate cancer progresses over the course of decades, so there is ample opportunity for prevention earlier in life. Epidemiological and laboratory studies point to vitamin D_3 as a promising chemopreventative agent for prostate cancer. Vitamin D_3 metabolites and analogs have been shown to induce cell cycle arrest, differentiation, and senescence in normal prostate cells and prostate cancer cells. Ongoing studies are interrogating the mechanistic effects behind vitamin D_3 actions in the prostate. Additionally, clinical trials aim to investigate the potential chemopreventative and therapeutic effects of vitamin D_3 metabolites and analogs, both alone and in combination with taxol-based chemotherapeutic agents. Herein we will summarize the epidemiological, laboratory, and clinical studies with vitamin D_3 and the prostate and discuss how the current data supports a role for vitamin D_3 in the prevention and treatment of prostate cancer.

2. Prostate cancer treatment and prevention

If prostate cancer is thought to be localized to the prostate and is classified as low-grade, "watchful waiting" is an option, since some prostate tumors do not become life-threatening. Otherwise, a prostatectomy or external beam radiation is the first line of therapy (or in some cases, brachytherapy). Both prostatectomy and radiation therapy can damage the nerves that rest along the prostate, so side effects include impotence and incontinence that may or may not reverse over time. If the cancer is thought to have spread beyond the prostate, then a more systematic therapeutic approach is needed.

Since androgens are required for growth of both normal prostate cells and most prostate cancer cells, androgen ablation therapy is standard in the forms of surgical or chemical castration. Castration has significant side effects, but it reduces tumor burden and metastatses and it can help ease pain from metastatic outgrowths. However, androgen deprivation therapy inherently selects for prostate cancer cells that can grow in the absence of androgens, which often leads to tumor recurrence in 18 to 24 months in the form of castration-resistant prostate cancer (Feldman & Feldman, 2001). The median survival time for patients with castration-resistant prostate cancer is only 12-18 months. There is no standard successful treatment for castration-resistant prostate cancer, but therapies include docetaxel or pacilaxel-based chemotherapy, which are palliative at best. The impacts on quality of life and the success rates of current treatment options for prostate cancer (especially for castration-resistant prostate cancer) highlight the need for improved therapeutic approaches and the importance of chemoprevention, especially in men who are at higher risks for prostate cancer.

The American Cancer Society states that some cases of prostate cancer may be prevented by maintaining a healthy lifestyle and by hormonal control. Men who take Finasteride, a 5-alpha reductase inhibitor, which is a treatment for benign prostatic hyperplasia (BPH) and male-pattern baldness, have a lower incidence of prostate cancer, but this drug is not widely used for its chemopreventative properties (Hamilton et al., 2010). Dietary sources of chemoprevention are promising, but clinical studies are lacking due to the time and funds required to carry them out (Thompson et al., 2005). One of the most promising dietary chemopreventative agents for prostate cancer is vitamin D_3, which we will discuss in detail below.

3. Prostate cancer risk factors

The major risk factors for prostate cancer include age, race, family history, and geographic location. Prostate cancer develops over the course of decades, so its incidence and detection rates increase with age. Men of African-American descent are almost twice as likely to get prostate cancer as Caucasian men, and the prostate cancer mortality rate is more than twice as high for African-American men (Jemal, et al., 2010). Conversely, Asian men have among the lowest prostate cancer incidence and mortality rates in the world. Interestingly, prostate cancer risk increases in Asian men who relocate to the United States, which emphasizes the contributions of diet and lifestyle to prostate cancer risk (Severson et al., 1989; Luo et al., 2004). Prostate cancer can also have a strong heritable component. The estimated lifetime risk for prostate cancer increases with the number of family members diagnosed, with up to a 45% increase for men with three or more relatives with prostate cancer (Bratt, 2002). The heritable component of prostate cancer is attributed to a number of heritable genetic and epigenetic aberrations, reviewed elsewhere (Nelson et al., 2003).

3.1 Prostate cancer risk factors and vitamin D_3

Of the major risk factors for prostate cancer, age, race, and geographic location are closely tied to vitamin D_3 status. Older men get less sun exposure and have a thinner epidermis (in which UV light synthesizes vitamin D_3) than younger men, which are two reasons why older men have lower serum vitamin D_3 levels (MacLaughlin & Holick, 1985; Lips, 2001). Studies have shown inverse correlations between prostate cancer incidence and geographical regions with less exposure to UV radiation (Hanchette & Schwartz, 1992). Prostate cancer risk and mortality rates are at least twice as high in African-American men than in Caucasian men, and one reason for this may be the high levels of melanin in the skin that blocks UV-induced synthesis of vitamin D_3 (Matsuoka et al., 1991). Japanese men have very low risks for prostate cancer and have among the highest serum vitamin D_3 levels in the world due to the traditional vitamin D_3-rich diet (Nakamura et al., 2000).

These and other epidemiological studies support a role for vitamin D_3 in prostate cancer prevention.

4. Vitamin D_3 metabolism

Vitamin D was discovered in 1920 and characterized as a vitamin that is necessary for skeletal development and calcium homeostasis (Mellanby, 1921). Its chemical structure later revealed that vitamin D is not a vitamin, but a seco-steroid hormone belonging to the steroid hormone family that can be synthesized in the body or obtained from the diet (Brockmann, 1936; Lawson et al., 1971). Vitamin D_3 can be synthesized upon exposure to sunlight or obtained from dietary sources such as oily fish, eggs, and fortified milk. Upon exposure to UV radiation, 7-dehydrocholesterol in the skin is converted to vitamin D_3, also known as cholecalciferol (Figure 1). Vitamin D_3 is the natural form of vitamin D obtained from the diet (DeLuca, 2004). Vitamin D_3 travels to the liver where vitamin D_3 25-hydroxylase (25-OHase, encoded by the cytochrome P450 enzyme CYP27A1) hydroxylates it to become 25-hydroxyvitamin D_3 ($25OHD_3$) (Blunt et al., 1968). $25OHD_3$ then enters the kidney where 25 hydroxyvitamin D_3 1α-hydroxylase (1α-OHase, encoded by CYP27B1) hydroxylates it at the 1α position, generating the hormonally active form 1,25 dihydroxyvitamin D_3 ($1,25(OH)_2D_3$) (Fraser & Kodicek, 1970). $1,25(OH)_2D_3$ then travels to target tissues to carry out its effects such as regulating mineral homeostasis. Tissues other than the kidney express endogenous 1α-OHase such as the bone, liver, placenta, macrophages, skin, breast, colon, and prostate, so $25OHD_3$ can be activated directly in these tissues (Schwartz et al., 1998; Zehnder et al., 2001).

Once activated, $1,25(OH)_2D_3$ (also known as calcitriol) can bind the vitamin D receptor (VDR) within the cytosol (Figure 2). Upon binding, conformational changes occur that expose the retinoid X receptor (RXR) dimerization domains and the nuclear localization domains, allowing the VDR and the RXR to heterodimerize and enter the nucleus (Yasmin et al., 2005). Nuclear receptor co-activators such as DRIP/Mediator and SRC/p160 associate with the $1,25(OH)_2D_3$ -VDR-RXR complex and regulate its transcriptional activity (Rachez & Freedman, 2000; MacDonald et al., 2001). The conformational change also causes the release of co-repressors such as nuclear co-repressors (NCoRs) and the silencing mediator for retinoid and thyroid hormone receptors (SMRT) histone deacetylase complex, allowing histones to be released and the $1,25(OH)_2D_3$ -VDR-RXR complex to bind the vitamin D response element (VDRE) in the promoters of target genes (Tagami et al., 1998). RNA polymerase II (RNA Pol II) is recruited to the transcriptional machinery complex and transcribes $1,25(OH)_2D_3$ target genes.

Plasma $1,25(OH)_2D_3$ levels are tightly regulated by a negative feedback loop because high levels of $1,25(OH)_2D_3$ can be toxic. One of the universal $1,25(OH)_2D_3$ -VDR-RXR target genes is CYP24A1, which encodes 24-hydroxylase (24-OHase). 24-OHase hydroxylates $1,25(OH)_2D_3$ at the 24 position, which targets it for further oxidation to C23 carboxylic acid which is catabolized to calcitroic acid and excreted from the body (Figure 1) (Prosser & Jones, 2004). Normal serum circulation levels of $25OHD_3$ are 30-50 ng/mL, while normal serum levels of $1,25(OH)_2D_3$ are only ~30 pg/mL (Shepard et al., 1979; Horst & Littledike, 1982). $1,25(OH)_2D_3$ circulates bound to the vitamin D binding protein (DBP) from which it disassociates before entering the cell (Arnaud & Constans, 1993). Responses to vitamin D_3 intake differ among individuals and among tissue-types due to variables including CYP24A1 levels, kidney function, and genetic and epigenetic differences in vitamin D_3 metabolic proteins.

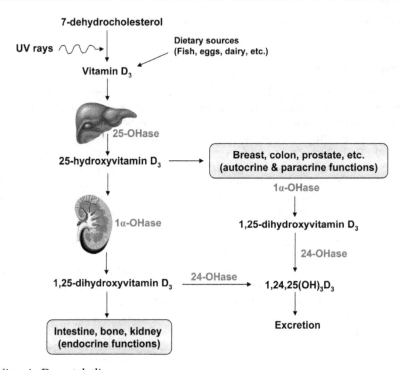

Fig. 1. Vitamin D₃ metabolism.

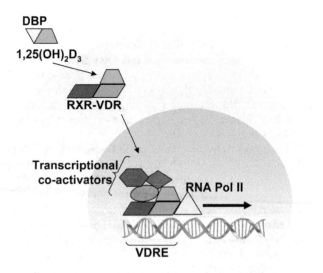

Fig. 2. Intracellular trafficking of 1,25(OH)₂D₃.

5. Vitamin D_3 epidemiology

There is an established association between increased prostate cancer risk and mortality and low serum $25OHD_3$ levels (Ahonen et al., 2000; Tretli et al., 2009), as well as an association between prostate cancer risk and genetic polymorphisms of the VDR (Ingles et al., 1997). However, other studies report no association or even a positive association between serum $25OHD_3$ and prostate cancer risk (Nomura et al., 1998; Park et al., 2010). The inconsistencies among reports warrant improved investigation and evaluation methods (reviewed in (Trottier et al., 2010)). One reason for the inconsistencies could be the apparent impact on prostate cancer risk of vitamin D_3 exposure over the course of a lifetime as opposed to the impact of serum levels of $25OHD_3$ over a defined time period (John et al., 2004; John et al., 2007); studies have shown that childhood sunburn frequency and UV exposure correlates with lower prostate cancer risks (Luscombe et al., 2001; Bodiwala et al., 2003). Another reason could be that, since prostate cancer develops over the course of decades, some patients' cancer cells may have lost the ability to activate $25OHD_3$ to $1,25(OH)_2D_3$ (Guileyardo et al., 1980; J. Y. Hsu et al., 2001; Chen et al., 2003). Studies with follow-up periods greater than 10 years are better for evaluating the implications of vitamin D_3 status in prostate cancer development (Ahonen, et al., 2000; Li et al., 2007). Additionally, intermittent high doses (>100,000 IU) of vitamin D_3 may be metabolized differently from lower daily doses (Rosen, 2011). There is no standardization for vitamin D_3, $25OHD_3$ or $1,25(OH)_2D_3$ administration, which has hampered clinical studies. Overall, the epidemiological studies encourage more laboratory and clinical investigations into a therapeutic role for vitamin D_3 and its metabolites in the prevention and treatment of prostate cancer.

6. *In vitro* and *in vivo* studies

As mentioned above, prostate cells express endogenous 1α-OHase and can synthesize $1,25(OH)_2D_3$ from $25(OH)D_3$, which suggests an important role for $1,25(OH)_2D_3$ in prostate biology (Schwartz, et al., 1998). We and others have shown that $25OHD_3$ inhibits prostate epithelial cell growth and induces p21 and p27 (common downstream targets of $1,25(OH)_2D_3$) to the same extents as does $1,25(OH)_2D_3$ (Barreto et al., 2000). This supports the application of $25OHD_3$ as a therapeutic that targets prostate tissue. Interestingly, 1α-OHase activity is lost and 24-OHase expression is elevated in prostate cancer cells compared to normal prostate cells, which supports a correlation between decreased $1,25(OH)_2D_3$ levels and prostate cancer (Miller et al., 1995; Whitlatch et al., 2002).

One of the ways that $1,25(OH)_2D_3$ is thought to maintain prostate homeostasis is by keeping cell growth in check. $1,25(OH)_2D_3$-induced apoptosis is rarely observed. LNCaP cells treated with $1,25(OH)_2D_3$ undergo cell cycle arrest at G1 as a result of increased p21 and p27 levels and decreased CDK2 activity followed by dephosphorylation of retinoblastoma (pRB) and subsequent suppression of E2F transcriptional activity (Figure 3) (Zhuang & Burnstein, 1998; Yang & Burnstein, 2003). Two of the most common downstream targets of $1,25(OH)_2D_3$ are CDKN1A (which encodes p21) and CDKN1B (which encodes p27). $25OHD_3$, $1,25(OH)_2D_3$, and its analogs have been shown to elevate p21 and p27 expression in several tissue types in conjunction with cell growth inhibition (Kawa et al., 1997; Barreto, et al., 2000; Colston & Hansen, 2002). CDKN1A contains a VDRE, so its transcription can be directly regulated by $1,25(OH)_2D_3$. $1,25(OH)_2D_3$ can also elevate p21 indirectly through direct transcriptional induction of insulin-like growth factor binding protein-3 (IGFBP-3), an upstream mediator of p21 transcription (Boyle et al., 2001; Peng et al., 2004; Peng et al., 2008). CDKN1B does not contain a VDRE, so p27 is regulated indirectly by 1,25(OH)$_2$D$_3$. CDK2 activates SKP2-mediated degradation of p27, so 1,25(OH)$_2$D$_3$-mediated induction of p27 is likely due to inhibition of CDK2 and p27 protein stabilization (Yang & Burnstein, 2003).

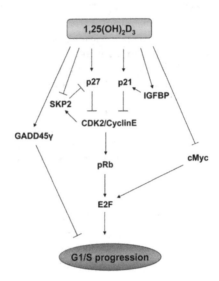

Fig. 3. 1,25(OH)$_2$D$_3$ signaling leading to G1 cell cycle arrest in prostate cancer cells.

More recently, 1,25(OH)$_2$D$_3$ has been shown to inhibit E2F and/or induce G1 arrest independently from pRB (Figure 3). In the C4-2 prostate cancer cell line, 1,25(OH)$_2$D$_3$ inhibited cMYC which subsequently suppressed E2F activity and cell cycle progression regardless of pRB status (Washington et al., 2011). We have reported that 1,25(OH)$_2$D$_3$ induces cell cycle arrest independently from pRB in prostate progenitor/stem cells (Maund et al., 2011). Flores and Burnstein recently reported that the cell cycle inhibitory protein GADD45γ mediates 1,25(OH)$_2$D$_3$-induced accumulation of LNCaP cells in G1 (Flores & Burnstein, 2010). Cell cycle arrest in G1 is a common downstream effect of 1,25(OH)$_2$D$_3$ treatment, and additional mechanisms of cell cycle regulation by 1,25(OH)$_2$D$_3$ are still being uncovered.

1,25(OH)$_2$D$_3$ can induce differentiation of several cell types including prostate stem cells, prostate epithelial cells and prostate cancer cells (Miller et al., 1992; Tokar & Webber, 2005; Maund, et al., 2011). Differentiated prostate cells do not normally divide, so 1,25(OH)$_2$D$_3$ may slow or halt any aberrant cell division. 1,25(OH)$_2$D$_3$-induced differentiation of the LNCaP prostate cancer cell line is evidenced by increased levels of prostate-specific antigen (PSA), kallikrein 2, E-cadherin, and androgen receptor (AR) (Esquenet et al., 1996; Campbell et al., 1997; Zhao et al., 1997; Darson et al., 1999; Zhao et al., 1999; Tokar & Webber, 2005).

AR signaling plays critical roles in prostate development, function, and pathogenesis. We reported that prostate progenitor/stem cells are AR-negative but, upon treatment with 1,25(OH)$_2$D$_3$, they become AR-positive (Barclay et al., 2008; Maund, et al., 2011). AR is not a direct transcriptional target of 1,25(OH)$_2$D$_3$ because it does not contain a VDRE, but we did observe increased AR mRNA in response to 1,25(OH)₂D₃; its mechanism of upregulation is unclear (Zhao, et al., 1999). Since AR signaling can contribute to prostate tumor growth, the induction of AR by 1,25(OH)₂D₃ may not be considered an anti-tumor effect. However, the induction of AR by 1,25(OH)₂D₃ signifies a transition from a less-differentiated prostate cell toward a more-differentiated prostate cell that is either less likely to become cancerous or, if already transformed, more responsive to therapeutic intervention such as castration. These hypotheses have yet to be tested *in vivo*. In LNCaP cells, growth inhibition by 1,25(OH)₂D₃ has been shown to be dependent on AR (Miller, et al., 1992; Zhao, et al., 1997; Zhao et al., 2000). AR-mediated induction of IGFBP-3 has been implicated in this process (Peng, et al., 2008). The exact mechanism(s) of 1,25(OH)₂D₃-induced differentiation is unknown, though differentiation is often preceded by an enrichment of cells in the G1 phase of the cell cycle (Studzinski & Harrison, 1999). Upregulation of p21 and p27 are implicated in differentiation of LNCaP and PC3 cells, and p27 is involved in senescence in a mouse model of prostate cancer (Campbell, et al., 1997; Majumder et al., 2008). This suggests that accumulation of prostate cells in G1 may precede 1,25(OH)₂D₃-induced differentiation and/or senescence, but the mechanisms remain unknown.

Our group recently reported that 1,25(OH)₂D₃ can induce senescence of prostate cancer cells *in vitro* (Axanova et al., 2010). Senescence is defined as a terminally-arrested state in which cells are metabolically active but cannot resume cell cycle progression (Muller, 2009), so induction of senescence is an additional form of 1,25(OH)₂D₃-mediated growth suppression. Senescence has been observed in cases of PIN that do not progress to prostate cancer (Majumder, et al., 2008), so it is possible that additional senescence induced by 1,25(OH)₂D₃ may impede prostate cancer progression. This has yet to be tested *in vivo*.

Another way that 1,25(OH)₂D₃ may impede prostate cancer progression and metastasis is through inhibition of cellular invasion and migration. *In vitro* studies have shown that 1,25(OH)₂D₃ decreases expression of alpha-6 and beta-4 integrins to inhibit the invasive capacities of prostate cancer cell lines (Sung & Feldman, 2000). 1,25(OH)₂D₃ is known to induce E-cadherin in prostate cancer cells (Campbell, et al., 1997), and E-cadherin was recently reported to mediate 1,25(OH)₂D₃-induced cellular adhesion that mitigates the metastatic capabilities of prostate cancer cells (J. W. Hsu et al., 2011). 1,25(OH)₂D₃ has also been shown to regulate a range of matrix metalloproteinases (MMPs) and tissue inhibitors of matrix metalloproteinases (TIMPs), also thought to mediate the effects of 1,25(OH)₂D₃ on invasion of prostate cancer cells (Bao et al., 2006).

In vivo studies with 1,25(OH)₂D₃ have been carried out primarily in xenograft models of prostate cancer as well as in the Dunning rat model of prostate cancer and, more recently, the Nkx3.1+/-PTEN+/- mouse model (Getzenberg et al., 1997; Lokeshwar et al., 1999; Banach-Petrosky et al., 2006; Trump et al., 2006). In the rat Dunning model, 1,25(OH)₂D₃ and 1,25(OH)₂D₃ analogs decreased tumor volumes and lung metastases, but the animals developed hypercalcemia. Use of 1,25(OH)₂D₃ analogs alone, however, were sufficient to reduce PC3 and LNCaP xenograft volumes without inducing hypercalcemia (Schwartz et al., 1995; Blutt et al., 2000). Nkx3.1+/-PTEN+/- mutant mice develop high-grade PIN with the capacity for progression to advanced metastatic and androgen-independent prostate cancer (Kim et al., 2002; Abate-Shen et al., 2003). Sustained intravenous delivery of 46 ng/kg/day of 1,25(OH)₂D₃ or vehicle control were administered to Nkx3.1+/-PTEN+/- pre-cancerous and cancerous cohorts of mice for 4 months (Banach-Petrosky, et al., 2006). Interestingly, 1,25(OH)₂D₃ suppressed PIN formation in the pre-cancerous cohort, but it did not affect prostate cancer progression in the cancerous cohort. Furthermore, increased levels of the

VDR were observed in the pre-cancerous cohort after $1,25(OH)_2D_3$ administration, while there was only a modest increase in VDR in the cancerous cohort, which could account for the ineffectiveness of $1,25(OH)_2D_3$ on tumor progression in the cancerous cohort. These results suggest that prostate cancer cells may have aberrations in the vitamin D_3 response pathway. Therefore, vitamin D_3 may be more effective as a chemopreventative agent than as a chemotherapeutic.

6.1 Prostate stem cells and vitamin D_3

Accumulating evidence supports the presence of adult prostate-specific stem cells, which undergo self-renewal into an identical prostate stem cell and multi-lineage differentiation into the multiple epithelial cell types of the prostate (Burger et al., 2005; Barclay, et al., 2008; Goldstein et al., 2010). They serve to maintain prostate tissue homeostasis and to stimulate tissue regeneration after injury. There are many similarities between the signalling pathways found to regulate stem cell processes and those that regulate cancer progression, which has led to the cancer stem cell hypothesis (Reya et al., 2001; Maund & Cramer, 2009; Mimeault & Batra, 2010). The prostate cancer stem cell hypothesis proposes that a transformed prostate stem cell can give rise to a heterogeneous prostate tumor, and that the tumor cannot be ablated unless the cancer stem cells are eliminated.

The aim of chemoprevention is to impede tumor development at the earliest point in its progression. According to the cancer stem cell hypothesis, the target cell population for prostate cancer prevention would be the prostate stem/progenitor cells (Maund & Cramer, 2010). Stem cells intrinsically have an extended replicative capacity. Agents that limit this capacity and promote differentiation are promising chemopreventative agents. We have recently reported that $1,25(OH)_2D_3$ is growth-inhibitory in adult prostate stem/progenitor cells (Maund, et al., 2011). $1,25(OH)_2D_3$ can induce G1 and G2 cell cycle arrest, stimulate differentiation toward a luminal epithelial cell type, and trigger senescence in this cell population, supporting a relevant role for vitamin D_3 in prostate chemoprevention (particularly in light of the cancer stem cell hypothesis). We found that the cytokine interleukin-1 alpha is highly upregulated by $1,25(OH)_2D_3$ and is a novel mediator of $1,25(OH)_2D_3$-induced growth inhibition of prostate stem/progenitor cells. In addition, microarray data revealed that $1,25(OH)_2D_3$ can impact gene expression and signalling pathways involved in stem cell self-renewal and multilineage differentiation including Hedgehog, Wnt, and TGFβ signaling (Maund, et al., 2011). $1,25(OH)_2D_3$ regulates components of these pathways in other cell types as well (Sarkar et al., 2010; Tang et al., 2011). This work is just beginning to reveal the cellular and genomic impacts of $1,25(OH)_2D_3$ in the stem cell population. Furthermore, $1,25(OH)_2D_3$ has been shown to exert anti-proliferative and pro-differentiating effects on hematopoietic and skin progenitor cells (Liu et al., 1996; Lehmann et al., 2010). The identification of tissue-specific stem cells and their potential contributions to cancer initiation and progression is changing the way we approach cancer prevention and treatment. A major aim is to identify compounds that effectively target the stem cell population, and $1,25(OH)_2D_3$ is a promising candidate for further investigation.

7. Clinical studies

Most clinical trials involving $1,25(OH)_2D_3$ and $1,25(OH)_2D_3$ analogs are carried out in combination with chemotherapeutic agents, particularly the taxanes, and are tested in patients with castration-resistant prostate cancer. $1,25(OH)_2D_3$ analogs such as EB1089 and

22-oxacalcitriol (OCT) are VDR ligands designed to recapitulate the anti-proliferative effects of $1,25(OH)_2D_3$ while minimizing the effects on calcium homeostasis that often lead to hypercalcemia (Steddon et al., 2001). To date, no $1,25(OH)_2D_3$ analog has fared significantly better than $1,25(OH)_2D_3$ alone. There are still many studies missing that are necessary for designing accurate clinical trials with $1,25(OH)_2D_3$ and $1,25(OH)_2D_3$ analogs including determination of the maximum-tolerated and optimal doses, definitions of phase II single-agent and combination doses, and randomized phase II trials that compare $1,25(OH)_2D_3$ alone versus $1,25(OH)_2D_3$ in combination with a single chemotherapeutic agent. These issues must be resolved in order to generate accurate phase II and phase III clinical trial data (Trump et al., 2010).

A high-dose formulation of $1,25(OH)_2D_3$ called DN-101 was tested for safety and efficacy in the ASCENT I (Androgen-independent prostate cancer Study of Calcitriol Enhancement of Taxotere) phase II trial in combination with docetaxel (Brawer, 2007). DN-101 administration was associated with improved survival but it did not impact PSA response (Beer et al., 2007). A large phase III trial (ASCENT II) was terminated in 2007 due to greater death rates in the experimental arm (docetaxel, prednisone, and DN-101) than the control arm (docetaxel, prednisone, and placebo). However, ASCENT II was not accurately designed to test the efficacy of DN-101 versus the placebo (Trump, et al., 2010). The docetaxel administration schedule and the DN-101 dosages were not consistent with those previously established. Since the optimal dose and maximum-tolerated dose for oral $1,25(OH)_2D_3$ remain undefined, the DN-101 doses used in the ASCENT trials were based on convenience: a weekly oral dose of 0.5 µg/kg. In pre-clinical trials, however, intravenous administration of >1 µg/kg $1,25(OH)_2D_3$ was required for anti-tumor effects (Trump, et al., 2010). Although the results from the ASCENT II trial were ambiguous, they highlighted several questions that need to be resolved before designing new $1,25(OH)_2D_3$ clinical trials.

Vitamin D_3 oral supplementation doses are still being defined; they vary depending on the desired endpoint and on individual vitamin D_3 metabolic capacity (Bischoff-Ferrari, 2009). Individuals with serum $25OHD_3$ levels less than 30 ng/mL are considered to be vitamin D_3 deficient. A recent retrospective analysis measured the impact of 8,000 IU/day vitamin D_3 supplementation on $25OHD_3$ levels in 2198 cancer patients (Vashi et al., 2010). They found that patients with baseline $25OHD_3$ levels between 20 and 32 ng/mL responded to supplementation better than those with baseline levels <20 ng/mL. Additionally, patients with prostate cancer were the most responsive to vitamin D_3 supplementation, in terms of the number of individuals whose $25OHD_3$ levels were >32 ng/mL after 8 weeks of supplementation. This finding supports further clinical investigations of vitamin D_3 in prostate cancer prevention and treatment. This study reported that 8,000 IU/day for 8 weeks was a safe and effective regimen for prostate and lung cancer patients, and they suggested that supplementation levels should be higher in colorectal and pancreatic cancer patients (Vashi, et al., 2010). Further studies are required to define maximum-tolerated and optimal doses for patients with different types of cancers.

The range of serum $25OHD_3$ associated with cancer prevention is 60-80 ng/mL (CF Garland et al., 2009). A recent community-based study of voluntary vitamin D_3 supplementation sought to define the doses necessary to reach serum $25OHD_3$ levels in this range (C. F. Garland et al., 2011). They reported that total vitamin D_3 intake from 9,400 to 17,400 IU/day would be necessary to achieve serum $25OHD_3$ levels of 30-50 ng/mL in this population. Additionally, they reported no toxicity from up to 40,000 IU/day. They proposed that most individuals should supplement their vitamin D_3 intake by 4,000-8,000 IU/day in order to reach serum 25OHD$_3$ levels associated with cancer prevention. This study will help shape additional clinical trials for vitamin D$_3$-based chemoprevention, and in the meantime it will help inform the public about the importance of sufficient vitamin D$_3$ supplementation. However, there is much controversy over the recommended vitamin D$_3$ supplementation doses. In 2010 the Institute of Medicine recommended a daily dose of 600 IU vitamin D$_3$, with a tolerable upper limit of 4,000 IU/day. However, the long-term benefits of vitamin D$_3$ doses in this range are unknown, and others (such as C.F. Garland et al., 2011 and Vashi et al., 2010) argue that 600 IU is insufficient for significant clinical benefits and that the tolerable upper limit exceeds 4,000 IU/day. It is becoming clear that the optimal daily vitamin D$_3$ dose is dependent on 1) the individual's baseline serum 25OHD$_3$ level, 2) the individual's vitamin D$_3$ metabolic capacity, and 3) the individual's health status and lifestyle (diabetic, prostate cancer vs. colorectal cancer patient, etc.). For these reasons and for the lack of definititve clinical studies there is controversy surrounding universal recommended vitamin D$_3$ doses. Future work should focus on resolving this continuing controversy.

8. Conclusion

Further understanding of the mechanisms of action behind 1,25(OH)$_2$D$_3$ signaling in the prostate and a deeper understanding of prostate stem cell biology will help potentiate the chemopreventative effects of vitamin D$_3$ and promote its concomitant use in primary and adjuvant prostate cancer therapies. Prostate cancer is a slow-growing disease that develops over the course of decades and typically affects men late in life. Treatment decisions are based on tumor severity and rate of PSA change, and some prostate tumors do not even progress to stages necessary for therapeutic intervention. The aim of prostate cancer chemoprevention is to delay tumor onset and progression. Chemopreventative strategies that delay prostate tumor onset or progression by even five years will drastically decrease the incidence of clinically-relevant prostate cancer and will reduce the need for prostate cancer treatment. Current findings that 1,25(OH)$_2$D$_3$, the metabolically active form of naturally-derived and FDA-approved vitamin D$_3$, is effective in regulating prostate progenitor/stem cell growth and differentiation supports the use of vitamin D$_3$ as a safe and effective chemopreventative agent for prostate cancer. Thorough studies assessing the efficacy of vitamin D$_3$ or its analogs in the clinical therapeutic setting are still needed.

9. References

Abate-Shen, C., Banach-Petrosky, W.A., Sun, X., Economides, K.D., Desai, N., Gregg, J.P., Borowsky, A.D., Cardiff, R.D. & Shen, M.M. (2003). Nkx3.1; Pten Mutant Mice Develop Invasive Prostate Adenocarcinoma and Lymph Node Metastases. *Cancer Res*, Vol.63, No.14, (Jul 15), pp. 3886-3890, 0008-5472

Ahonen, M.H., Tenkanen, L., Teppo, L., Hakama, M. & Tuohimaa, P. (2000). Prostate Cancer Risk and Prediagnostic Serum 25-Hydroxyvitamin D Levels (Finland). *Cancer Causes Control*, Vol.11, No.9, (Oct), pp. 847-852, 0957-5243

Arnaud, J. & Constans, J. (1993). Affinity Differences for Vitamin D Metabolites Associated with the Genetic Isoforms of the Human Serum Carrier Protein (Dbp). *Hum Genet*, Vol.92, No.2, (Sep), pp. 183-188, 0340-6717

Axanova, L.S., Chen, Y.Q., McCoy, T., Sui, G. & Cramer, S.D. (2010). 1,25-Dihydroxyvitamin D(3) and Pi3k/Akt Inhibitors Synergistically Inhibit Growth and Induce Senescence in Prostate Cancer Cells. *Prostate,* Vol.70, No.15, (Nov 1), pp. 1658-1671, 1097-0045

Banach-Petrosky, W., Ouyang, X., Gao, H., Nader, K., Ji, Y., Suh, N., DiPaola, R.S. & Abate-Shen, C. (2006). Vitamin D Inhibits the Formation of Prostatic Intraepithelial Neoplasia in Nkx3.1;Pten Mutant Mice. *Clin Cancer Res,* Vol.12, No.19, (Oct 1), pp. 5895-5901, 1078-0432

Bao, B.Y., Yeh, S.D. & Lee, Y.F. (2006). 1alpha,25-Dihydroxyvitamin D3 Inhibits Prostate Cancer Cell Invasion Via Modulation of Selective Proteases. *Carcinogenesis,* Vol.27, No.1, (Jan), pp. 32-42, 0143-3334

Barclay, W.W., Axanova, L.S., Chen, W., Romero, L., Maund, S.L., Soker, S., Lees, C.J. & Cramer, S.D. (2008). Characterization of Adult Prostatic Progenitor/Stem Cells Exhibiting Self-Renewal and Multilineage Differentiation. *Stem Cells,* Vol.26, No.3, (Mar), pp. 600-610, 1549-4918

Barreto, A.M., Schwartz, G.G., Woodruff, R. & Cramer, S.D. (2000). 25-Hydroxyvitamin D3, the Prohormone of 1,25-Dihydroxyvitamin D3, Inhibits the Proliferation of Primary Prostatic Epithelial Cells. *Cancer Epidemiol Biomarkers Prev,* Vol.9, No.3, (Mar), pp. 265-270, 1055-9965

Beer, T.M., Ryan, C.W., Venner, P.M., Petrylak, D.P., Chatta, G.S., Ruether, J.D., Redfern, C.H., Fehrenbacher, L., Saleh, M.N., Waterhouse, D.M., Carducci, M.A., Vicario, D., Dreicer, R., Higano, C.S., Ahmann, F.R., Chi, K.N., Henner, W.D., Arroyo, A. & Clow, F.W. (2007). Double-Blinded Randomized Study of High-Dose Calcitriol Plus Docetaxel Compared with Placebo Plus Docetaxel in Androgen-Independent Prostate Cancer: A Report from the Ascent Investigators. *J Clin Oncol,* Vol.25, No.6, (Feb 20), pp. 669-674, 1527-7755

Bischoff-Ferrari, H. (2009). Vitamin D: What Is an Adequate Vitamin D Level and How Much Supplementation Is Necessary? *Best Pract Res Clin Rheumatol,* Vol.23, No.6, (Dec), pp. 789-795, 1532-1770

Blunt, J.W., DeLuca, H.F. & Schnoes, H.K. (1968). 25-Hydroxycholecalciferol. A Biologically Active Metabolite of Vitamin D3. *Biochemistry,* Vol.7, No.10, (Oct), pp. 3317-3322, 0006-2960

Blutt, S.E., Polek, T.C., Stewart, L.V., Kattan, M.W. & Weigel, N.L. (2000). A Calcitriol Analogue, Eb1089, Inhibits the Growth of Lncap Tumors in Nude Mice. *Cancer Res,* Vol.60, No.4, (Feb 15), pp. 779-782, 0008-5472

Bodiwala, D., Luscombe, C.J., Liu, S., Saxby, M., French, M., Jones, P.W., Fryer, A.A. & Strange, R.C. (2003). Prostate Cancer Risk and Exposure to Ultraviolet Radiation: Further Support for the Protective Effect of Sunlight. *Cancer Lett,* Vol.192, No.2, (Mar 31), pp. 145-149, 0304-3835

Boyle, B.J., Zhao, X.Y., Cohen, P. & Feldman, D. (2001). Insulin-Like Growth Factor Binding Protein-3 Mediates 1 Alpha,25-Dihydroxyvitamin D(3) Growth Inhibition in the Lncap Prostate Cancer Cell Line through P21/Waf1. *J Urol,* Vol.165, No.4, (Apr), pp. 1319-1324, 0022-5347

Bratt, O. (2002). Hereditary Prostate Cancer: Clinical Aspects. *J Urol*, Vol.168, No.3, (Sep), pp. 906-913, 0022-5347

Brawer, M.K. (2007). Recent Progress in the Treatment of Advanced Prostate Cancer with Intermittent Dose-Intense Calcitriol (Dn-101). *Rev Urol*, Vol.9, No.1, (Winter), pp. 1-8, 1523-6161

Brockmann, H. (1936). Die Isolierung Des Antirachitischen Vitamins Aus Thunfischleberol. *Hoppe Seylers Z Physiol Chem*, Vol.241, No., pp. 104-115,

Burger, P.E., Xiong, X., Coetzee, S., Salm, S.N., Moscatelli, D., Goto, K. & Wilson, E.L. (2005). Sca-1 Expression Identifies Stem Cells in the Proximal Region of Prostatic Ducts with High Capacity to Reconstitute Prostatic Tissue. *Proc Natl Acad Sci U S A*, Vol.102, No.20, (May 17), pp. 7180-7185, 0027-8424

Campbell, M.J., Elstner, E., Holden, S., Uskokovic, M. & Koeffler, H.P. (1997). Inhibition of Proliferation of Prostate Cancer Cells by a 19-nor-Hexafluoride Vitamin D3 Analogue Involves the Induction of P21waf1, P27kip1 and E-Cadherin. *J Mol Endocrinol*, Vol.19, No.1, (Aug), pp. 15-27, 0952-5041

Chen, T.C., Wang, L., Whitlatch, L.W., Flanagan, J.N. & Holick, M.F. (2003). Prostatic 25-Hydroxyvitamin D-1alpha-Hydroxylase and Its Implication in Prostate Cancer. *J Cell Biochem*, Vol.88, No.2, (Feb 1), pp. 315-322, 0730-2312

Colston, K.W. & Hansen, C.M. (2002). Mechanisms Implicated in the Growth Regulatory Effects of Vitamin D in Breast Cancer. *Endocr Relat Cancer*, Vol.9, No.1, (Mar), pp. 45-59, 1351-0088

Darson, M.F., Pacelli, A., Roche, P., Rittenhouse, H.G., Wolfert, R.L., Saeid, M.S., Young, C.Y., Klee, G.G., Tindall, D.J. & Bostwick, D.G. (1999). Human Glandular Kallikrein 2 Expression in Prostate Adenocarcinoma and Lymph Node Metastases. *Urology*, Vol.53, No.5, (May), pp. 939-944, 0090-4295

DeLuca, H.F. (2004). Overview of General Physiologic Features and Functions of Vitamin D. *Am J Clin Nutr*, Vol.80, No.6 Suppl, (Dec), pp. 1689S-1696S, 0002-9165

Esquenet, M., Swinnen, J.V., Heyns, W. & Verhoeven, G. (1996). Control of Lncap Proliferation and Differentiation: Actions and Interactions of Androgens, 1alpha,25-Dihydroxycholecalciferol, All-Trans Retinoic Acid, 9-Cis Retinoic Acid, and Phenylacetate. *Prostate*, Vol.28, No.3, (Mar), pp. 182-194, 0270-4137

Feldman, B.J. & Feldman, D. (2001). The Development of Androgen-Independent Prostate Cancer. *Nat Rev Cancer*, Vol.1, No.1, (Oct), pp. 34-45, 1474-175X

Flores, O. & Burnstein, K.L. (2010). Gadd45gamma: A New Vitamin D-Regulated Gene That Is Antiproliferative in Prostate Cancer Cells. *Endocrinology*, Vol.151, No.10, (Oct), pp. 4654-4664, 1945-7170

Fraser, D.R. & Kodicek, E. (1970). Unique Biosynthesis by Kidney of a Biological Active Vitamin D Metabolite. *Nature*, Vol.228, No.5273, (Nov 21), pp. 764-766, 0028-0836

Garland, C., Gorham, E., Mohr, S. & Garland, F. (2009). Vitamin D for Cancer Prevention: Global Perspective. *Ann Epidemiol*, Vol.19, No.7, (Jul), pp. 468-483, 1873-2585

Garland, C.F., French, C.B., Baggerly, L.L. & Heaney, R.P. (2011). Vitamin D Supplement Doses and Serum 25-Hydroxyvitamin D in the Range Associated with Cancer Prevention. *Anticancer Res*, Vol.31, No.2, (Feb), pp. 607-611, 1791-7530

Getzenberg, R.H., Light, B.W., Lapco, P.E., Konety, B.R., Nangia, A.K., Acierno, J.S., Dhir, R., Shurin, Z., Day, R.S., Trump, D.L. & Johnson, C.S. (1997). Vitamin D Inhibition of Prostate Adenocarcinoma Growth and Metastasis in the Dunning Rat Prostate Model System. *Urology*, Vol.50, No.6, (Dec), pp. 999-1006, 0090-4295

Goldstein, A.S., Stoyanova, T. & Witte, O.N. (2010). Primitive Origins of Prostate Cancer: In Vivo Evidence for Prostate-Regenerating Cells and Prostate Cancer-Initiating Cells. *Mol Oncol*, Vol.4, No.5, (Oct), pp. 385-396, 1878-0261

Guileyardo, J.M., Johnson, W.D., Welsh, R.A., Akazaki, K. & Correa, P. (1980). Prevalence of Latent Prostate Carcinoma in Two U.S. Populations. *J Natl Cancer Inst*, Vol.65, No.2, (Aug), pp. 311-316, 0027-8874

Hamilton, R.J., Kahwati, L.C. & Kinsinger, L.S. (2010). Knowledge and Use of Finasteride for the Prevention of Prostate Cancer. *Cancer Epidemiol Biomarkers Prev*, Vol.19, No.9, (Sep), pp. 2164-2171, 1538-7755

Hanchette, C.L. & Schwartz, G.G. (1992). Geographic Patterns of Prostate Cancer Mortality. Evidence for a Protective Effect of Ultraviolet Radiation. *Cancer*, Vol.70, No.12, (Dec 15), pp. 2861-2869, 0008-543X

Horst, R.L. & Littledike, E.T. (1982). Comparison of Plasma Concentrations of Vitamin D and Its Metabolites in Young and Aged Domestic Animals. *Comp Biochem Physiol B*, Vol.73, No.3, pp. 485-489, 0305-0491

Hsu, J.W., Yasmin-Karim, S., King, M.R., Wojciechowski, J.C., Mickelsen, D., Blair, M.L., Ting, H.J., Ma, W.L. & Lee, Y.F. (2011). Suppression of Prostate Cancer Cell Rolling and Adhesion to Endothelium by 1alpha,25-Dihydroxyvitamin D3. *Am J Pathol*, Vol.178, No.2, (Feb), pp. 872-880, 1525-2191

Hsu, J.Y., Feldman, D., McNeal, J.E. & Peehl, D.M. (2001). Reduced 1alpha-Hydroxylase Activity in Human Prostate Cancer Cells Correlates with Decreased Susceptibility to 25-Hydroxyvitamin D3-Induced Growth Inhibition. *Cancer Res*, Vol.61, No.7, (Apr 1), pp. 2852-2856, 0008-5472

Ingles, S.A., Ross, R.K., Yu, M.C., Irvine, R.A., La Pera, G., Haile, R.W. & Coetzee, G.A. (1997). Association of Prostate Cancer Risk with Genetic Polymorphisms in Vitamin D Receptor and Androgen Receptor. *J Natl Cancer Inst*, Vol.89, No.2, (Jan 15), pp. 166-170, 0027-8874

Jemal, A., Siegel, R., Xu, J. & Ward, E. (2010). Cancer Statistics, 2010. *CA Cancer J Clin*, Vol.60, No.5, (Sep-Oct), pp. 277-300, 1542-4863

John, E.M., Dreon, D.M., Koo, J. & Schwartz, G.G. (2004). Residential Sunlight Exposure Is Associated with a Decreased Risk of Prostate Cancer. *J Steroid Biochem Mol Biol*, Vol.89-90, No.1-5, (May), pp. 549-552, 0960-0760

John, E.M., Koo, J. & Schwartz, G.G. (2007). Sun Exposure and Prostate Cancer Risk: Evidence for a Protective Effect of Early-Life Exposure. *Cancer Epidemiol Biomarkers Prev*, Vol.16, No.6, (Jun), pp. 1283-1286, 1055-9965

Kawa, S., Nikaido, T., Aoki, Y., Zhai, Y., Kumagai, T., Furihata, K., Fujii, S. & Kiyosawa, K. (1997). Vitamin D Analogues up-Regulate P21 and P27 During Growth Inhibition of Pancreatic Cancer Cell Lines. *Br J Cancer*, Vol.76, No.7, pp. 884-889, 0007-0920

Kim, M.J., Cardiff, R.D., Desai, N., Banach-Petrosky, W.A., Parsons, R., Shen, M.M. & Abate-Shen, C. (2002). Cooperativity of Nkx3.1 and Pten Loss of Function in a Mouse

Model of Prostate Carcinogenesis. *Proc Natl Acad Sci U S A,* Vol.99, No.5, (Mar 5), pp. 2884-2889, 0027-8424

Lawson, D.E., Fraser, D.R., Kodicek, E., Morris, H.R. & Williams, D.H. (1971). Identification of 1,25-Dihydroxycholecalciferol, a New Kidney Hormone Controlling Calcium Metabolism. *Nature,* Vol.230, No.5291, (Mar 26), pp. 228-230, 0028-0836

Lehmann, B., Schättiger, K. & Meurer, M. (2010). Conversion of Vitamin D(3) to Hormonally Active 1alpha,25-Dihydroxyvitamin D(3) in Cultured Keratinocytes: Relevance to Cell Growth and Differentiation. *J Steroid Biochem Mol Biol,* Vol., No., (Feb), 1879-1220

Li, H., Stampfer, M.J., Hollis, J.B., Mucci, L.A., Gaziano, J.M., Hunter, D., Giovannucci, E.L. & Ma, J. (2007). A Prospective Study of Plasma Vitamin D Metabolites, Vitamin D Receptor Polymorphisms, and Prostate Cancer. *PLoS Med,* Vol.4, No.3, (Mar), pp. e103, 1549-1676

Lips, P. (2001). Vitamin D Deficiency and Secondary Hyperparathyroidism in the Elderly: Consequences for Bone Loss and Fractures and Therapeutic Implications. *Endocr Rev,* Vol.22, No.4, (Aug), pp. 477-501, 0163-769X

Liu, M., Lee, M.H., Cohen, M., Bommakanti, M. & Freedman, L.P. (1996). Transcriptional Activation of the Cdk Inhibitor P21 by Vitamin D3 Leads to the Induced Differentiation of the Myelomonocytic Cell Line U937. *Genes Dev,* Vol.10, No.2, (Jan 15), pp. 142-153, 0890-9369

Lokeshwar, B.L., Schwartz, G.G., Selzer, M.G., Burnstein, K.L., Zhuang, S.H., Block, N.L. & Binderup, L. (1999). Inhibition of Prostate Cancer Metastasis in Vivo: A Comparison of 1,23-Dihydroxyvitamin D (Calcitriol) and Eb1089. *Cancer Epidemiol Biomarkers Prev,* Vol.8, No.3, (Mar), pp. 241-248, 1055-9965

Luo, W., Birkett, N.J., Ugnat, A.M. & Mao, Y. (2004). Cancer Incidence Patterns among Chinese Immigrant Populations in Alberta. *J Immigr Health,* Vol.6, No.1, (Jan), pp. 41-48, 1096-4045

Luscombe, C.J., Fryer, A.A., French, M.E., Liu, S., Saxby, M.F., Jones, P.W. & Strange, R.C. (2001). Exposure to Ultraviolet Radiation: Association with Susceptibility and Age at Presentation with Prostate Cancer. *Lancet,* Vol.358, No.9282, (Aug 25), pp. 641-642, 0140-6736

MacDonald, P.N., Baudino, T.A., Tokumaru, H., Dowd, D.R. & Zhang, C. (2001). Vitamin D Receptor and Nuclear Receptor Coactivators: Crucial Interactions in Vitamin D-Mediated Transcription. *Steroids,* Vol.66, No.3-5, (Mar-May), pp. 171-176, 0039-128X

MacLaughlin, J. & Holick, M.F. (1985). Aging Decreases the Capacity of Human Skin to Produce Vitamin D3. *J Clin Invest,* Vol.76, No.4, (Oct), pp. 1536-1538, 0021-9738

Majumder, P.K., Grisanzio, C., O'Connell, F., Barry, M., Brito, J.M., Xu, Q., Guney, I., Berger, R., Herman, P., Bikoff, R., Fedele, G., Baek, W.K., Wang, S., Ellwood-Yen, K., Wu, H., Sawyers, C.L., Signoretti, S., Hahn, W.C., Loda, M. & Sellers, W.R. (2008). A Prostatic Intraepithelial Neoplasia-Dependent P27 Kip1 Checkpoint Induces Senescence and Inhibits Cell Proliferation and Cancer Progression. *Cancer Cell,* Vol.14, No.2, (Aug 12), pp. 146-155, 1878-3686

Matsuoka, L.Y., Wortsman, J., Haddad, J.G., Kolm, P. & Hollis, B.W. (1991). Racial Pigmentation and the Cutaneous Synthesis of Vitamin D. *Arch Dermatol*, Vol.127, No.4, (Apr), pp. 536-538, 0003-987X

Maund, S.L., Barclay, W.W., Hover, L.D., Axanova, L.S., Sui, G., Hipp, J.D., Fleet, J.C., Thorburn, A. & Cramer, S.D. (2011). Interleukin-1 Alpha Mediates the Anti-Proliferative Effects of 1,25 Dihydroxyvitamin D3 in Prostate Progenitor/Stem Cells. *Cancer Res* Vol. 71, No. 15 (Aug 1):pp. 5276-5286

Maund, S.L. & Cramer, S.D. (2009). Translational Implications of Stromal-Epithelial Interactions in Prostate Cancer and the Potential Role of Prostate Cancer Stem/Progenitor Cells. *The Handbook of Cell Signaling,* Vol. 3, No., pp. 2773-2782 978-0-12-374145-5

Maund, S.L. & Cramer, S.D. (2010). The Tissue-Specific Stem Cell as a Target for Chemoprevention. *Stem Cell Rev,* Vol., No., (Nov 18), 1558-6804

Mellanby, E. (1921). Experimental Rickets. *Spec Rep Ser Med Res Council (GB),* Vol.SRS61, No.4,

Miller, G.J., Stapleton, G.E., Ferrara, J.A., Lucia, M.S., Pfister, S., Hedlund, T.E. & Upadhya, P. (1992). The Human Prostatic Carcinoma Cell Line Lncap Expresses Biologically Active, Specific Receptors for 1 Alpha,25-Dihydroxyvitamin D3. *Cancer Res,* Vol.52, No.3, (Feb 1), pp. 515-520, 0008-5472

Miller, G.J., Stapleton, G.E., Hedlund, T.E. & Moffat, K.A. (1995). Vitamin D Receptor Expression, 24-Hydroxylase Activity, and Inhibition of Growth by 1alpha,25-Dihydroxyvitamin D3 in Seven Human Prostatic Carcinoma Cell Lines. *Clin Cancer Res,* Vol.1, No.9, (Sep), pp. 997-1003, 1078-0432

Mimeault, M. & Batra, S.K. (2010). New Advances on Critical Implications of Tumor- and Metastasis-Initiating Cells in Cancer Progression, Treatment Resistance and Disease Recurrence. *Histol Histopathol,* Vol.25, No.8, (Aug), pp. 1057-1073, 1699-5848

Muller, M. (2009). Cellular Senescence: Molecular Mechanisms, in Vivo Significance, and Redox Considerations. *Antioxid Redox Signal,* Vol.11, No.1, (Jan), pp. 59-98, 1557-7716

Nakamura, K., Nashimoto, M., Hori, Y. & Yamamoto, M. (2000). Serum 25-Hydroxyvitamin D Concentrations and Related Dietary Factors in Peri- and Postmenopausal Japanese Women. *Am J Clin Nutr,* Vol.71, No.5, (May), pp. 1161-1165, 0002-9165

Nelson, W.G., De Marzo, A.M. & Isaacs, W.B. (2003). Prostate Cancer. *N Engl J Med,* Vol.349, No.4, (Jul 24), pp. 366-381, 1533-4406

Nomura, A.M., Stemmermann, G.N., Lee, J., Kolonel, L.N., Chen, T.C., Turner, A. & Holick, M.F. (1998). Serum Vitamin D Metabolite Levels and the Subsequent Development of Prostate Cancer (Hawaii, United States). *Cancer Causes Control,* Vol.9, No.4, (Aug), pp. 425-432, 0957-5243

Park, S.Y., Cooney, R.V., Wilkens, L.R., Murphy, S.P., Henderson, B.E. & Kolonel, L.N. (2010). Plasma 25-Hydroxyvitamin D and Prostate Cancer Risk: The Multiethnic Cohort. *Eur J Cancer,* Vol.46, No.5, (Mar), pp. 932-936, 1879-0852

Peng, L., Malloy, P.J. & Feldman, D. (2004). Identification of a Functional Vitamin D Response Element in the Human Insulin-Like Growth Factor Binding Protein-3 Promoter. *Mol Endocrinol*, Vol.18, No.5, (May), pp. 1109-1119, 0888-8809

Peng, L., Wang, J., Malloy, P.J. & Feldman, D. (2008). The Role of Insulin-Like Growth Factor Binding Protein-3 in the Growth Inhibitory Actions of Androgens in Lncap Human Prostate Cancer Cells. *Int J Cancer*, Vol.122, No.3, (Feb 1), pp. 558-566, 1097-0215

Prosser, D.E. & Jones, G. (2004). Enzymes Involved in the Activation and Inactivation of Vitamin D. *Trends Biochem Sci*, Vol.29, No.12, (Dec), pp. 664-673, 0968-0004

Rachez, C. & Freedman, L.P. (2000). Mechanisms of Gene Regulation by Vitamin D(3) Receptor: A Network of Coactivator Interactions. *Gene*, Vol.246, No.1-2, (Apr 4), pp. 9-21, 0378-1119

Reya, T., Morrison, S.J., Clarke, M.F. & Weissman, I.L. (2001). Stem Cells, Cancer, and Cancer Stem Cells. *Nature*, Vol.414, No.6859, (Nov 1), pp. 105-111, 0028-0836

Rosen, C.J. (2011). Clinical Practice. Vitamin D Insufficiency. *N Engl J Med*, Vol.364, No.3, (Jan 20), pp. 248-254, 1533-4406

Sarkar, F.H., Li, Y., Wang, Z. & Kong, D. (2010). The Role of Nutraceuticals in the Regulation of Wnt and Hedgehog Signaling in Cancer. *Cancer Metastasis Rev*, Vol.29, No.3, (Sep), pp. 383-394, 1573-7233

Schwartz, G.G., Hill, C.C., Oeler, T.A., Becich, M.J. & Bahnson, R.R. (1995). 1,25-Dihydroxy-16-Ene-23-Yne-Vitamin D3 and Prostate Cancer Cell Proliferation in Vivo. *Urology*, Vol.46, No.3, (Sep), pp. 365-369, 0090-4295

Schwartz, G.G., Whitlatch, L.W., Chen, T.C., Lokeshwar, B.L. & Holick, M.F. (1998). Human Prostate Cells Synthesize 1,25-Dihydroxyvitamin D3 from 25-Hydroxyvitamin D3. *Cancer Epidemiol Biomarkers Prev*, Vol.7, No.5, (May), pp. 391-395, 1055-9965

Severson, R.K., Nomura, A.M., Grove, J.S. & Stemmermann, G.N. (1989). A Prospective Study of Demographics, Diet, and Prostate Cancer among Men of Japanese Ancestry in Hawaii. *Cancer Res*, Vol.49, No.7, (Apr 1), pp. 1857-1860, 0008-5472

Shepard, R.M., Horst, R.L., Hamstra, A.J. & DeLuca, H.F. (1979). Determination of Vitamin D and Its Metabolites in Plasma from Normal and Anephric Man. *Biochem J*, Vol.182, No.1, (Jul 15), pp. 55-69, 0264-6021

Steddon, S.J., Schroeder, N.J. & Cunningham, J. (2001). Vitamin D Analogues: How Do They Differ and What Is Their Clinical Role? *Nephrol Dial Transplant*, Vol.16, No.10, (Oct), pp. 1965-1967, 0931-0509

Studzinski, G.P. & Harrison, L.E. (1999). Differentiation-Related Changes in the Cell Cycle Traverse. *Int Rev Cytol*, Vol.189, No., pp. 1-58, 0074-7696

Sung, V. & Feldman, D. (2000). 1,25-Dihydroxyvitamin D3 Decreases Human Prostate Cancer Cell Adhesion and Migration. *Mol Cell Endocrinol*, Vol.164, No.1-2, (Jun), pp. 133-143, 0303-7207

Tagami, T., Lutz, W.H., Kumar, R. & Jameson, J.L. (1998). The Interaction of the Vitamin D Receptor with Nuclear Receptor Corepressors and Coactivators. *Biochem Biophys Res Commun*, Vol.253, No.2, (Dec 18), pp. 358-363, 0006-291X

Tang, J.Y., Xiao, T.Z., Oda, Y., Chang, K.S., Shpall, E., Wu, A., So, P.L., Hebert, J., Bikle, D. & Epstein, E.H., Jr. (2011). Vitamin D3 Inhibits Hedgehog Signaling and Proliferation in Murine Basal Cell Carcinomas. *Cancer Prev Res (Phila)*, Vol.4, No.5, (May), pp. 744-751, 1940-6215

Thompson, I.M., Tangen, C.M., Klein, E.A. & Lippman, S.M. (2005). Phase Iii Prostate Cancer Prevention Trials: Are the Costs Justified? *J Clin Oncol*, Vol.23, No.32, (Nov 10), pp. 8161-8164, 0732-183X

Tokar, E.J. & Webber, M.M. (2005). Chemoprevention of Prostate Cancer by Cholecalciferol (Vitamin D3): 25-Hydroxylase (Cyp27a1) in Human Prostate Epithelial Cells. *Clin Exp Metastasis*, Vol.22, No.3, pp. 265-273, 0262-0898

Tretli, S., Hernes, E., Berg, J.P., Hestvik, U.E. & Robsahm, T.E. (2009). Association between Serum 25(Oh)D and Death from Prostate Cancer. *Br J Cancer*, Vol.100, No.3, (Feb 10), pp. 450-454, 1532-1827

Trottier, G., Bostrom, P.J., Lawrentschuk, N. & Fleshner, N.E. (2010). Nutraceuticals and Prostate Cancer Prevention: A Current Review. *Nat Rev Urol*, Vol.7, No.1, (Jan), pp. 21-30, 1759-4820

Trump, D.L., Deeb, K.K. & Johnson, C.S. (2010). Vitamin D: Considerations in the Continued Development as an Agent for Cancer Prevention and Therapy. *Cancer J*, Vol.16, No.1, (Jan-Feb), pp. 1-9, 1540-336X

Trump, D.L., Muindi, J., Fakih, M., Yu, W.D. & Johnson, C.S. (2006). Vitamin D Compounds: Clinical Development as Cancer Therapy and Prevention Agents. *Anticancer Res*, Vol.26, No.4A, (Jul-Aug), pp. 2551-2556, 0250-7005

Vashi, P.G., Trukova, K., Lammersfeld, C.A., Braun, D.P. & Gupta, D. (2010). Impact of Oral Vitamin D Supplementation on Serum 25-Hydroxyvitamin D Levels in Oncology. *Nutr J*, Vol.9, No., pp. 60, 1475-2891

Washington, M.N., Kim, J.S. & Weigel, N.L. (2011). 1alpha,25-Dihydroxyvitamin D3 Inhibits C4-2 Prostate Cancer Cell Growth Via a Retinoblastoma Protein (Rb)-Independent G1 Arrest. *Prostate*, Vol.71, No.1, (Jan 1), pp. 98-110, 1097-0045

Whitlatch, L.W., Young, M.V., Schwartz, G.G., Flanagan, J.N., Burnstein, K.L., Lokeshwar, B.L., Rich, E.S., Holick, M.F. & Chen, T.C. (2002). 25-Hydroxyvitamin D-1alpha-Hydroxylase Activity Is Diminished in Human Prostate Cancer Cells and Is Enhanced by Gene Transfer. *J Steroid Biochem Mol Biol*, Vol.81, No.2, (Jun), pp. 135-140, 0960-0760

Yang, E.S. & Burnstein, K.L. (2003). Vitamin D Inhibits G1 to S Progression in Lncap Prostate Cancer Cells through P27kip1 Stabilization and Cdk2 Mislocalization to the Cytoplasm. *J Biol Chem*, Vol.278, No.47, (Nov 21), pp. 46862-46868, 0021-9258

Yasmin, R., Williams, R.M., Xu, M. & Noy, N. (2005). Nuclear Import of the Retinoid X Receptor, the Vitamin D Receptor, and Their Mutual Heterodimer. *J Biol Chem*, Vol.280, No.48, (Dec 2), pp. 40152-40160, 0021-9258

Zehnder, D., Bland, R., Williams, M.C., McNinch, R.W., Howie, A.J., Stewart, P.M. & Hewison, M. (2001). Extrarenal Expression of 25-Hydroxyvitamin D(3)-1 Alpha-Hydroxylase. *J Clin Endocrinol Metab*, Vol.86, No.2, (Feb), pp. 888-894, 0021-972X

Zhao, X.Y., Ly, L.H., Peehl, D.M. & Feldman, D. (1997). 1alpha,25-Dihydroxyvitamin D3 Actions in Lncap Human Prostate Cancer Cells Are Androgen-Dependent. *Endocrinology*, Vol.138, No.8, (Aug), pp. 3290-3298, 0013-7227

Zhao, X.Y., Ly, L.H., Peehl, D.M. & Feldman, D. (1999). Induction of Androgen Receptor by 1alpha,25-Dihydroxyvitamin D3 and 9-Cis Retinoic Acid in Lncap Human Prostate Cancer Cells. *Endocrinology*, Vol.140, No.3, (Mar), pp. 1205-1212, 0013-7227

Zhao, X.Y., Peehl, D.M., Navone, N.M. & Feldman, D. (2000). 1alpha,25-Dihydroxyvitamin D3 Inhibits Prostate Cancer Cell Growth by Androgen-Dependent and Androgen-Independent Mechanisms. *Endocrinology*, Vol.141, No.7, (Jul), pp. 2548-2556, 0013-7227

Zhuang, S.H. & Burnstein, K.L. (1998). Antiproliferative Effect of 1alpha,25-Dihydroxyvitamin D3 in Human Prostate Cancer Cell Line Lncap Involves Reduction of Cyclin-Dependent Kinase 2 Activity and Persistent G1 Accumulation. *Endocrinology*, Vol.139, No.3, (Mar), pp. 1197-1207, 0013-7227

7

Highlights of Natural Products in Prostate Cancer Drug Discovery

Jorge A. R. Salvador[1,2*] and Vânia M. Moreira[1,3]

[1]*Laboratório de Química Farmacêutica, Faculdade de Farmácia da*
Universidade de Coimbra Pólo das Ciências da Saúde
Azinhaga de Santa Comba, Coimbra
[2]*Centro de Neurociências e Biologia Celular*
Universidade de Coimbra, Coimbra
[3]*Centro de Química de Coimbra, Faculdade de Ciências e Tecnologia*
da Universidade de Coimbra Rua Larga, Coimbra
Portugal

1. Introduction

The remarkable impact of natural products (NPs) in the quest for new agents and new directions in medicinal discovery is well established. The exploration of Nature as a source of novel active agents that may serve as leads and scaffolds for drugs targeting a myriad of diseases and the use of synthetic organic chemistry to modify them have been a driving force for drug discovery. Worldwide, prostate cancer (PC) is the second leading cause of death after lung cancer on both USA and Australia, and the third after lung and colo-rectal cancers in Europe. The heavy burden of PC is further exemplified by the fact that it accounts for about 1 in 4 newly diagnosed cancers each year among USA men, and in 2010, approximately 32,050 men are expected to die from this disease in the USA alone whereas in Europe 2.5 million cases of PC are freshly diagnosed every year, 9% of which prove fatal. PC is a slow progressing disease found to be primarily dependent on androgens which are involved in its development, growth and progression. Transition into a hormone-refractory state typically occurs in less than 2 years following the onset of the common androgen deprivation therapies available. Thus, a relevant issue on PC drug discovery is the ability to target both androgen-dependent and –independent cells in order to avoid recurrence phenomena which could be accomplished by multi-target agents. NPs from various sources have been tested on PC-related targets with promising results. Recent research has brought into light compounds such as iejimalide B, spisulosine, pristimerin, celastrol, withaferin A, and several other pentacyclic triterpenoids such as betulinic, ursolic, and boswellic acids which show promise for future drug development. Other examples include the synthetic epothilone ixabepilone A, the gossypol-derived AT-101, the triptolide derivative PG490-88Na, irofulven, trabectedin, the rapamycin derivative temsirolimus, and docetaxel which is currently first-line therapy for castration-resistant PC combined with prednisone. This

---

* Corresponding author

chapter will highlight significant contributions of NPs and NP-derived agents on PC drug discovery starting from their action on PC-related targets and focusing on molecules which have proceeded into clinical trials.

2. Natural products and cancer

Over the course of millennia, natural compounds have evolved into specific scaffolds that interact with cellular macromolecules (Clardy & Walsh, 2004). Such scaffolds can be used as templates and fine-tuned by medicinal chemists to produce novel compounds with therapeutic applications. Indeed, about 40% of drugs used today are derived from natural plant, animal or microbial sources (Carlson, 2010). A total of 13 NPs and NP-derived drugs were approved for marketing worldwide from 2005 to 2007, out of which ziconotide (Prialt®, Elan), exanetide (Byetta®, Eli Lilly and Amylin Pharmaceuticals), retapamulin (Altabax® or Altargo®, GSK), trabectedin (Yondelis®, ET-743, J&J), and ixabepilone (Ixempra®, BMS-247750, Bristol-Meyers Squibb) were members of new human drug classes (Butler, 2008). These compounds are depicted on Figure 1.

Historically, the development of a NP lead has been limited by availability and structural complexity of the parent natural compounds (Cragg *et al.*, 2009). NPs are often produced in trace quantities, and biomass is limited or, in the case of microbial sources, unculturable. To circumvent such difficulties as extraction, assay-based functional fractionation, isolation, characterization, and target validation, classical drug-discovery has been gradually replaced by molecular target-based drug discovery (Ojima, 2008). This approach uses high-throughput screening of large libraries of compounds, lead identification from hits, and lead optimization, computational and structural biology, and has become a main stream in the past two decades. Nonetheless, sorafenib mesylate remains the only *de novo* combinatorial drug approved by the Food and Drug Administration (FDA) to date and is used for the treatment of advanced renal cancer (Newman & Cragg, 2007).

It is therefore clear that Nature will continue to be a major source of new drug leads, including anticancer agents. Newman & Cragg have recently reported that in the period of 1981 to 2006, out of 100 new chemical anticancer entities only 22.2% were totally synthetic (Newman & Cragg, 2007). Expressed as a proportion of the nonbiologicals/vaccines, 77.8% were either NPs *per se* or were based thereon, or mimicked NPs in one form or another. Recent success examples of NP-derived anticancer agents approved for marketing worldwide include temsirolimus (Torisel®, CCI-779, Fig.1), a semi-synthetic derivative of sirolimus (rapamycin, rapamune) which is an immunosuppressant first isolated from the bacterium *Streptomyces hygroscopicus* (Butler, 2008). It was approved in the US in May 2007 and Europe in November 2007 for the treatment of advanced renal cell carcinoma. Temsirolimus is the first mammalian target of rapamycin (mTOR) inhibitor approved for use in oncology. Trabectedin (Fig.1), a tetrahydroisoquinoline alkaloid produced by the ascidian *Ecteinascidia turbinata* was approved by the European Medicines Agency (EMA) in September 2007 for the treatment of advanced soft tissue sarcoma. Trabectedin is in Phase III clinical trials for the treatment of ovarian cancer and other ongoing Phase II trials include paediatric sarcomas, breast and prostate cancers (Butler, 2008). Also, ixabepilone (Fig. 1), a semi-synthetic derivative of epothilone B (Fig. 1) was approved in October 2007 by the FDA for the treatment of breast cancer, either as monotherapy or in combination with capecitabine (Butler, 2008, Toppmeyer & Goodin, 2010).

H_2N — CKGKGAKCSRLMYDCCTGSCRSGKC — CONH_2

Ziconotide (Prialt®)
Synthetic analogue of w-conotoxin MVIIA isolated from Cognus Magnus
PAIN

HGEGTFTSDLSKQMEEEAVRLFIEWLKNGGPSSGAPPPS

Exanatide (Byetta®)
Heloderma suspectum
TYPE II DIABETES

R =

Retapamulin (Altabax® or Altargo®)
ANTIMICROBIAL

R = OH **Pleuromutilin**
Pleurotus mutilus

Trabectedin (Yondelis®)
Ecteinascidia turbinata
CANCER

$R_1 = O; R_2 = Me$ **Epothilone B (patupilone)**
$R_1 = NH; R_2 = Me$ **Ixabepilone (Ixempra®)**
Sorangium cellulosum
CANCER

R =

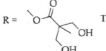

Temsirolimus (Torisel®)
CANCER

R = OH **Sirolimus (Rapamycin)**
Streptomyces hygroscopicus

Fig. 1. NPs approved for marketing which constitute new human drug classes (2005-2007).

3. Prostate cancer worldwide

PC is a common disease worldwide. Apart from skin cancer, PC is one of the most common cancers in men in developed countries such as the USA and Australia, as well as in the European Union (Black *et al.*, 1997, Greenlee *et al.*, 2000, Jemal *et al.*, 2011, Jemal *et al.*, 2010). It is also a leading cause of mortality and the second most common cause of cancer-related death in both the USA and Australia, and the third most common cause of cancer-related death in the European Union (Jemal *et al.*, 2011, Jemal *et al.*, 2010).

PC is a hormone-sensitive cancer that is influenced by androgens such as testosterone, produced from cholesterol mainly in the testis but also in the adrenal glands as well as in other tissues including prostate tissue (Moreira *et al.*, 2008, Schrijvers *et al.*, 2010). Dihydrotestosterone, the main metabolite of testosterone, is the principal ligand for the androgen receptor (AR). After transfer from the cytoplasm to the nucleus, this ligand-receptor complex activates different pathways involved in cell cycle progression and cell division. Huggins & Hodges introduced androgen deprivation as therapy (ADT) for advanced and metastatic PC in 1941 (Huggins & Hodges, 1941, Huggins *et al.*, 1941) and ever since this strategy has been applied for advanced PC treatment. Thus, in patients with metastatic PC which are symptomatic and have rapidly increasing levels of prostate-specific antigen (PSA), standard first-line treatment is castration either by bilateral orchietomy or by biochemical methods using luteinizing hormone-releasing hormone (LHRH) agonists (Antonarakis & Carducci, 2010, Harzstark & Small, 2010). This procedure is effective in about 80 to 90% of patients. However, transition into a hormone-refractory state will typically occur in less than 2 years following the onset of the common ADTs. There is evidence that AR-mediated signaling and gene expression can persist in metastatic castrate-resistant PC (mCRPC), even in the face of castrate levels of androgen (Chatterjee, 2003, Debes & Tindall, 2004, Sartor, 2011). This may be due in part to the upregulation of enzymes involved in androgen synthesis, the overexpression of AR, or the emergence of mutant ARs with promiscuous recognition of various steroidal ligands. Patients with castrate-resistant PC (CRPC) can be offered antiandrogens in addition to castration which results in response in 33% of individuals (Harzstark & Small, 2010). In case of progression, antiandrogen withdrawal results in response in about 5 to 20% of patients (Harzstark & Small, 2010). Other options include secondary hormonal therapy using mainly ketoconazole due to its ability to inhibit cytochrome P450 17α-hydroxylase $C_{17,20}$-lyase (CYP17), one of the enzymes responsible for the biosynthesis of androgen precursors in the human body (Moreira *et al.*, 2008). Despite its efficacy and ease of administration, ketoconazole bears several side effects (De Felice *et al.*, 1981, Lake-Bakaar *et al.*, 1987). Patients with CRPC are currently treated with docetaxel (Fig. 5) chemotherapy and prednisone which improves survival time in about 18 months (Mancuso *et al.*, 2007, Harzstark & Small, 2010). Nonetheless, patients with CRPC will die of their cancer and thus new treatments are required (Lassi & Dawson, 2010, Sartor, 2011). Two additional treatment options for mCRPC patients have been recently established in the "post-docetaxel space." Therapy with cabazitaxel (Fig. 5) and prednisone or treatment with the CYP17 inhibitor and antiandrogen abiraterone (also combined with prednisone) has been shown to improve survival in patients with mCRPC following docetaxel therapy (Sartor, 2011). Compared with mitoxantrone/prednisone, cabazitaxel/prednisone significantly improved overall survival, with a 30% reduction in rate of death, in patients with progression of mCRPC. Similarly, abiraterone acetate plus prednisone significantly decreased the rate of death by 35% compared with placebo plus prednisone in mCRPC patients progressing after prior docetaxel therapy (Sartor, 2011).

A relevant issue on PC drug discovery is the ability to target both androgen-sensitive and androgen-insensitive cells in order to avoid recurrence phenomena, which could be accomplished by multi-target drugs. In addition, androgen-insensitive PC cells have a very low rate of proliferation (Nemoto et al., 1990). Less than 10% of such cells proliferate during a given day thus leaving an extremely small therapeutic index for anti-proliferation drugs. The development of new drugs that can delay the onset and/or progression of human PC is therefore bound to have a significant impact on disease-related cost, morbidity and mortality for a large fraction of the world population.

4. Natural products and prostate cancer

4.1 Marine compounds

The preclinical pipeline continues to supply several hundred novel marine compounds every year and those continue to feed the clinical pipeline with potentially valuable compounds (Singh et al., 2008, Mayer et al., 2010). Thus, in the US there are three FDA approved marine-derived drugs, namely cytarabine (Cytosar-U®, Depocyt®, Fig. 2), vidarabine (Vira-A®, Fig. 2) and ziconotide (Fig. 1). The current clinical pipeline includes 13 marine-derived compounds that are either in Phase I, Phase II or Phase III clinical trials. Several key Phase III studies are ongoing and there are seven marine-derived compounds now in Phase II trials (Mayer et al., 2010).

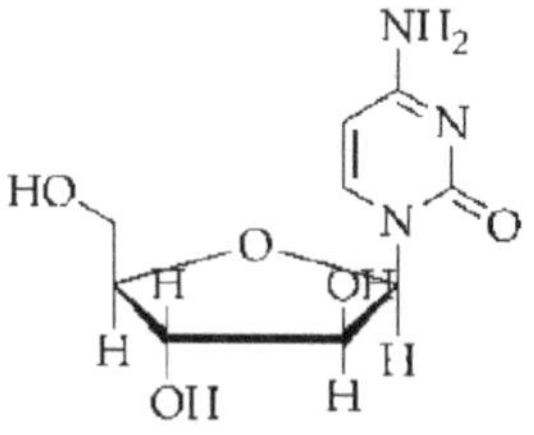

Cytarabine (Cytosar-U®)
Developed from spongothymidine from Tethya crypta
CANCER

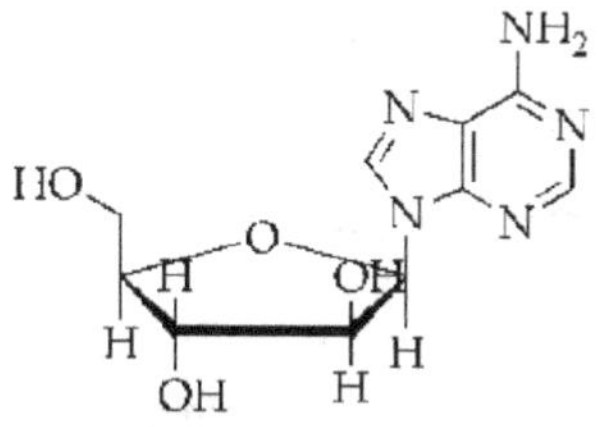

Vidarabine (Vira-A®)
Developed from spongouridine from Tethya crypta
ANTIVIRAL, OPHTHALMIC

Fig. 2. FDA-approved marine-derived products

Several marine-derived products have been tested on PC targets. Iejimalides A-D (Fig. 3), 24-membered ring lactones bearing an *N*-formyl serine terminated side chain, are a class of marine macrolides found in the tunicate *Eudistoma cf. rigida*, a species of marine tunicate native to coral reefs in the vicinity of Ie Island (Iejima) near Okinawa in Japan, which have been found to be cytotoxic against a wide range of cancer cells at low nanomolar concentrations (Schweitzer et al., 2007, McHenry et al., 2010). The effects of iejimalide B were studied on LNCaP and PC-3 cells (Wang *et al.*, 2008). On LNCaP cells, the compound induced a dose-dependent G0/G1 arrest and apoptosis, after 48 hours of treatment. Iejimalide B was found to modulate the steady-state levels of many gene products associated with the cell cycle and death, however, the same concentrations of compound initially induced a G0/G1 arrest followed by S phase arrest on PC-3 cells, without triggering apoptosis (Wang *et al.*, 2008). Increased expression of the cyclin kinase inhibitor p21[WAF1/CIP1] and downregulation of cyclin A expression were also observed with no modulation of the genes associated with cell death. Comparison of the effects of iejimalide B on the two cell lines suggested that the compound induced cell cycle arrest by two different mechanisms and that the induction of apoptosis on LNCaP cells was p53-dependent (Wang *et al.*, 2008).

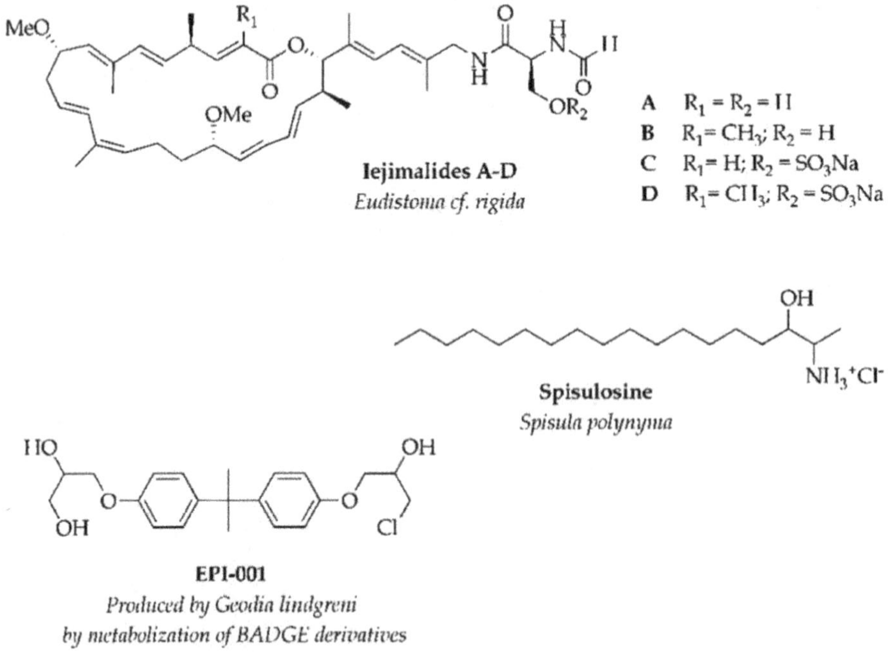

Iejimalides A-D
Eudistoma cf. rigida

A $R_1 = R_2 = H$
B $R_1 = CH_3; R_2 = H$
C $R_1 = H; R_2 = SO_3Na$
D $R_1 = CHI_3; R_2 = SO_3Na$

Spisulosine
Spisula polynyma

EPI-001
Produced by Geodia lindgreni
by metabolization of BADGE derivatives

Fig. 3. Marine-derived compounds with impact on PC

Spisulosine (PharmaMar, ES-285, Fig. 3) is a novel anti-cancer agent recently isolated from the sea mollusc *Spisula polynyma* which inhibits the growth of several solid tumor cell lines (Padron & Peters, 2006) including human prostate PC-3 and LNCaP cells with an IC_{50} of 1-10 μM, through intracellular accumulation of ceramide and activation of the atypical protein kinase isoform PKCζ (Sanchez *et al.*, 2008). Thus, intracellular ceramide levels were increased after 48 hours of treatment with spisulosine. Both fumonisin B1, a mycotoxin produced by *Fusarium verticillioides* and a reported inhibitor of ceramide synthase, and myriocin, a potent fungal inhibitor of serine palmitoyltransferase, prevented this effect pointing to a *de novo* synthesis of ceramide in the mechanism of action of spisulosine on PC cells. The same effect was not observed with specific inhibitors of the stress-related mitogen activated protein (MAP) kinases as well as of the peroxisome proliferator-activated receptor (PPARγ), phosphatidylinositol 3-kinase (PI3K)/protein kinase B (Akt), and classical protein kinases C (PKCs) pathways, rulling out interference of these pathways in the mechanism of action of spisulosine (Sanchez *et al.*, 2008). Spisulosine entered Phase I clinical trials in patients with solid tumors. A dose-escalation study evaluated the safety, pharmacokinetics, pharmacogenomics, and efficacy of ES-285 in adult cancer patients (Baird *et al.*, 2009). ES-285 showed an acceptable safety profile at doses up to 128 mg/m². At this dose level, pharmacokinetic data indicated that pharmacologically relevant concentrations had been achieved, and pharmacogenomic studies indicated consistent, dose-responsive changes in expression of genes of potential biological relevance. This study identified transaminitis and neurotoxicity as the dose-limiting toxicities associated with a 24-hour infusion of ES-285 given once every 3 weeks (Baird *et al.*, 2009). These schedule independent hepato- and neuro-toxicity events caused the discontinuation of the clinical development of ES-285 (Vilar *et al.*, 2010, Schoffski *et al.*, 2011).

As previously mentioned, trabectedin (Fig. 1) is currently under phase II/III development in breast cancer, hormone-resistant PC (HRPC), sarcomas, and ovarian cancer (Bayes *et al.*, 2004, Michaelson *et al.*, 2005, Zelek *et al.*, 2006, Carter & Keam, 2007). Trabectedin binds to the minor groove of DNA and forms covalent bonds at the N2 position of guanidine (Marco *et al.*, 2006). Two of the tetrahydroisoquinoline rings recognize and bind to the minor groove of the DNA double helix whereas the other ring protrudes out of the minor groove and interacts directly with transcription factors. Trabectedin bends DNA towards the major groove rather than towards the site of interaction, unlike other compounds that bind to the minor groove (Carter & Keam, 2007). The cytotoxicity of this compound towards cancer cells has been explained mostly by its interference with the transcription-coupled nucleotide excision repair (TC-NER) pathway (Carter & Keam, 2007). Sensitization of the death receptor pathway has been recently reported to be essential in amplifying the cytotoxic properties of trabectedin and to account for the hepatotoxicity observed in patients treated with this drug (Martinez-Serra *et al.*, 2011). Both *in vitro* and *in vivo* activities have been found for trabectedin against a range of tumor cells lines, human xenografts, and human tumor explants, including STS, ovarian, breast, prostate and renal cancers, melanoma, and non-small cell lung cancer (NSCLC) (Li *et al.*, 2001, Carter & Keam, 2007). Unlike most anticancer drugs, the mechanism of resistance to trabectedin does not appear to involve P-glycoprotein (Carter & Keam, 2007).

Recently, a specific inhibitor of AR-dependent tumour growth that does not exhibit toxicity at a therapeutic dose range has been identified (Skinner, 2010, Thompson, 2010). EPI-001 (Fig. 3) has a new mode of action, as it targets the transactivation of AR regardless of the presence of androgen, and is a promising therapy to delay the progression of CRPC. This compound was first isolated from the marine sponge *Geodia lindgreni* by Sadar *et al.* which immediately identified its similarity to BADGE (bisphenol A diglycidic ether) and realized that it must be of industrial origin (Andersen *et al.*, 2010). The collected sponge presumably bioaccumulated the BADGE derivatives from contaminated seawater. EPI-001 was first isolated and purified and afterwards synthesized in order to be tested on PC targets. Thus, EPI-001 blocked transactivation of the amino-terminal domain of the AR and was specific for its inhibition without attenuating transcriptional activities of related steroid receptors

(Andersen *et al.*, 2010). EPI-001 interacted with the AF-1 region, inhibited protein-protein interactions with AR, and reduced AR interaction with androgen-response elements on target genes. Importantly, EPI-001 blocked androgen-induced proliferation and caused cytoreduction of CRPC in xenografts dependent on AR for growth and survival without causing toxicity (Andersen *et al.*, 2010).

4.2 Microbial compounds
Due to the current ability to cultivate only a vanishingly small number of naturally occurring microorganisms, the study of either terrestrial or marine natural microbial ecosystems has been severely limited (Cragg *et al.*, 2009). Nonetheless, a most impressive number of highly effective microbially derived chemotherapeutic agents has been discovered and developed (Cragg *et al.*, 2009, Newman & Cragg, 2009), examples of which are temsirolimus and ixabepilone (Fig. 1) (Butler, 2008, Toppmeyer & Goodin, 2010). The microbial universe thus presents a vast untapped resource for drug discovery and the advent of genetic techniques that permit the isolation and expression of biosynthetic cassettes will most likely place microbes at the frontier for NPs lead discovery.

4.2.1 Epothilones
Ixabepilone or aza-epothilone B (BMS-247550, Bristol-Myers-Squibb Co., Fig. 1) is a semi-synthetic analogue of patupilone (epothilone B, EPO906, Fig. 1) which is FDA-approved for the treatment of breast cancer (Butler, 2008, Toppmeyer & Goodin, 2010). The epothilones are 16-membered macrolides isolated from the myxobacterium *Sorangium cellulosum* (Hofle *et al.*, 1996, Gerth *et al.*, 1996) which bind to tubulin heterodimers and prevent the depolymerization of microtubules with subsequent mitotic arrest and apoptotic cell death, in a fashion analogous to plant-derived taxanes such as paclitaxel (Fig. 5) (Wartmann & Altmann, 2002, Cheng *et al.*, 2008). The main difference resides in the fact that taxanes are substrates for P-glycoprotein and epothilones are not, and this ability together with ease of formulation have been considered advantages for overcoming taxane resistance of tumor cells (Wartmann & Altmann, 2002, Cheng *et al.*, 2008). Moreover, whereas the synthesis of paclitaxel relies on 10-deacetylbaccatin III which is available from the needles of various *Taxus* species (Cragg *et al.*, 2009), total synthesis of patupilone B has been accomplished (Su *et al.*, 1997). The progress of epothilones in the PC setting has been extensively reviewed (Lee & Kelly, 2009, Lassi & Dawson, 2010, Cheng *et al.*, 2008, Bystricky & Chau, 2011).
Patupilone inhibits the proliferation of DU145 and TSU-Pr1 PC cells in the low nanomolar range causing mitotic arrest (Sepp-Lorenzino *et al.*, 1999). Inhibition of proliferation appears to be dependent on the p53 status of the tumor cells (Ioffe *et al.*, 2004). Patupilone is active *in vivo* against human PC xenografts (O'Reilly *et al.*, 2005). It produced transient to long-lasting tumor regressions, including apparent cures, in s.c. transplanted DU145 and PC-3M PC xenografts in mice, with the 2.5 mg/kg regimen twice every 7 days being superior to a single dose of 4 mg/kg patupilone (O'Reilly *et al.*, 2005). The anti-tumor activity was superior to that of paclitaxel, which failed to produce tumor regressions, although displaying a better tolerability profile. Despite the enthusiastic *in vivo* results, an objective tumor response rate of only 20% has been reported for patupilone on HRPC in which 78% of patients had received one (unspecified) prior line of chemotherapy, a number comparable to

the 12% objective tumor response obtained with docetaxel (Fig. 5) and prednisone combined treatment, in the phase III TAX 327 study (Larkin, 2007). In phase I trials, patupilone has been considered generally safe and well tolerated, with patients experiencing no severe neuropathy or hematologic toxicity (Rubin et al., 2005). Therefore, the safety and efficacy of weekly patupilone 2.5 mg/m^2 were investigated in patients with CRPC in a multicenter phase II trial (Hussain et al., 2009). Modest response rates were observed with 2.5 mg/m^2 of patupilone weekly for 3 weeks of a 4-week cycle and therefore development of patupilone in advanced PC at the dose and schedule tested was not warranted. A once every 3 weeks schedule with proactive antidiarrhea management appeared to be the most promising schedule (Hussain et al., 2009).

Ixabepilone has demonstrated activity in patients with chemotherapy-naive metastatic HRPC (Hussain et al., 2005). Phase I clinical trials of ixabepilone administered i.v. as a 1 hour infusion daily, for 5 consecutive days every 21 days, at doses of 1.5 mg/m^2/day, displayed antitumor responses in patients with prior taxane treatment against solid tumors (Mancuso et al., 2007). Major adverse effects were neutropenia and neuropathy. Ixabepilone was also evaluated as a single agent in two first line studies. PSA response was observed in 30-35% of cases with an objective clinical response rate of over 15% in patients with measurable disease (Mancuso et al., 2007). When combined with estramustine phosphate (ixabepilone 35 mg/m^2 i.v. on day 2 with a 280 mg oral dose of estramustine, 3 times/day, on days 1-5, every 3 weeks), it was found to be well tolerated and have antitumor activity in patients with castrate-metastatic PC (Rosenberg et al., 2006, Rivera et al., 2008). Second-line taxane chemotherapy after ixabepilone resulted in a substantial frequency of PSA declines. Although patients with ixabepilone-refractory disease were less likely to respond to second-line taxane chemotherapy, 36% did achieve a PSA response. For patients with taxane-resistant HRPC, a randomized phase II study compared ixabepilone to mitoxantrone/ prednisone (Mancuso et al., 2007). A PSA decline of over 50% was seen in 20% of patients and median survival of 13 months was found for patients on the mitoxantrone arm, as compared to a PSA decline of over 50% in 17% and median survival of 12 months for ixabepilone treatment (Mancuso et al., 2007, Rivera et al., 2008). A recent phase II clinical trial concluded that the combination of ixabepilone and mitoxantrone with prednisone appears to have greater activity than either mitoxantrone or ixabepilone alone in the second-line setting for CRPC, and suggests at least additive if not synergistic activity (Harzstark et al., 2011). The combination is well tolerated, although some hematologic toxicity is present and dosing with pegfilgrastim is required. The results of this study suggest that it is appropriate to study further the ixabepilone and mitoxantrone with prednisone regimen in patients with docetaxel resistant CRPC (Harzstark et al., 2011).

The fully synthetic epothilone sagopilone (Fig.4) (ZK-EPO, Bayer Schering Pharma AG) is undergoing initial testing in PC with promising results (Galmarini, 2009). In preclinical studies, sagopilone inhibited cell growth in a wide range of human cancer cell lines. Moreover, sagopilone was not recognized by multidrug-resistant (MDR) cellular efflux mechanisms, and maintained its activity in MDR tumor models. Phase I clinical trials established that the sagopilone side-effect profile was similar to that reported for taxanes, with neuropathy and neutropenia being the most commonly reported toxicities (Arnold et al., 2009, Schmid et al., 2010). A recommended dose for phase II studies was established at 16.53 mg/m^2, once every 3 weeks (Schmid et al., 2010). Proof-of-concept has already been established in patients with platinum-resistant ovarian cancer and androgen-independent PC, and clinical responses have been shown in patients with melanoma and small-cell lung cancer. Results are awaited from other ongoing trials (Schmid *et al.*, 2010).

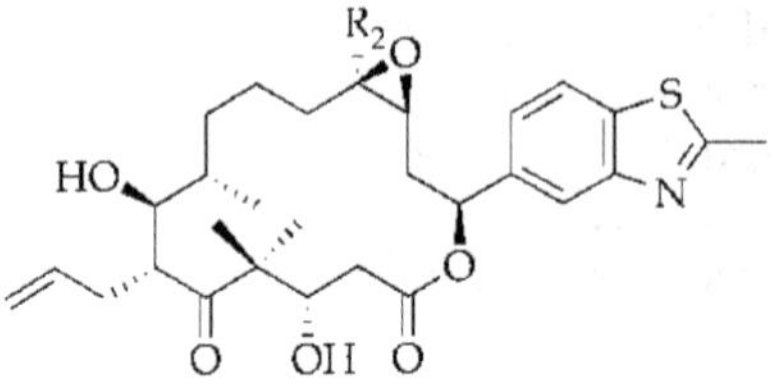

Sagopilone (ZK-EPO)

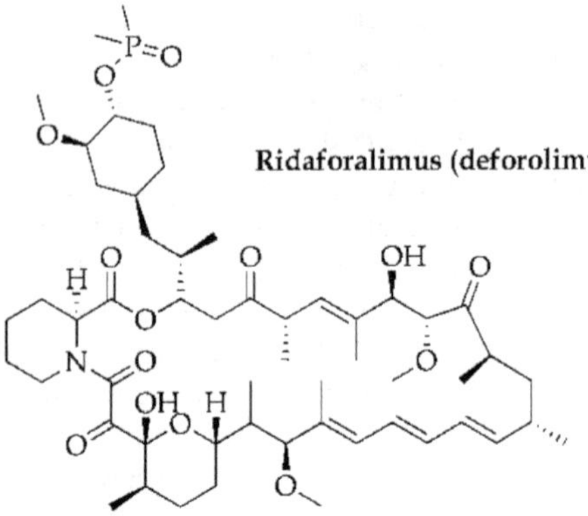

Ridaforalimus (deforolimus)

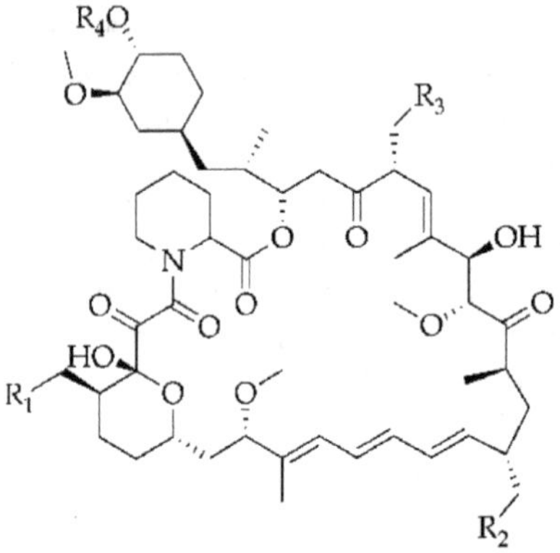

HHMP = 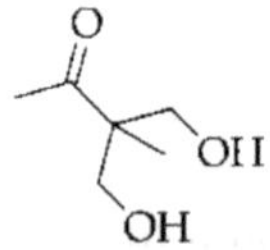

$R_1 = R_2 = R_3 = H; R_4 = CH_2CH_2OH$ **Everolimus (Zortress®)**
$R_1 = CH_3; R_2 = R_3 = H, R_4 = HHMP$ **Homotemsirolimus A**
$R_1 = R_3 = H; R_2 = CH_3; R_4 = HHMP$ **Homotemsirolimus B**
$R_1 = R_2 = H; R_3 = CH_3; R_4 = HHMP$ **Homotemsirolimus C**

Fig. 4. Microbial-derived compounds with impact on PC.

4.2.2 mTOR inhibitors

The protein kinase mTOR regulates protein translation, cell growth, and apoptosis (Garcia & Danielpour, 2008, Seeliger *et al.*, 2007). Alterations in the pathway regulating this kinase occur in many solid malignancies including prostate, bladder, and kidney cancer. *In vitro* and *in vivo* models of prostate and bladder cancer have established the importance of the mTOR pathway in control of cancer progression and metastasis (Garcia & Danielpour, 2008, Opdenaker & Farach-Carson, 2009). The mTOR inhibitors temsirolimus (Fig. 1) and everolimus (RAD001, Zortress®, Novartis, Fig.4), two ester analogues of sirolimus (rapamycin, Fig. 1), as well as rapamycin itself have clear antitumor activity in *in vitro* and *in vivo* models and are under clinical trial investigations for prostate and bladder cancers (Seeliger *et al.*, 2007, Armstrong *et al.*, 2010). Ridaforulimus (deforolimus, AP23573, MK-

8669, Merck and ARID Pharmaceuticals, Fig. 4), yet another mTOR inhibitor and a derivative of rapamycin is also undergoing clinical trials for PC (Gross et al., 2006, Squillace et al., 2008).

Genetic alterations, including loss of phosphatase and tensin homolg (PTEN), mutation of the PI3K, and amplification of AKT1 and AKT2 leading to activation of Akt kinase activity have been linked with the development of castrate progressive PC (Seeliger et al., 2007, Majumder et al., 2004). It is also known that alterations of the Akt signaling cascade (mTOR dependent) can lead to the development of prostate intraepithelial neoplasia (Majumder et al., 2004). Repopulation of PTEN-negative cancer cells between courses of chemotherapy has been reported to be inhibited by temsirolimus on PC-3 and DU145 PC xenografts with only mild myelosuppression, thus suggesting its role on minimization of drug resistance in patients (Wu et al., 2005). In addition, the effects of concurrent and sequential administration of docetaxel and temsirolimus on PC-3 and LnCaP tumor cells and xenografts were studied (Fung et al., 2009). Temsirolimus originated greater growth delay of PC-3 xenografts than docetaxel alone. This effect was greater than that expected from the in vitro sensitivity, and differed from the general experience in treatment of human PC, where chemotherapy has shown greater activity than molecular-targeted agents. In contrast, for LnCaP cells, temsirolimus had similar inhibitory effects to those observed with PC-3 cells in culture, but no significant effect on LnCaP xenografts (Fung et al., 2009). Despite similar cell cycle effects between concurrent and sequential treatments in in vitro experiments, in vivo growth delay studies showed better delay of tumor regrowth with concurrent temsirolimus and docetaxel treatment compared to sequential treatment in the prostate xenografts (Fung et al., 2009). As previously mentioned, temsirolimus is the first mTOR inhibitor approved for use in oncology (Butler, 2008). Further results from ongoing clinical trials should help to establish whether a role exits for this drug on the PC setting.

Deforolimus alone was shown to inhibit proliferation of several prostate cell lines by 20–60% (maximal inhibition) and as expected, sensitivity was associated with loss of PTEN (Squillace et al., 2008). The anti-proliferative activity of deforolimus and bicalutamide, alone and in combination, was determined in three cell lines representing different stages of PC progression. The combination was strongly synergistic in both androgen-dependent LNCaP and androgen-independent C4–2 cells but only additive in RWPE-1 (normal prostate epithelium) cells. The data provided support for the clinical testing of deforolimus in combination with bicalutamide to treat androgen-dependent and -independent PC (Squillace et al., 2008). Also, a phase II clinical trial of deforolimus in patients with taxane-resistant HRPC concluded that the compound is well tolerated and promotes disease stabilization (Gross et al., 2006).

The ability of everolimus to enhance the cytotoxic effects of radiation on PC-3 and DU145 cells has been reported (Cao et al., 2006). Both cell lines became more vulnerable to irradiation after treatment with everolimus, with the PTEN-deficient PC-3 cell line showing the greater sensitivity. This increased susceptibility to radiation was found to be associated with induction of autophagy (Cao et al., 2006). Treatment with everolimus resulted in growth inhibition of C4-2 cells in bone, an effect augmented by addition of docetaxel and zoledronic acid (Morgan et al., 2008). Moreover it had a significant impact on maintenance of body weight. A single phase II study evaluated the effect of everolimus in patients with newly diagnosed, localized PC (Lerut et al., 2005). The most frequently observed adverse events are common toxicity criteria grade 1 to 2 stomatitis and rash. Recently, three temsirolimus analogues, homotemsirolimuses A-C (Fig. 4), were isolated from a temsirolimus preparation made from rapamycin and found to inhibit mTOR as well as the proliferation of LNCaP cells with potency comparable to that of rapamycin and temsirolimus (Kong *et al.*, 2011).

4.3 Plant compounds
Plant-derived NPs have been an important source of several clinically useful anti-cancer agents (Grothaus *et al.*, 2010, Cragg *et al.*, 2009, Butler, 2008, Ojima, 2008). Plants continue to play a major role in drug discovery as evidenced by the number of promising new agents in clinical development based on selective activity against cancer-related molecular targets. One of the most noteworthy contributions of plants to this field has been the isolation of tubulin interactive agents such as the *Vinca* alkaloids and the taxanes which are the basis of the majority of the currently available anticancer therapies.

4.3.1 Taxanes
Paclitaxel (Taxol®, Bristol-Myers Squibb, Fig. 5) was first isolated from the bark of the Western yew tree in 1971 and found to possess unique pharmacological actions as an inhibitor of mitosis, differing from the *Vinca* alkaloids and colchicine derivatives in that it promotes rather than inhibits microtubule formation (Hardman & Limbird, 2001). It binds specifically to the β-tubulin subunit of microtubules and antagonizes the disassembly of this key cytoskeletal protein causing mitotic arrest. Resistance to paclitaxel is associated to high levels of P-glycoprotein expressed by tumor cells (Hardman & Limbird, 2001). Paclitaxel is currently used to treat multiple cancers such as lung, ovarian, head and neck, breast, and advanced stages of Kaposi's sarcoma. Modification of the side chain of paclitaxel resulted in the more potent analogue docetaxel (Taxotere®, Sanofi-Aventis, Fig. 5) which has clinical activity against breast, ovarian and NSCLC (Hardman & Limbird, 2001). The present status and perspectives of taxane-based regimens for cancer treatment have been thoroughly reviewed (Mancuso *et al.*, 2007, Sartor, 2011).

In 2004, the results of the two major phase III clinical trials TAX 327 and SWOG 9916 established docetaxel as a primary chemotherapeutic option for patients with mCRPC (Berthold *et al.*, 2008, Tannock *et al.*, 2004). Outcomes of TAX 327 demonstrated that chemotherapy with docetaxel was a viable option that prolonged survival for patients with mCRPC and in addition with an extended follow-up, the survival benefit of docetaxel in the TAX 327 trial has persisted. In SWOG 9916, a regimen of docetaxel and estramustine was compared with mitoxantrone and prednisone (Petrylak *et al.*, 2004). In this study, the docetaxel regimen also conferred a significant survival benefit and increased median survival. At present, docetaxel/prednisone remains the first-line chemotherapy of choice for patients with CRPC (Sartor, 2011). Combinations of docetaxel and different drug classes, including tyrosine kinase inhibitors, antiangiogenesis agents, and immunologic agents, have been the object of several studies for CRPC. Nonetheless, phase III data for combination therapy with docetaxel has not produced any viable therapeutic options (Sartor, 2011).

Cabazitaxel (XRP-6258, Jevtana®, Sanofi-Aventis, Fig. 5) is a novel taxane-class cytotoxic agent in which two hydroxyl groups have been replaced by methoxy groups, that has shown efficacy in model system tumors that are resistant to paclitaxel and docetaxel (Kumar *et al.*, 2010, Sartor, 2011). Multiple cases of complete regression were observed with cabazitaxel in studies using human tumor xenografts. Notably, long-term tumor-free survival (exceeding 133 days) and complete tumor regression were seen in pancreatic xenografts (MIA PaCa-2), head and neck xenografts (SR475), and prostate DU145 xenografts (Kumar et al., 2010). In a recently published, randomized, multicenter, phase III trial (TROPIC), the efficacy and safety of cabazitaxel and prednisone were compared with those of mitoxantrone and prednisone for the treatment of mCRPC that had progressed following docetaxel-based chemotherapy (De Bono et al., 2010). Tumor response and PSA response significantly favored cabazitaxel, as did median time to tumor progression and median time to PSA progression. Pain response and time to pain progression were similar between the treatment groups (De Bono et al., 2010). Neutropenia, leukopenia, and anemia were the predominant toxicities associated with cabazitaxel in the study. The findings of TROPIC study established cabazitaxel as the first agent to prolong survival after docetaxel treatment, with a 30% reduction in death over mitoxantrone (De Bono et al., 2010). On the basis of these data, cabazitaxel has been approved by the FDA for use in patients with mCRPC who have progressed after docetaxel (Galsky et al., 2010, Sartor, 2011).

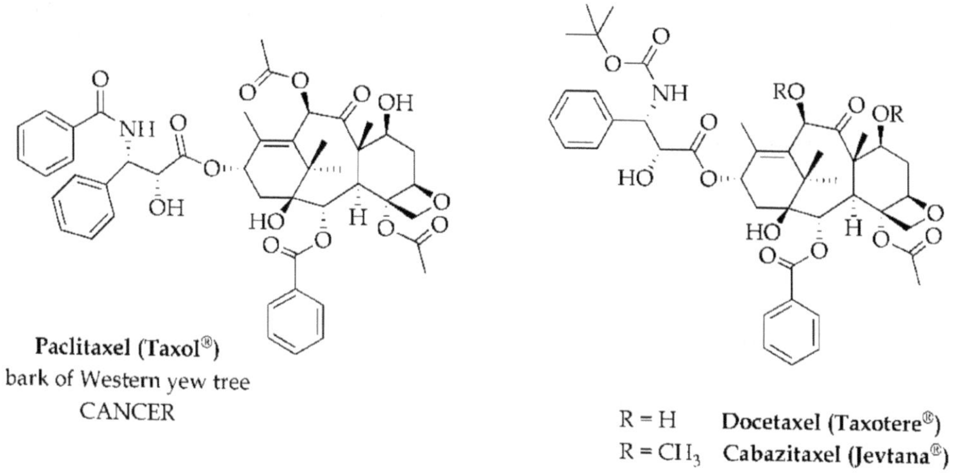

Paclitaxel (Taxol®)
bark of Western yew tree
CANCER

R = H   Docetaxel (Taxotere®)
R = CH₃   Cabazitaxel (Jevtana®)

Fig. 5. Taxanes.

4.3.2 Irofulven

Irofulven (MGI 114, NSC 683863, Pharma, Inc., Fig. 6), an anticancer agent derived from the mushroom natural product illudin S has been found to inhibit DU145, PC-3, and LNCaP cell proliferation with IC$_{50}$ values of 100, 200, and 700 nM, respectively (Poindessous et al., 2003). The cytotoxicity of irofulven is not affected by loss of p53 or mismatch repair function, and the drug is not a substrate for multidrug transporters such as P-glycoprotein and MDR-1. Irofulven acts by alkylating cellular macromolecular targets (Liang et al., 2004). The drug is a potent inducer of apoptosis in various types of tumor cells, whereas it is nonapoptotic in normal cells. Irofulven-induced signaling was studied on LnCaP-Pro5 cells and was found to be integrated at the level of mitochondrial dysfunction. The induction of both caspase-dependent and caspase-independent death pathways was consistent with pleiotropic effects, which include targeting of cellular DNA and proteins (Liang et al., 2004). The effect of irofulven on apoptosis was also reported to be largely Bcl-2 independent, a highly desirable property seeing that elevated levels of this protein correlate with an increased metastatic potencial of cancer cells (Herzig *et al.*, 2003). Irofulven has demonstrated activity against PC-3 and DU145 cells as monotherapy and enhanced efficacy was displayed in combination with mitoxantrone or docetaxel (Van Laar *et al.*, 2004) and these results highlighted its potential to be used in combination regimens in clinical trials. Thus a phase I and pharmacokinetic study of irofulven (0.4 mg/kg) and cisplatin (30 mg/m²) in patients with solid tumors concluded that the regimen was adequately tolerated with substantial evidence of antitumor activity observed (Hilgers *et al.*, 2006). Combination regiments of the same dosage of irofulven with capecitabine (2,000mg/m²/day) were also found safe on phase I clinical trials in patients with solid tumors (Alexandre *et al.*, 2007). Other combination regimens with oxaliplatin were reported to be effective on docetaxel-resistant HRPC patients (Tchen *et al.*, 2005). Irofulven was also reported to be active as a single agent against HPRC on a phase II trial (Senzer *et al.*, 2005). Based on evidence of irofulven activity in HRPC observed in these prior Phase I/II studies, a randomized Phase II study in docetaxel-refractory HRPC patients was initiated using irofulven/prednisone or irofulven/capecitabine/predisone versus mitoxantrone/prednisone (Hart *et al.*, 2006). Preliminary results suggested a longer survival and time to progression, a higher PSA response, and an acceptable safety profile for irofulven/prednisone and irofulven/capecitabine/predisone compared to mitoxantrone/prednisone. Based on these data, irofulven may have a role in treating docetaxel-resistant HRPC patients (Hart *et al.*, 2006).

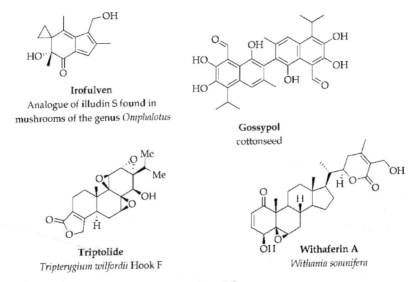

Irofulven
Analogue of illudin S found in
mushrooms of the genus *Omphalotus*

Gossypol
cottonseed

Triptolide
Tripterygium wilfordii Hook F

Withaferin A
Withania somnifera

Fig. 6. Plant-derived compounds with impact on PC

4.3.3 Gossypol

Gossypol (Fig. 6), a polyphenolic compound present in cottonseed (Huang *et al.*, 2006), was originally identified as a male antifertility agent. Gossypol treatment resulted in a marked reduction of the prostate weight of guinea-pigs and adult rats as well as induction of structural and functional changes of the gland somewhat similar to the ones observed after castration (Moh *et al.*, 1992, Wong & Tam, 1989). Antiproliferative and antimetastatic activities in androgen-independent Dunning R3327-MAT-LyLu PC cell-bearing Copenhagen rats have been reported with gossypol (Chang *et al.*, 1993). The compound has also been reported to potently inhibit both isoforms of 5α-reductase (Chang *et al.*, 1993). Gossypol inhibited the proliferation without affecting the viability of PC-3 cells with an IC_{50} value of lower than 1 µM, and induced a dose- and time-dependent accumulation of cells at the G0/G1 phase of the cell cycle (Shidaifat *et al.*, 1996). On DU145 cells gossypol significantly enhanced apoptosis through downregulation of Bcl-2 and Bcl-xL and upregulation of Bax at the mRNA and protein levels (Huang *et al.*, 2006). Activation of caspases 3, 8, and 9 was also found to occur as well as increased PARP cleavage. Thus, gossypol is a natural BH3 mimetic and small molecule inhibitor of Bcl-2/Bcl-xL/Mcl-1 that potently induces apoptosis in various cancer cell lines (Meng *et al.*, 2008). It also significantly enhances the antitumor activity of docetaxel in human PC both *in vitro* and *in vivo*. Gossypol effectively reduced the viability of LAPC4, PC-3, and DU145 PC cells and inhibited tumor growth in a NOD/SCID xenograft model (Volate *et al.*, 2010). The growth of prostate tumor initiating cells (pTICs) isolated from DU145 (CD44+/hi) were also inhibited. The inhibitory effects of gossypol have been attributed to the induction of DNA damage, which consequently leads to the stabilization of p53 and the activation of the mitochondrial pathway of apoptosis (Volate *et al.*, 2010). In addition, gossypol was recently reported to induce autophagy in human androgen-independent PC with a high level of Bcl-2 both *in vitro* and *in vivo* (Lian *et al.*, 2011).

A derivative of gossypol, R-(–)-gossypol acetic acid (AT-101, Ascenta Therapeutics, Inc.) has been evaluated on a phase I/II trial as a single-agent in men with chemotherapy-naive castrate-resistant PC (Liu *et al.*, 2009). The compound was well tolerated when administered at 20 mg/day for 21 of 28 days. Evidence of single-agent clinical activity was observed with PSA declines in some patients. Further investigation of AT-101 in PC thus is warranted and trials combining AT-101 with androgen deprivation, as well as with docetaxel chemotherapy are ongoing (Liu *et al.*, 2009).

4.3.4 Triptolide

Triptolide (PG 490, Fig. 6) is a diterpene triepoxide purified from *Tripterygium wilfordii* Hook F (Kupchan *et al.*, 1972) that was found to attenuate activation of p53 in response to γ-irradiation or other stresses such as hypoxia or DNA damaging drugs, in primary cultures of normal and malignant PC epithelial cells, despite the presence of the wild-type p53 gene (Girinsky *et al.*, 1995). Moreover, triptolide inhibited LNCaP growth with an IC_{50} value of 10 ng/ml (Shamona *et al.*, 1997). Half-maximal growth inhibition of five PC cell strains, E-PZ-10 and four cell lines derived from prostatic adenocarcinomas of Gleason grade 3/3 (E-CA-11), 30% intraductal carcinoma / 70% Gleason grade 4 (E-CA-12) and 3/4 (E-CA-13 and E-CA-14), was observed with 0.1 ng/ml triptolide (Kiviharju *et al.*, 2002). Whereas low concentrations of triptolide induced senescence of cells with G1 arrest, higher concentrations (50-100 ng/ml) triggered apoptosis. However, in contrast with the previous findings, protein levels of p53 were significantly increased and predominantly accumulated in the nuclei of prostatic epithelial cells (Kiviharju *et al.*, 2002). Nonetheless, downregulation of p53 target gene products such as Hdm-2 and p21WAF1/CIP1 and Bcl-2 was also found to occur. It was suggested that triptolide may use multiple signaling pathways, some of which involve p53 in cells with wild-type p53, growth arrest and induction of apoptosis (Kiviharju *et al.*, 2002). Clinical and experimental studies have demonstrated that triptolide has anti-inflammatory and immunosuppressive activities, and effectively prolongs allograft survival in organ transplantation including bone marrow, cardiac, renal and skin transplantation (Liu, 2011).

PG490-88Na (Pharmagenesis Inc.), a water-soluble prodrug of triptolide (14-succinyl sodium salt) that is converted into triptolide in the serum, has been elucidated as a new immunosuppressant (Fidler *et al.*, 2003). It effectively prevents acute and chronic rejection in organ transplantation and shows potent antitumor activity. The compound has been approved for phase I clinical trials for PC (Fidler *et al.*, 2003, Kiviharju *et al.*, 2002). However, the safety and side effects of triptolide for PC therapy need to be further elucidated. Further development of triptolide derivatives may produce promising anticancer drug candidate (Liu, 2011).

4.3.5 Withaferin A

Withaferin A (Fig. 6), a steroidal lactone purified from the medicinal plant "Indian Winter Cherry" or *Withania somnifera*, has been widely studied for its antitumor effects (Glotter *et al.*, 1966). Withaferin A was inhibits the chymotrypsin-like activity of purified rabbit 20S proteasome (IC_{50} of 4.5 µM) and of 26S proteasome in cultured PC-3 cells, with an IC_{50} value of 10-20 µM, and tumors (Yang *et al.*, 2007). Inhibition of PC tumor cellular proteasome both *in vitro* and *in vivo* by withaferin A was accompanied by accumulation of Bax, IκB-α and p27, and induction of apoptosis (Yang *et al.*, 2007). Proteasome inhibition occurred before the apoptotic events of caspase-3 activation with PARP cleavage and the expected morphological changes (rounding and condensation), on PC-3 cells, at 10 µM of withaferin A. On LNCaP cells, AR protein levels were decreased by withaferin A and apoptosis triggered by the same mechanisms seen on PC-3 cells (Yang *et al.*, 2007). Treatment of human PC-3 xenografts with withaferin A at 4.0 and 8.0 mg/kg/day for 24 days caused 54 to 70% inhibition of tumor growth, as compared to control, that was associated with a 28 to 56% inhibition of proteasomal chymotrypsin-like activity. Induction of apoptosis by withaferin A on PC cells bears additional interest because it has been shown to be mediated by the cancer specific target protein (Par-4) (El-Guendy *et al.*, 2003). Moreover, treatment of androgen-responsive PC cells with antiandrogens such as flutamide or bicalutamide which do not induce apoptosis on their own, rendered these cells amenable to apoptosis triggered by withaferin A. Apoptosis by withaferin A required upregulation of Par-4 expression for inhibition of NF-κB activity and activation of the caspase cascade (Srinivasan *et al.*, 2007). Therefore, withaferin A shows promise for HRPC treatment seeing that it not only seems to suppress the growth of metastatic cells but can also be exploited in combination regimens with antiandrogens to target resistant clones.

4.3.6 Pentacyclic triterpenoids

Terpenoids, among which are pentacyclic triterpenoids such as betulinic, ursolic, oleanolic, and boswellic acids as well as pristimerin and celastrol (Fig. 7), are extensively found in fruits, vegetables and medicinal plants (Salvador, 2010). This category of compounds exhibits multiple properties including antioxidation, anti-inflammation, anti-HIV, and anticancer activities (Shah *et al.*, 2009, Petronelli *et al.*, 2009).

In vitro and *in vivo* studies indicate that pentacyclic triterpenoids caused inhibition on cell proliferation and tumor growth in a variety of human cancers (Salvador, 2010). Structurally some of the terpenoids are similar to human hormones and thus bear interest in the development of drugs that target hormone-dependent cancers such as breast and prostate cancers (Yang & Dou, 2010). The mechanisms by which these compounds exhibit their anticancer activity include inhibition of the proteasome, NF-κB, and the antiapoptotic protein Bcl-2 (Yang & Dou, 2010, Wang & Fang, 2009).

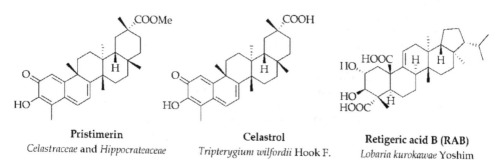

Betulinic acid (BA)
Synthesized form betulin
extracted from birch bark

Ursolic acid (UA)
Salvia officinalis and *Ocimum sanctum*

Boswellic acids (ABA and ABKA)
Boswellia gum resins

Pristimerin
Celastraceae and *Hippocrateaceae*

Celastrol
Tripterygium wilfordii Hook F.

Retigeric acid B (RAB)
Lobaria kurokawae Yoshim

Fig. 7. Pentacyclic triterpenoids

Betulinic acid (BA, Fig. 7) is a NP identified in various bark extracts and is readily synthesized from betulin, a major constituent of the bark of birch trees (Aggarwal & Shishodia, 2006). It is currently undergoing development as a therapeutic agent against melanoma (Tan *et al.*, 2003). BA inhibited the proliferation of several PC cells and triggered apoptosis probably due to AR downregulation that led to decreased expression of vascular endothelial growth factor (VEGF) and survivin, and caspase-dependent PARP cleavage (Chintharlapalli et al., 2007, Kessler et al., 2007). BA was shown to induce proteasome-dependent degradation of Sp proteins in LNCaP cells (Chintharlapalli et al., 2007, Yao et al., 2004, Wang et al., 2003). In vivo, BA (10 and 20 mg/kg/day) inhibited tumor growth in athymic nude mice bearing LNCaP cell xenografts, which was accompanied by decreased expression of Sp1, Sp3 and Sp4 proteins and VEGF, and increased apoptosis in tumors from BA-treated mice (Chintharlapalli et al., 2007). In androgen-refractory PC-3 cells, BA effectively inhibited NF-κB binding to DNA and its translocation to the nucleus, IκBα phosphorylation, and IκB kinase complex (IKK) activation, and in addition sensitized cells to TNFα-induced apoptosis through suppression of NF-κB (Rabi et al., 2008). A major advantage in using BA for cancer therapy is its low toxicity. Doses as high as 500 mg/kg, administered every 4th day for 6 weeks to athymic mice carrying human melanomas have been shown to have no detectable toxic side effects (Pisha et al., 1995). However, a study demonstrated that BA cannot be used to potentiate cell death in combination with most anticancer drugs that induce apoptosis via formation of topoisomerase I-DNA cleavable complexes such as camptothecin, staurosporine and etoposide (Ganguly et al., 2007). Thus, the compound inhibits all types of topoisomerase-I DNA cleavable complexes formation irrespective of the process of initiation, therefore disrupting the series of events that leads to cell death.

Ursolic acid (UA, Fig. 7) is present in many plants such as Salvia officinalis and Basil (Ocimum sanctum) and also a constituent of several herbal medicines marketed in Asia and worlwide for inflammatory conditions (Aggarwal & Shishodia, 2006, Kondo et al., 2011, Kwon et al., 2010). UA inhibits the proliferation of PC-3 and LNCaP cells with IC_{50} values of 32.6 and 15.7 μM, respectively (Kassi et al., 2007). At 55 μM, induction of apoptosis is seen on PC-3 cells with a decrease on bcl-2 gene levels. UA-induced apoptosis on human prostate epithelial cells has been suggested to involve caspase activation through downregulation of cellular inhibitor of apoptosis proteins (c-IAPs) family proteins and without mitochondrial dysfunction (Choi et al., 2000). On DU145 cells UA-induced apoptosis was reported to occur via JNK-mediated Bcl-2 phosphorylation and degradation (Zhang et al., 2009). Also, UA was found to overcome Bcl-2-mediated resistance to apoptosis in LNCaP androgen-independent cells (Zhang, Kong, Wang et al., 2010). UA inhibits cell invasion by downregulating matrix metalloproteinase-9 via inhibition of Akt in PC-3 cells (Zhang, Kong, Zeng et al., 2010).

Boswellic acids, particularly acetyl-boswellic acids such as acetyl-β-boswellic acid (ABA) and acetyl-11-keto-β-boswellic acid (ABKA, Fig. 7), can be isolated to chemical homogeneity from the gum resins of various Boswellia species and are well-known for their anti-inflammatory and antitumor activities (Aggarwal & Shishodia, 2006, Moussaieff & Mechoulam, 2009, Shah et al., 2009). It has been reported that acetyl-boswellic acids promote apoptosis of PC-3 cells both in vitro and in vivo by intercepting IKK activity (Syrovets et al., 2005). In particular, AKBA has the ability to induce cell growth arrest and reduce the AR expression and transcriptional activity in LNCaP cells via inhibition of the Sp1 binding activity (Yuan et al., 2008). Both PC-3 and LNCaP cells were sensitive to AKBA-induced apoptosis that correlated with the activation of caspase-8 and the upregulation of death-receptor 5 (DR5) protein most likely by induced expression of CCAAT/enhancer binding protein homologous protein (CHOP) protein (Lu et al., 2008). In addition, AKBA potently inhibits human prostate tumor growth through inhibition of angiogenesis induced by VEGFR2 signaling pathways (Pang et al., 2009).

Pristimerin (Fig. 7) is a natural compound found in the *Celastraceae* and *Hippocrateaceae* families that are rich in quinone-methide triterpenes (Filho *et al.*, 2002). Pristimerin targets the proteasome to induce apoptosis in human PC-3 and AR-positive C4-2B cells (Yang, Landis-Piwowar *et al.*, 2008). Proliferation of PC-3 cells was inhibited by pristimerin (Chang *et al.*, 2003) with induction of apoptosis that correlated with inhibition proteasome activity (Yang, Landis-Piwowar *et al.*, 2008). The IC_{50} value for the inhibition of purified rabbit 20S proteasome with pristimerin was 2.2 µM. Similarly, pristimerin also potently inhibited 26S proteasome chymotrypsin-like activity in a extract prepared from exponentially grown PC-3 cells, with an IC_{50} of 3.0 µM (Yang, Landis-Piwowar *et al.*, 2008). About 40% inhibition of cellular proteasome activity occurred in C4-2B cells with 5 µM of pristimerin and was accompanied by AR suppression with consequent apoptosis induction. Computational modeling showed that pristimerin interacts with the catalytically active amino acid N-Thr of the proteasome β5 subunit (Yang, Landis-Piwowar *et al.*, 2008). Celastrol (Fig. 7), an active compound extracted from the root bark of the Chinese medicine "Thunder of God Vine" (*Tripterygium wilfordii Hook F.*), has been used for years as a natural remedy for inflammatory conditions (Kannaiyan *et al.*, 2011). The anti-inflammatory effects of this triterpene have been demonstrated in animal models of different inflammatory diseases, including arthritis, Alzheimer's disease, asthma, and systemic lupus erythematosus. Celastrol has also been found to inhibit the proliferation of a variety of tumor cells and suppress tumor initiation, promotion and metastasis in various cancer models *in vivo* (Salminen *et al.*, 2010, Kannaiyan *et al.*, 2011). Celastrol potently and preferentially inhibits the chymotrypsin-like activity of human PC cellular 26S proteasome at 1-5 µM (Yang *et al.*, 2006). Inhibition of the proteasome activity by celastrol is accompanied by suppression of AR protein expression and induction of apoptosis. The involvement of calpain in AR breakdown during celastrol-induced apoptosis in PC cells has been demonstrated (Yang, Murthy *et al.*, 2008). By inhibiting proteasomal activity, celastrol suppresses proliferation, invasion and angiogenesis by inducing the apoptotic machinery and attenuating constitutive NF-kB activity, both *in vitro* and *in vivo*, in androgen-independent PC cell lines (Dai *et al.*, 2010). Angiogenesis-mediated tumor growth is also suppressed by celastrol by targeting the AKT/mTOR/P70S6K pathway, (Pang *et al.*, 2010). Celastrol sensitizes PC-3 cells to radiation both *in vitro* and *in vivo* by impairing DNA damage processing and augmenting apoptosis (Dai *et al.*, 2009). It also potentiated the apoptotic effects of TRAIL through down-regulation of cell survival proteins and up-regulation of death receptors via the ROS-mediated up-regulation of CHOP pathway on several tumor cell lines including PC (Sung *et al.*, 2010).
Recent research has brought into light the effects of retigeric acid B (RAB, Fig. 7), a NP isolated from the lichen *Lobaria kurokawae* Yoshim and previously exploited for its antifungal activity, on PC cells (Liu *et al.*, 2010). Thus, RB was able to suppress AR expression and transcriptional activity in LNCaP cells, and inhibition of PC-3 cell growth was accompanied by induction of the S-phase cell cycle arrest as well as apoptosis.

5. Conclusion

Outstanding contributions from Nature have paved the way in drug discovery and allowed the establishment of conventional therapies for the treatment of the majority of human diseases, including cancer. Whereas plants have been the most common source of active molecules throughout the centuries, the now unraveling potential of marine and microbial sources is bound to provide highly active compounds with a myriad of biological activities which may improve the therapeutic options available for many human diseases in a nearby future. Many compounds from plant, marine and microbial sources have been studied on PC targets. Therapies which target both androgen-dependent and –independent PC cells and can thus circumvent the mechanisms of PC recurrence have been exhaustively investigated. In this setting, molecules such as AT-101, EPI-001, trabectedin, temsirolimus and everolimus, ixabepilone A and sagupilone, docetaxel and cabazitaxel, irofulven, PG490-88Na, as well as several pentacyclic triterpenoids, which have been discussed herein, are excellent examples of NPs with an impact on PC.

6. Acknowledgment

Jorge A. R. Salvador thanks Universidade de Coimbra for financial support. Vânia M. Moreira acknowledges Fundação para a Ciência e a Tecnologia for financial support (SFRH/BPD/45037/2008).

7. References

Aggarwal, B. B. & Shishodia, S. (2006). Molecular targets of dietary agents for prevention and therapy of cancer. *Biochem. Pharmacol.* Vol. 71, pp. 1397-1421.

Alexandre, J., Kahatt, C., Bertheault-Cvitkovic, F., Faivre, S., Shibata, S., Hilgers, W., Goldwasser, F., Lokiec, F., Raymond, E., Weems, G., Shah, A., MacDonald, J. R. & Cvitkovic, E. (2007). A phase I and pharmacokinetic study of irofulven and capecitabine administered every 2 weeks in patients with advanced solid tumors. *Invest. New Drugs.* Vol. 25, pp. 453-462.

Andersen, R. J., Mawji, N. R., Wang, J., Wang, G., Haile, S., Myung, J. K., Watt, K., Tam, T., Yang, Y. C., Banuelos, C. A., Williams, D. E., McEwan, I. J., Wang, Y. & Sadar, M. D. (2010). Regression of castrate-recurrent prostate cancer by a small-molecule inhibitor of the amino-terminus domain of the androgen receptor. *Cancer Cell.* Vol. 17, pp. 535-546.

Antonarakis, E. S. & Carducci, M. A. (2010). Future directions in castrate-resistant prostate cancer therapy. *Clin. Genitourin. Cancer.* Vol. 8, pp. 37-46.

Armstrong, A. J., Netto, G. J., Rudek, M. A., Halabi, S., Wood, D. P., Creel, P. A., Mundy, K., Davis, S. L., Wang, T., Albadine, R., Schultz, L., Partin, A. W., Jimeno, A., Fedor, H., Febbo, P. G., George, D. J., Gurganus, R., De Marzo, A. M. & Carducci, M. A. (2010). A pharmacodynamic study of rapamycin in men with intermediate- to high-risk localized prostate cancer. *Clin. Cancer Res.* Vol. 16, pp. 3057-3066.

Arnold, D., Voigt, W., Kiewe, P., Behrmann, C., Lindemann, S., Reif, S., Wiesinger, H., Giurescu, M., Thiel, E. & Schmoll, H. J. (2009). Weekly administration of sagopilone (ZK-EPO), a fully synthetic epothilone, in patients with refractory solid tumours: results of a phase I trial. *Br. J. Cancer.* Vol. 101, pp. 1241-1247.

Baird, R. D., Kitzen, J., Clarke, P. A., Planting, A., Reade, S., Reid, A., Welsh, L., Lazaro, L. L., Heras, B. D. L., Judson, I. R., Kaye, S. B., Eskens, F., Workman, P., deBono, J. S. & Verweij, J. (2009). Phase I safety, pharmacokinetic, and pharmacogenomic trail of ES-285, a novel marine cytotoxic agent, administered to adult patients with advanced solid tumors. *Mol. Cancer Ther.* Vol. 8, pp. 1430-1437.

Bayes, M., Rabasseda, X. & Prous, J. R. (2004). Gateways to clinical trials. *Meth. Findings Exp. Clin. Pharmacol.* Vol. 26, pp. 473-503.

Berthold, D., Pond, G., Soban, F., de Wit, R., Eisenberger, M. & Tannock, I. (2008). Docetaxel plus prednisone or mitoxantrone plus prednisone for advanced prostate cancer: updated survival in the TAX 327 study. *J. Clin. Oncol.* Vol. 26, pp. 242-245.

Black, R. J., Bray, F., Ferlay, J. & Parkin, D. M. (1997). Cancer incidence and mortality in the european union: cancer registry data and estimates of national incidence for 1990. *Eur. J.Cancer.* Vol. 33, pp. 1075-1107.

Butler, M. S. (2008). Natural products to drugs: natural product-derived compounds in clinical trials. *Nat. Prod. Rep.* Vol. 25, pp. 475-516.

Bystricky, B. & Chau, I. (2011). Patupilone in cancer treatment. *Expert Opin. Invest. Drugs.* Vol. 20, pp. 107-117.

Cao, C., Subhawong, T., Albert, J. M., Kim, K. W., Geng, L., Sekhar, K. R., Gi, Y. J. & Lu, B. (2006). Inhibition of mammalian target of rapamycin or apoptotic pathway induces autophagy and radiosensitizes PTEN null prostate cancer cells. *Cancer Res.* Vol. 66, pp. 10040-10047.

Carlson, E. E. (2010). Natural products as chemical probes. *ACS Chem. Biol.* Vol. 5, pp. 639-653.

Carter, N. J. & Keam, S. J. (2007). Trabectedin- a review of its use in the management of soft tissue sarcoma and ovarian cancer. *Drugs.* Vol. 67, pp. 2257-2276.

Chang, C. J. G., Ghosh, P. K., Hu, Y. F., Brueggemeier, R. W. & Lin, Y. C. (1993). Antiproliferative and antimetastatic effects of gossypol on dunning prostate cell-bearing copenhagen rats. *Res. Commun. Chem. Pathol. Pharmacol.* Vol. 79, pp. 293-312.

Chang, F. R., Hayashi, K., Chen, I. H., Liaw, C. C., Bastow, K. F., Nakanishi, Y., Nozaki, H., Cragg, G. A., Wu, Y. C. & Lee, K. H. (2003). Antitumor agents. 228. Five new agarofurans, reissantins A-E, and cytotoxic principles from Reissantia buchananiii. *J. Nat. Prod.* Vol. 66, pp. 1416-1420.

Chatterjee, B. (2003). The role of the androgen receptor in the development of prostatic hyperplasia and prostate cancer. *Mol. Cell. Biochem.* Vol. 253, pp. 89-101.

Cheng, K. L., Bradley, T. & R, B. D. (2008). Novel microtubule-targeting agents – the epothilones. *Biologics.* Vol. 2, pp. 789-881.

Chintharlapalli, S., Papineni, S., Ramaiah, S. K. & Safe, S. (2007). Betulinic acid inhibits prostate cancer growth through inhibition of specificity protein transcription factors. *Cancer Res.* Vol. 67, pp. 2816-2823.

Choi, Y. H., Baek, J. H., Yoo, M. A., Chung, H. Y., Kim, N. D. & Kim, K. W. (2000). Induction of apoptosis by ursolic acid through activation of caspases and down-regulation of c-IAPs in human prostate epithelial cells. *Int. J. Oncol.* Vol. 17, pp. 565-571.

Clardy, J. & Walsh, C. (2004). Lessons from natural molecules. *Nature.* Vol. 432, pp. 829-837.

Cragg, G. M., Grothaus, P. G. & Newman, D. J. (2009). Impact of natural products on developing new anti-cancer agents. *Chemical Reviews.* Vol. 109, pp. 3012-3043.

Dai, Y., DeSano, J., Tang, W. H., Meng, X. J., Meng, Y., Burstein, E., Lawrence, T. S. & Xu, L. A. (2010). Natural proteasome inhibitor celastrol suppresses androgen-independent prostate cancer progression by modulating apoptotic proteins and NF-κB. *Plos One.* Vol. 5, pp. e14153.

Dai, Y., DeSano, J. T., Meng, Y., Ji, Q., Ljungman, M., Lawrence, T. S. & Xu, L. (2009). Celastrol potentiates radiotherapy by impairment of DNA damage processing in human prostate cancer. *Int. J. Rad. Oncol. Biol. Phys.* Vol. 74, pp. 1217-1225.

De Bono, J., Oudard, S., Ozguroglu, M., Hansen, S., Machiels, J., Kocak, I., Gravis, G., Bodrogi, I., Mackenzie, M., Shen, L., Roessner, M., Gupta, S. & Sartor, A. (2010).

TROPIC investigators: prednisone plus cabazitaxel or mitoxantrone for metastatic castration-resistant prostate cancer progressing after docetaxel treatment: a randomised open-label trial. *Lancet* Vol. 376, pp. 1147-1154.

De Felice, R., Johnson, D. G. & Galgiani, J. N. (1981). Gynecomastia with ketoconazole. *Antimicrob. Agents Chemother.* Vol. 19, pp. 1073-1074.

Debes, J. D. & Tindall, D. J. (2004). Mechanisms of androgen-refractory prostate cancer. *N. Engl. J. Med.* Vol. 351, pp. 1488-1490.

El-Guendy, N., Zhao, Y., Gurumurthy, S., Burikhanov, R. & Rangnekar, V. M. (2003). Identification of a unique core domain of Par-4 sufficient for selective apoptosis induction in cancer cells. *Mol. Cell. Biol.* Vol. 23, pp. 5516-5525.

Fidler, J. M., Li, K., Chung, C., Wei, K., Ross, J. A., Gao, M. & Rosen, G. D. (2003). PG490-88, a derivative of triptolide, causes tumor regression and sensitizes tumors to chemotherapy. *Mol. Cancer Ther.* Vol. 2, pp. 855-862.

Filho, W. B., Corsino, J., Bolzani, V. S., Furlan, M., Pereira, A. M. S. & França, S. C. (2002). Quantitative determination of cytotoxic friedo-*nor*-oleanane derivatives from five morphological types of *Maytenus ilicifolia* (Celastraceae) by reverse-phase high performance liquid chromatography. *Phytochemical Anal.* Vol. 13, pp. 75-78.

Fung, A. S., Wu, L. C. & Tannock, I. F. (2009). Concurrent and sequential administration of chemotherapy and the mammalian target of rapamycin inhibitor temsirolimus in human cancer cells and xenografts. *Clin. Cancer Res.* Vol. 15, pp. 5389-5395.

Galmarini, C. M. (2009). Sagopilone, a microtubule stabilizer for the potential treatment of cancer. *Curr. Opin. Invest. Drugs.* Vol. 10, pp. 1359-1371.

Galsky, M., Dritselis, A., Kirkpatrick, P. & Oh, W. (2010). Cabazitaxel. *Nat. Rev. Drug Discov.* Vol. 9, pp. 677-678.

Ganguly, A., Das, B., Roy, A., Sen, N., Dasgupta, S. B., Mukhopadhayay, S. & Majumder, H. K. (2007). Betulinic acid, a catalytic inhibitor of topoisomerase I, inhibits reactive oxygen species-mediated apoptotic topoisomerase I-DNA cleavable complex formation in prostate cancer cells but does not affect the process of cell death. *Cancer Res.* Vol. 67, pp. 11848-11858.

Garcia, J. A. & Danielpour, D. (2008). Mammalian target of rapamycin inhibition as a therapeutic strategy in the management of urologic malignancies. *Mol. Cancer Ther.* Vol. 7, pp. 1347-1354.

Gerth, K., Bedorf, N., Hofle, G., Irschik, H. & Reichenbach, H. (1996). Epothilons A and B : antifungal and cytotoxic compounds from *Sorangium cellulosum* (Myxobacteria). Production, physico-chemical and biological properties. *J. Antibiotics.* Vol. 49, pp. 560-563.

Girinsky, T., C, K., Graeber, T. G., Peehl, D. M. & Giaccia, A. J. (1995). Attenuated response of p53 and p21 in primary cultures of human prostatic epithelial cells exposed to DNA-damaging agents. *Cancer Res.* Vol. 55, pp. 3726-3731.

Glotter, E., Waitman, R. & Lavie, D. (1966). Constituents of *Withania Somnifera Dun* .8. A new steroidal lactone 27-deoxy-14-hydroxy-withaferin A. *J. Chem. Soc. C.* pp. 1765-1767.

Greenlee, R. T., Murray, T., Bolden, S. & Wingo, P. A. (2000). Cancer statistics, 2000. *CA Cancer J Clin.* Vol. 50, pp. 7-33.

Gross, M. E., Amato, R. J., Mushtaq, M., Wilding, G., Bubley, G., Trudeau, C., Rivera, V. M., Bedrosian, C. L. & Agus, D. B. (2006). A phase 2 trial of AP23573, an mTOR inhibitor, in patients (pts) with taxane-resistant androgen-independent prostate cancer (AIPC). *EJC Suppl.* Vol. 4, pp. 362.

Grothaus, P. G., Cragg, G. M. & Newman, D. J. (2010). Plant natural products in anticancer drug discovery. *Curr. Org. Chem.* Vol. 14, pp. 1781-1791.

Hardman, J. G. & Limbird, L. E. (Ed)(s).). (2001). *The pharmacological basis of therapeutics,* McGraw-Hill, ISBN: 0-07-135469-7, New York.

Hart, L., Hainsworth, J., Ciuleanu, T., Oudard, S., Berger, E., Alexandre, J., Chi, K., Ruether, D., Kahatt, C. & MacDonald, J. (2006). Randomized phase II trial of irofulven/prednisone, irofulven/ capecitabine/ prednisone, or mitoxantrone/ prednisone in hormone refractory prostate cancer (HRPC) patients failing first-line docetaxel: preliminary results. *EJC Suppl.* Vol. 4, pp. 299.

Harzstark, A. L., Rosenberg, J. E., Weinberg, V. K., Sharib, J., Ryan, C. J., Smith, D. C., Pagliaro, L. C., Beer, T. M., Liu, G. & Small, E. J. (2011). Ixabepilone, mitoxantrone, and prednisone for metastatic castration-resistant prostate cancer after docetaxel-based therapy. *Cancer.* Vol. 117, pp. 2419-2425.

Harzstark, A. L. & Small, E. J. (2010). Castrate-resistant prostate cancer: therapeutic strategies. *Expert Opin. Pharmacother.* Vol. 11, pp. 937-945.

Herzig, M. C. S., Trevino, A. V., Liang, H. Y., Salinas, R., Waters, S. J., MacDonald, J. R., Woynarowska, B. A. & Woynarowski, J. M. (2003). Apoptosis induction by the dual-action DNA- and protein-reactive antitumor drug irofulven is largely Bcl-2-independent. *Biochem. Pharmacol.* Vol. 65, pp. 503-513.

Hilgers, W., Faivre, S., Chieze, S., Alexandre, J., Lokiec, F., Goldwasser, F., Raymond, E., Kahatt, C., Taamma, A., Weems, G., MacDonald, J. R., Misset, J. L. & Cvitkovic, E. (2006). A phase I and pharmacokinetic study of irofulven and cisplatin administered in a 30-min infusion every two weeks to patients with advanced solid tumors. *Invest. New Drugs.* Vol. 24, pp. 311-319.

Hofle, G., Bedorf, N., Steinmetz, H., Schomburg, D., Gerth, K. & Reichenbach, H. (1996). Epothilone A and B - novel 16-membered macrolides with cytotoxic activity: isolation, crystal structure, and conformation in solution. *Angew. Chem. Int. Ed. Engl.* Vol. 35, pp. 1567-1569.

Huang, Y. W., Wang, L. S., Chang, H. L., Ye, W. P., Dowd, M. K., Wan, P. J. & Lin, Y. C. (2006). Molecular mechanisms of (-)-gossypol-induced apoptosis in human prostate cancer cells. *Anticancer Res.* Vol. 26, pp. 1925-1933.

Huggins, C. & Hodges, C. V. (1941). Studies on Prostatic Cancer. I. The effect of castration, of estrogen and of androgen injection on serum phosphatases in metastatic carcinoma of the prostate. *Cancer Res.* Vol. 1, pp. 293-297.

Huggins, C., Stevens, R. E. & Hodges, C. V. (1941). Studies on prostatic cancer. II. The effect of castration on clinical patients with carcinoma of the prostate. *Arch. Surg.* Vol. 43, pp. 209-223.

Hussain, A., DiPaola, R. S., Baron, A. D., Higano, C. S., Tchekmedyian, N. S. & Johri, A. R. (2009). Phase II trial of weekly patupilone in patients with castration-resistant prostate cancer. *Ann. Oncol.* Vol. 20, pp. 492-497.

Hussain, M., Tangen, C. M., Lara, P. N., Vaishampayan, U. N., Petrylak, D. P., Colevas, A. D., Sakr, W. A. & Crawford, E. D. (2005). Ixabepilone (epothilone B analogue BMS-247550) is active in chemotherapy-naive patients with hormone-refractory prostate cancer: A southwest oncology group trial S0111. *J. Clin. Oncol.* Vol. 23, pp. 8724-8729.

Ioffe, M. L., White, E., Nelson, D. A., Dvorzhinski, D. & DiPaola, R. S. (2004). Epothilone induced cytotoxicity is dependent on p53 status in prostate cells. *Prostate.* Vol. 61, pp. 243-247.

Jemal, A., Bray, F., Center, M. M., Ferlay, J., Ward, E. & Forman, D. (2011). Global cancer statistics. *CA Cancer J. Clin.* Vol. 61, pp. 69-90.

Jemal, A., Siegel, R., Xu, J. Q. & Ward, E. (2010). Cancer statistics, 2010. *CA Cancer J. Clin.* Vol. 60, pp. 277-300.

Kannaiyan, R., Shanmugam, M. K. & Sethi, G. (2011). Molecular targets of celastrol derived from Thunder of God Vine: potential role in the treatment of inflammatory disorders and cancer. *Cancer Lett.* Vol. 303, pp. 9-20.

Kassi, E., Papoutsi, Z., Pratsinis, H., Aligiannis, N., Manoussakis, M. & Moutsatsou, P. (2007). Ursolic acid, a naturally occurring triterpenoid, demonstrates anticancer activity on human prostate cancer cells. *J. Cancer Res. Clin. Oncol.* Vol. 133, pp. 493-500.

Kessler, J. H., Mullauer, F. B., de Roo, G. M. & Medema, J. P. (2007). Broad *in vitro* efficacy of plant-derived betulinic acid against cell lines derived from the most prevalent human cancer types. *Cancer Lett.* Vol. 251, pp. 132-145.

Kiviharju, T. M., Lecane, P. S., Sellers, R. G. & Peehl, D. M. (2002). Antiproliferative and proapoptotic activities of triptolide (PG490), a natural product entering clinical trials, on primary cultures of human prostatic epithelial cells. *Clin. Cancer Res.* Vol. 8, pp. 2666-2674.

Kondo, M., MacKinnon, S. L., Craft, C. C., Matchett, M. D., Hurta, R. A. R. & Neto, C. C. (2011). Ursolic acid and its esters: occurrence in cranberries and other Vaccinium fruit and effects on matrix metalloproteinase activity in DU145 prostate tumor cells. *J. Sci. Food Agric.* Vol. 91, pp. 789-796.

Kong, F. M., Zhu, T. M., Yu, K., Pagano, T. G., Desai, P., Radebaugh, G. & Fawzi, M. (2011). Isolation and structure of homotemsirolimuses A, B, and C. *J. Nat. Prod.* Vol. 74, pp. 547-553.

Kumar, S., Twardowski, P. & Sartor, O. (2010). Critical appraisal of cabazitaxel in the management of advanced prostate cancer. *Clin. Interv. Aging.* Vol. 5, pp. 395-402.

Kupchan, S. M., Coutr, W. A., Dailey, R. G., Gilmore, C. J. & Bryan, R. F. (1972). Triptolide and tripdiolide, novel antileukemic diterpenoid triepoxides from *Tripterygium wilfordii. J. Am. Chem. Soc.* Vol. 94, pp. 7194-7195.

Kwon, S. H., Park, H. Y., Kim, J. Y., Jeong, I. Y., Lee, M. K. & Seo, K. I. (2010). Apoptotic action of ursolic acid isolated from Corni fructus in RC-58T/h/SA#4 primary human prostate cancer cells. *Bioorg. Med. Chem. Lett.* Vol. 20, pp. 6435-6438.

Lake-Bakaar, G., Scheuer, P. J. & Sherlock, S. (1987). Hepatic reactions associated with ketoconazole in the United Kingdom. *BMJ.* Vol. 294, pp. 419-422.

Larkin, J. M. G. (2007). Patupilone. *Drugs Future.* Vol. 32, pp. 323-336.

Lassi, K. & Dawson, N. A. (2010). Update on castrate-resistant prostate cancer: 2010. *Curr. Opin. Oncol.* Vol. 22, pp. 263-267.

Lee, J. J. & Kelly, W. K. (2009). Epothilones: tubulin polymerization as a novel target for prostate cancer therapy. *Nat. Clin. Pract. Oncol.* Vol. 6, pp. 85-92.

Lerut, E., Roskams, T., Goossens, E., Bootle, D., Dimitrijevic, S., Stumm, M., Shand, N. & van Poppel, H. (2005). Molecular pharmacodynamic (MPD) evaluation of dose and schedule of RAD001 (everolimus) in patients with operable prostate carcinoma (PC). *J. Clin. Oncol.* Vol. 23, pp. 209S-209S.

Li, W. W., Takahashi, N., Jhanwar, S., Cordon-Cardo, C., Elisseyeff, Y., Jimeno, J., Faircloth, G. & Bertino, J. R. (2001). Sensitivity of soft tissue sarcoma cell lines to chemotherapeutic agents: Identification of ecteinascidin-743 as a potent cytotoxic agent. *Clin. Cancer Res.* Vol. 7, pp. 2908-2911.

Lian, J., Wu, X., He, F., Karnak, D., Tang, W., Meng, Y., Xiang, D., Ji, M., Lawrence, T. S. & Xu, L. (2011). A natural BH3 mimetic induces autophagy in apoptosis-resistant prostate cancer via modulating Bcl-2-Beclin1 interaction at endoplasmic reticulum. *Cell Death Differ.* Vol. 18, pp. 60-71.

Liang, H. Y., Salinas, R. A., Leal, B. Z., Kosakowska-Cholody, T., Michejda, C. J., Waters, S. J., Herman, T. S., Woynarowski, J. M. & Woynarowska, B. A. (2004). Caspase-mediated apoptosis and caspase-independent cell death induced by irofulven in prostate cancer cells. *Mol. Cancer Ther.* Vol. 3, pp. 1385-1396.

Liu, G., Kelly, W. K., Wilding, G., Leopold, L., Brill, K. & Somer, B. (2009). An open-label, multicenter, phase I/II study of single-agent AT-101 in men with castrate-resistant prostate cancer. *Clin. Cancer Res.* Vol. 15, pp. 3172-3176.

Liu, H., Liu, Y. Q., Liu, Y. Q., Xu, A. H., Young, C. Y. F., Yuan, H. Q. & Lou, H. X. (2010). A novel anticancer agent, retigeric acid B, displays proliferation inhibition, S phase arrest and apoptosis activation in human prostate cancer cells. *Chem-Bio Inter.* Vol. 188, pp. 598-606.

Liu, Q. Y. (2011). Triptolide and its expanding multiple pharmacological functions. *Int. Immunopharmacol.* Vol. 11, pp. 377-383.

Lu, M., Xia, L. J., Hua, H. M. & Jing, Y. K. (2008). Acety-keto-β-boswellic acid induces apoptosis through a death receptor 5-mediated pathway in prostate cancer cells. *Cancer Res.* Vol. 68, pp. 1180-1186.

Majumder, P. K., Febbo, P. G., Bikoff, R., Berger, R., Xue, Q., McMahon, L. M., Manola, J., Brugarolas, J., McDonnell, T. J., Golub, T. R., Loda, M., Lane, H. A. & Sellers, W. R. (2004). mTOR inhibition reverses Akt-dependent prostate intraepithelial neoplasia through regulation of apoptotic and HIF-1-dependent pathways. *Nat. Med.* Vol. 10, pp. 594-601.

Mancuso, A., Oudard, S. & Sternberg, C. N. (2007). Effective chemotherapy for hormone-refractory prostate cancer (HRPC): present status and perspectives with taxane-based treatments. *Critical Rev.Oncol. Hematol.* Vol. 61, pp. 176-185.

Marco, E., David-Cordonnier, M.-H. l. n., Bailly, C., Cuevas, C. & Gago, F. (2006). Further insight into the DNA recognition mechanism of trabectedin from the differential affinity of its demethylated analogue ecteinascidin ET729 for the triplet DNA binding site CGA. *J. Med. Chem.* Vol. 49, pp. 6925-6929.

Martinez-Serra, J., Maffiotte, E., Martin, J., Bex, T., Navarro-Palou, M., Ros, T., Plazas, J. M., Vogler, O., Gutierrez, A., Amat, J. C., Ramos, R., Saus, C., Gines, J., Alemany, R., Diaz, M. & Besalduch, J. (2011). Yondelis (R) (ET-743, Trabectedin) sensitizes cancer cell lines to CD95-mediated cell death: new molecular insight into the mechanism of action. *Eur. J. Pharmacol.* Vol. 658, pp. 57-64.

Mayer, A. M. S., Glaser, K. B., Cuevas, C., Jacobs, R. S., Kem, W., Little, R. D., McIntosh, J. M., Newman, D. J., Potts, B. C. & Shuster, D. E. (2010). The odyssey of marine pharmaceuticals: a current pipeline perspective. *Trends Pharmacol. Sci.* Vol. 31, pp. 255-265.

McHenry, P., Wang, W. L. W., Devitt, E., Kluesner, N., Davisson, V. J., McKee, E., Schweitzer, D., Helquist, P. & Tenniswood, M. (2010). Iejimalides A and B inhibit lysosomal vacuolar H+-ATPase (V-ATPase) activity and induce S-phase arrest and apoptosis in MCF-7 Cells. *J. Cell. Biochem.* Vol. 109, pp. 634-642.

Meng, Y., Tang, W. H., Dai, Y., Wu, X. Q., Liu, M. L., Ji, G., Ji, M., Pienta, K., Lawrence, T. & Xu, L. (2008). Natural BH3 mimetic (-)-gossypol chemosensitizes human prostate cancer via Bcl-xL inhibition accompanied by increase of Puma and Noxa. *Mol. Cancer Ther.* Vol. 7, pp. 2192-2202.

Michaelson, M. D., Gilligan, T., Oh, W., Kantoff, P., Taplin, M. E., Izquierdo, M. A., Flores, L. & Smith, M. R. (2005). Phase II study of three hour, weekly infusion of trabectedin (ET-743) in men with metastatic, androgen-independent prostate carcinoma (AIPC). *J. Clin. Oncol.* Vol. 23, pp. 382S-382S.

Moh, P. P., Chang, C. J. G., Brueggemeier, R. W. & Lin, Y. C. (1992). Effect of gossypol (Gp) on 5α-reductase and 3α-hydroxysteroid dehydrogenase (3α-Hsd) in adult-rat testes. *Faseb J.* Vol. 6, pp. A2031-A2031.

Moreira, V. M., Salvador, J. A. R., Vasaitis, T. S. & Njar, V. C. (2008). CYP17 inhibitors for prostate cancer treatment - an update. *Curr. Med. Chem.* Vol. 15, pp. 868-899.

Morgan, T. M., Pitts, T. E. M., Gross, T. S., Poliachik, S. L., Vessella, R. L. & Corey, E. (2008). RAD001 (Everolimus) inhibits growth of prostate cancer in the bone and the inhibitory effects are increased in combination with docetaxel and zoledronic acid. *Prostate.* Vol. 68, pp. 861-871.

Moussaieff, A. & Mechoulam, R. (2009). Boswellia resin: from religious ceremonies to medical uses; a review of *in-vitro, in-vivo* and clinical trials. *J. Pharm. Pharmacol.* Vol. 61, pp. 1281-1293.

Nemoto, R., Hattori, K., Uchida, K., Shimazui, T., Nishijima, Y., Koiso, K. & Harada, M. (1990). S-Phase fraction of human prostate adenocarcinoma studied with *In vivo* bromodeoxyuridine labeling. *Cancer.* Vol. 66, pp. 509-514.

Newman, D. J. & Cragg, G. M. (2009). Microbial antitumor drugs: natural products of microbial origin as anticancer agents. *Curr. Opin. Invest. Drugs.* Vol. 10, pp. 1280-1296.

Newman, D. J. & Cragg, G. M. (2007). Natural products as sources of new drugs over the last 25 years. *J. Nat. Prod.* Vol. 70, pp. 461-477.

O'Reilly, T., McSheehy, P. M., Wenger, F., Hattenberger, M., Muller, M., Vaxelaire, J., Altmann, K. H. & Wartmann, M. (2005). Patupilone (epothilone B, EPO906) inhibits growth and metastasis of experimental prostate tumors *in vivo*. *Prostate.* Vol. 65, pp. 231-240.

Ojima, I. (2008). Modern natural products chemistry and drug discovery. *J. Med. Chem.* Vol. 51, pp. 2587-2588.

Opdenaker, L. M. & Farach-Carson, M. C. (2009). Rapamycin selectively reduces the association of transcripts containing complex 5 ' UTRs with ribosomes in C4-2B prostate cancer cells. *J. Cell. Biochem.* Vol. 107, pp. 473-481.

Padron, J. M. & Peters, G. J. (2006). Cytotoxicity of sphingoid marine compound analogs in mono- and multilayered solid tumor cell cultures. *Invest. New Drugs.* Vol. 24, pp. 195-202.

Pang, X. F., Yi, Z. F., Zhang, J., Lu, B. B., Sung, B., Qu, W. J., Aggarwal, B. B. & Liu, M. Y. (2010). Celastrol suppresses angiogenesis-mediated tumor growth through inhibition of AKT/mammalian target of rapamycin pathway. *Cancer Res.* Vol. 70, pp. 1951-1959.

Pang, X. F., Yi, Z. F., Zhang, X. L., Sung, B. K., Qu, W. J., Lian, X. Y., Aggarwal, B. B. & Liu, M. Y. (2009). Acetyl-11-keto-β-boswellic acid inhibits prostate tumor growth by suppressing vascular endothelial growth factor receptor 2-mediated angiogenesis. *Cancer Res.* Vol. 69, pp. 5893-5900.

Petronelli, A., Pannitteri, G. & Testa, U. (2009). Triterpenoids as new promising anticancer drugs. *Anti-Cancer Drugs.* Vol. 20, pp. 880-892.

Petrylak, D., Tangen, C., Hussain, M., Lara, P. J., Jones, J., Taplin, M., Burch, P., Berry, D., Moinpour, C., Kohli, M., Benson, M., Small, E., Raghavan, D. & Crawford, E. (2004). Docetaxel and estramustine compared with mitoxantrone and prednisone for advanced refractory prostate cancer. *N. Engl. J. Med.* Vol. 351, pp. 1513-1520.

Pisha, E., Chan, H., Lee, I. S., Chagwedera, T. E., Farnsworth, N. R., Cordell, G. A., Beecher, C. W. W., Fong, H. H. S., Kinghorn, A. D., Brown, D. M., Wani, M. C., Wall, M. E., Hieken, T. J., Gupta, T. K. & Pezzuto, J. M. (1995). Discovery of betulinic acid as a selective inhibitor of human melanoma that functions by induction of apoptosis. *Nat. Med.* Vol. 1, pp. 1046-1051.

Poindessous, V., Koeppel, F., Raymond, E., Comisso, M., Waters, S. J. & Larsen, A. K. (2003). Marked activity of irofulven toward human carcinoma cells: Comparison with cisplatin and ecteinascidin. *Clin. Cancer Res.* Vol. 9, pp. 2817-2825.

Rabi, T., Shukla, S. & Gupta, S. (2008). Betulinic acid suppresses constitutive and TNFα-induced NF-κB activation and induces apoptosis in human prostate carcinoma PC-3 cells. *Mol. Carcinogen.* Vol. 47, pp. 964-973.

Rivera, E., Lee, J. & Davies, A. (2008). Clinical development of ixabepilone and other epothilones in patients with advanced solid tumors. *Oncologist.* Vol. 13, pp. 1207-1223.

Rosenberg, J. E., Galsky, M. D., Rohs, N. C., Weinberg, V. K., Oh, W. K., Kelly, W. K. & Small, E. J. (2006). A retrospective evaluation of second-line chemotherapy response in hormone-refractory prostate carcinoma - Second-line taxane-based therapy after first-line epothilone-B analog ixabepilone (BMS-247550) therapy. *Cancer.* Vol. 106, pp. 58-62.

Rubin, E. H., Rothermel, J., Tesfaye, F., Chen, T., Hubert, M., Ho, Y. Y., Hsu, C. H. & Oza, A. M. (2005). Phase I dose-finding study of weekly single-agent patupilone in patients with advanced solid tumors. *J. Clin. Oncol.* Vol. 23, pp. 9120-9129.

Salminen, A., Lehtonen, M., Paimela, T. & Kaarniranta, K. (2010). Celastrol: molecular targets of Thunder God Vine. *Biochem. Biophys. Res. Commun.* Vol. 394, pp. 439-442.

Salvador, J. A. R. (Ed). (2010). *Pentacyclic triterpenes as promising agents in cancer*, Nova Science Publishers, ISBN: 978-1-60876-973-5, New York, USA.

Sanchez, A. M., Malagarie-Cazenave, S., Olea, N., Vara, D., Cuevas, C. & Diaz-Laviada, I. (2008). Spisulosine (ES-285) induces prostate tumor PC-3 and LNCaP cell death by *de novo* synthesis of ceramide and PKCξ activation. *Eur. J. Pharmacol.* Vol. 584, pp. 237-245.

Sartor, O. (2011). Progression of metastatic castrate-resistant prostate cancer: impact of therapeutic intervention in the post-docetaxel space. *J. Hematol Oncol.* Vol. 4, pp. 18.

Schmid, P., Kiewe, P., Possinger, K., Korfel, A., Lindemann, S., Giurescu, M., Reif, S., Wiesinger, H., Thiel, E. & Kunhardt, D. (2010). Phase I study of the novel, fully synthetic epothilone sagopilone (ZK-EPO) in patients with solid tumors. *Ann. Oncol.* Vol. 21, pp. 633-639.

Schoffski, P., Dumez, H., Ruijter, R., Miguel-Lillo, B., Soto-Matos, A., Alfaro, V. & Giaccone, G. (2011). Spisulosine (ES-285) given as a weekly three-hour intravenous infusion: results of a phase I dose-escalating study in patients with advanced solid malignancies. *Cancer Chemother. Pharmacol.* doi:10.1007/s00280-00011-01612-00281.

Schrijvers, D., Van Erps, P. & Cortvriend, J. (2010). Castration-refractory prostate cancer: new drugs in the pipeline. *Adv. Ther.* Vol. 27, pp. 285-296.

Schweitzer, D., Zhu, J., Jarori, G., Tanaka, J., Higa, T., Davisson, V. J. & Helquist, P. (2007). Synthesis of carbamate derivatives of iejimalides. Retention of normal antiproliferative activity and localization of binding in cancer cells. *Bioorg. Med. Chem.* Vol. 15, pp. 3208-3216.

Seeliger, H., Guba, M., Kleespies, A., Jauch, K. W. & Bruns, C. J. (2007). Role of mTOR in solid tumor systems: a therapeutical target against primary tumor growth, metastases, and angiogenesis. *Cancer Metast. Rev.* Vol. 26, pp. 611-621.

Senzer, N., Arsenau, J., Richards, D., Berman, B., MacDonald, J. R. & Smith, S. (2005). Irofulven demonstrates clinical activity against metastatic hormone-refractory prostate cancer in a phase 2 single-agent trial. *Am. J. Clin. Oncol. Cancer Clin. Trials.* Vol. 28, pp. 36-42.

Sepp-Lorenzino, L., Balog, A., Su, D. S., Meng, D., Timaul, N., Scher, H. I., Danishefsky, S. J. & Rosen, N. (1999). The microtubule-stabilizing agents epothilones A and B and their desoxy-derivatives induce mitotic arrest and apoptosis in human prostate cancer cells. *Prostate Cancer Prostatic Dis.* Vol. 2, pp. 41-52.

Shah, B. A., Qazi, G. N. & Taneja, S. C. (2009). Boswellic acids: a group of medicinally important compounds. *Nat. Prod. Rep.* Vol. 26, pp. 72-89.

Shamona, L. A., Pezzuto, J. M., Graves, J. M., Metha, R. R., Wangcharoentrakul, S., Sangsuwand, R., Chaichanad, S., Tuchindad, T., Cleasond, P. & Reutrakuld, V. (1997). Evaluation of the mutagenic, cytotoxic, and antitumor potential of triptolide, a highly oxygenated diterpene isolated from *Tripterygium wilfovdii*. *Cancer Lett.* Vol. 112, pp. 113-117.

Shidaifat, F., Canatan, H., Kulp, S. K., Sugimoto, Y., Chang, W. Y., Zhang, Y., Brueggemeier, R. W., Somers, W. J. & Lin, Y. C. (1996). Inhibition of human prostate cancer cells growth by gossypol is associated with stimulation of transforming growth factor β. *Cancer Lett.* Vol. 107, pp. 37-44.

Singh, R., Sharma, M., Joshi, P. & Rawat, D. S. (2008). Clinical status of anti-cancer agents derived from marine sources. *Anti Cancer Agents Med. Chem.* Vol. 8, pp. 603-617.

Skinner, M. (2010). Prostate Cancer: a new target. *Nat. Rev. Cancer.* Vol. 10, pp. 534-535.

Squillace, R., Miller, D., Wardwell, S., Wang, F., Clackson, T. & Rivera, V. (2008). Synergistic activity of the mTOR inhibitor deforolimus (AP23573; MK-8669) and the anti-androgen bicalutamide in prostate cancer models. *EJC Suppl.* Vol. 6, pp. 103-103.

Srinivasan, S., Ranga, R. S., Burikhanov, R., Han, S. S. & Chendil, D. (2007). Par-4-dependent apoptosis by the dietary compound withaferin A in prostate cancer cells. *Cancer Res.* Vol. 67, pp. 246-253.

Su, D.-S., Meng, D., Bertinato, P., Balog, A., Sorensen, E. J., Danishefsky, S. J., Zheng, Y. H., Chou, T. C., He, L. & Horwitz, S. B. (1997). Total synthesis of (-)-Epothilone B: an extension of the Suzuki coupling method and insights into structure-activity relationships of the epothilones. *Angew. Chem. Int. Ed. Engl.* Vol. 36, pp. 757-759.

Sung, B., Park, B., Yadav, V. R. & Aggarwal, B. B. (2010). Celastrol, a triterpene, enhances TRAIL-induced apoptosis through the down-regulation of cell survival proteins and up-regulation of death receptors. *J. Biol. Chem.* Vol. 285, pp. 11498-11507.

Syrovets, T., Gschwend, J. E., Buchele, B., Laumonnier, Y., Zugmaier, W., Genze, F. & Simmet, T. (2005). Inhibition of IkB kinase activity by acetyl-boswellic acids promotes apoptosis in androgen-independent PC-3 prostate cancer cells *in vitro* and *in vivo*. *J. Biol. Chem.* Vol. 280, pp. 6170-6180.

Tan, Y., Yu, R. & Pezzuto, J. M. (2003). Betulinic acid-induced programmed cell death in human melanoma cells involves mitogen-activated protein kinase activation. *Clin Cancer Res.* Vol. 9, pp. 2866-2875.

Tannock, I., de Wit, R., Berry, W., Horti, J., Pluzanska, A., Chi, K., Oudard, S., Théodore, C., James, N., Turesson, I., Rosenthal, M. & Eisenberger, M. (2004). TAX 327 investigators: docetaxel plus prednisone or mitoxantrone plus prednisone for advanced prostate cancer. *N. Engl. J. Med.* Vol. 351, pp. 1502-1512.

Tchen, N., Alexandre, J., Misset, J. L., Berthault-Cvitkovic, F., Kahatt, C., Benettaib, B., Weems, G., MacDonald, J. R. & Cvitkovic, E. (2005). A combination of irofulven and oxaliplatin is active in patients with hormone refractory prostate cancer (HRPC) with secondary resistance to docetaxel: phase I preliminary evidence. *Clin. Cancer Res.* Vol. 11, pp. 9057S-9058S.

Thompson, T. C. (2010). Grappling with the androgen receptor: a new approach for treating advanced prostate cancer. *Cancer Cell.* Vol. 17, pp. 525-526.

Toppmeyer, D. L. & Goodin, S. (2010). Ixabepilone, a new treatment option for metastatic breast cancer. *Am J. Clin. Oncol.* Vol. 33, pp. 516-521.

Van Laar, E. S., Weitman, S., MacDonald, J. R. & Waters, S. J. (2004). Antitumor activity of irofulven monotherapy and in combination with mitoxantrone or docetaxel against human prostate cancer models. *Prostate.* Vol. 59, pp. 22-32.

Vilar, E., Grünwald, V., Schöffski, P., Singer, H., Salazar, R., Iglesias, J. L., Casado, E., Cullell-Young, M., Baselga, J. & Tabernero, J. (2010). A phase I dose-escalating study of ES-285, a marine sphingolipid-derived compound, with repeat dose administration in patients with advanced solid tumors. *Invest. New Drugs.* Vol. pp. 1-7.

Volate, S. R., Kawasaki, B. T., Hurt, E. M., Milner, J. A., Kim, Y. S., White, J. & Farrar, W. L. (2010). Gossypol induces apoptosis by activating p53 in prostate cancer cells and prostate tumor-initiating cells. *Mol. Cancer Ther.* Vol. 9, pp. 461-470.

Wang, L., Wei, D., Huang, S., Peng, Z., Le, X., Wu, T. T., Yao, J., Ajani, J. & Xie, K. (2003). Transcription factor Sp1 expression is a significant predictor of survival in human gastric cancer. *Clin. Cancer Res.* Vol. 9, pp. 6371-6380.

Wang, S. R. & Fang, W. S. (2009). Pentacyclic triterpenoids and their saponins with apoptosis-inducing activity. *Curr. Topics Med. Chem.* Vol. 9, pp. 1581-1596.

Wang, W. L. W., McHenry, P., Jeffrey, R., Schweitzer, D., Helquist, P. & Tenniswood, M. (2008). Effects of iejimalide B, a marine macrolide, on growth and apoptosis in prostate cancer cell lines. *J. Cell. Biochem.* Vol. 105, pp. 998-1007.

Wartmann, M. & Altmann, K. H. (2002). The biology and medicinal chemistry of epothilones. *Curr. Med. Chem. Anti Cancer Agents.* Vol. 2, pp. 123-148.

Wong, Y. C. & Tam, C. C. (1989). Structural-changes of the guinea-pig prostatic epithelial-cells after gossypol treatment. *Acta Anat.* Vol. 134, pp. 18-25.

Wu, L., Birle, D. C. & Tannock, I. F. (2005). Effects of the mammalian target of rapamycin inhibitor CCI-779 used alone or with chemotherapy on human prostate cancer cells and xenografts. *Cancer Res.* Vol. 65, pp. 2825-2831.

Yang, H., Chen, D., Cui, D. C., Yuan, X. & Dou, Q. P. (2006). Celastrol, a triterpene extracted from the Chinese "Thunder of God Vine," is a potent proteasome inhibitor and suppresses human prostate cancer growth in nude mice. *Cancer Res.* Vol. 66, pp. 4758-4765.

Yang, H. J. & Dou, Q. P. (2010). Targeting apoptosis pathway with natural terpenoids: implications for treatment of breast and prostate cancer. *Curr. Drug Targets.* Vol. 11, pp. 733-744.

Yang, H. J., Landis-Piwowar, K. R., Lu, D., Yuan, P., Li, L. H., Reddy, G. P. V., Yuan, X. & Dou, Q. P. (2008). Pristimerin induces apoptosis by targeting the proteasome in prostate cancer cells. *J. Cell. Biochem.* Vol. 103, pp. 234-244.

Yang, H. J., Murthy, S., Sarkar, F. H., Sheng, S. J., Reddy, G. P. V. & Dou, Q. P. (2008). Calpain-mediated androgen receptor breakdown in apoptotic prostate cancer cells. *J. Cell. Physiol.* Vol. 217, pp. 569-576.

Yang, H. J., Shi, G. Q. & Dou, Q. P. (2007). The tumor proteasome is a primary target for the natural anticancer compound withaferin A isolated from "Indian Winter Cherry". *Mol. Pharmacol.* Vol. 71, pp. 426-437.

Yao, J. C., Wang, L., Wei, D., Gong, W. R., Hassan, M., Wu, T. T., Mansfield, P. & Xie, K. (2004). Association between expression of transcription factor Sp1 and increased vascular endothelial growth factor expression, advanced stage, and poor survival in patients with resected gastric cancer. *Clin. Cancer Res.* Vol. 10, pp. 4109-4117.

Yuan, H. Q., Feng, K., Wang, X. L., Young, C. Y. F., Hu, X. Y. & Lou, H. X. (2008). Inhibitory effect of acetyl-11-keto-β-boswellic acid on androgen receptor by interference of Sp1 binding activity in prostate cancer cells. *Biochem. Pharmacol.* Vol. 75, pp. 2112-2121.

Zelek, L., Yovine, A., Brain, E., Turpin, F., Taamma, A., Riofrio, M., Spielmann, M., Jimeno, J. & Misset, J. L. (2006). A phase II study of Yondelis (trabectedin, ET-743) as a 24-h continuous intravenous infusion in pretreated advanced breast cancer. *Br. J. Cancer.* Vol. 94, pp. 1610-1614.

Zhang, Y. X., Kong, C. Z., Wang, H. Q., Wang, L. H., Xu, C. L. & Sun, Y. H. (2009). Phosphorylation of Bcl-2 and activation of caspase-3 via the c-Jun N-terminal kinase pathway in ursolic acid-induced DU145 cells apoptosis. *Biochimie.* Vol. 91, pp. 1173-1179.

Zhang, Y. X., Kong, C. Z., Wang, L. H., Li, J. Y., Liu, X. K., Xu, B., Xu, C. L. & Sun, Y. H. (2010). Ursolic acid overcomes Bcl-2-mediated resistance to apoptosis in prostate cancer cells involving activation of JNK-induced Bcl-2 phosphorylation and degradation. *J. Cell. Biochem.* Vol. 109, pp. 764-773.

Zhang, Y. X., Kong, C. Z., Zeng, Y., Wang, L. H., Li, Z. H., Wang, H. Q., Xu, C. L. & Sun, Y. H. (2010). Ursolic acid induces PC-3 cell apoptosis via activation of JNK and inhibition of Akt pathways *In Vitro. Mol. Carcinogen.* Vol. 49, pp. 374-385.

8

Zinc Supplementation and Prostate Cancer

Wong Pooi-Fong[1] and AbuBakar Sazaly[2]
[1]Department of Pharmacology
[2]Department of Medical Microbiology
Faculty of Medicine, University of Malaya
Malaysia

1. Introduction

Prostate cancer continues to be one of the most common fatal cancers in men (Jemal et al., 2010). The comprehensive understanding of the etiology of this disease is however, far from complete because of multitude of genetics and environmental factors involved in the development of this disease (Deutsch et al., 2004; Giovannucci, 2001). One characteristic feature of the prostate gland is its unique ability to accumulate high concentrations of zinc, which may otherwise be toxic to other tissues (Costello & Franklin, 1998). For reasons primarily still unknown, cancerous prostate cells somehow lose its ability to accumulate intracellular zinc concentrations. This is based on consistent observations of low zinc concentrations in malignant prostate tissues as compared to normal prostate and benign prostatic hyperplasia tissues (Feustel & Wennrich, 1984; Ho, 2004; Vartsky et al., 2003; Zaichick et al., 1997). These findings thereby, imply a potential importance of zinc in the pathogenesis of prostate cancer.

It is suggested that dietary zinc supplementation protects against oxidative damage, reduces cancer risk (Ho, 2004) and has therapeutic potentials against prostate cancer (Franklin & Costello, 2007). Epidemiologic studies, however, provided contradictory findings on the effectiveness of zinc in prevention against prostate cancer. While there are studies that showed zinc reduces the risk of developing prostate cancer (Key et al., 1997; Kristal et al., 1999), others showed that advanced prostate cancer is associated with high intake of zinc and potentiate the development of benign prostate hyperplasia (BPH) and progression towards cancer (Gallus et al., 2007; Lagiou et al., 1999; Lawson et al., 2007; Leitzmann et al., 2003; Moyad, 2004). Various mechanisms have been proposed to explain how high zinc regulates prostate health and indirectly, how its absence or low concentration could have contributed to the occurrence of prostate cancer. Restoration of high zinc to cancerous prostate tissues has been shown to inhibit prostate cancer cells proliferation (Feng et al., 2002; Feng et al., 2000; Iguchi et al., 1998; Liang et al., 1999) and invasion (Ishii et al., 2004; Ishii et al., 2001a; Ishii et al., 2001b; Uzzo et al., 2006). In contrast, there are studies which showed that zinc under non-physiological conditions could promote cancer cell growth and invasion (Boissier et al., 2000; Nemoto et al., 2000; Wong & Abubakar, 2008a; Wong & Abubakar, 2010).

Because of the diverse roles of zinc in cell signaling, the exact pathways and genes affected by the absence or presence of high zinc concentrations in prostate cancer cells remain unraveled. In an attempt to further understand the complexity of the role of zinc in prostate cancer, this chapter will discuss issues related to the regulatory roles of zinc in normal prostate, the consequences of losing this regulatory role in the malignant cells and the implications of zinc supplementation in the cancer cells.

2. Zinc and human health

Zinc is an essential trace element, critical for diverse biological functions in the human body. Its importance in humans was not discovered until 1961 where zinc deficiency was found to be the cause of growth retardation and hypogonadism in Iranian and Egyptian patients (Prasad et al., 1961; Prasad et al., 1963). Meat, poultry, oyster, dairy products, legumes and cereals are food rich in zinc. However, phytates, which are present in some cereals and legumes can reduce the bioavailability of zinc by inhibiting absorption of zinc in the intestines (Sandstrom, 1997; Wise, 1995). The recommended dietary allowance (RDA) for daily intake of zinc in 97-98% healthy individuals is 8 mg/d for women, 11 mg/d for men, 11-12 mg/ml for pregnant and lactating women. Children from 1-3 years old, 4-8 years and 9-13 years old require 3, 5 and 8 mg/d of zinc, respectively (Food and Nutritional Board of Medicine, 2010a). The tolerable upper intake level (UL), defined as the maximal daily intake unlikely to cause adverse health effects is 40 mg/d for adults. For children of 1-3, 4-8 and 9-13 years old, ULs are 7 mg/d, 12 and 23 mg/d, respectively, (Food and Nutritional Board of Medicine, 2010b).

Deficiency of zinc is associated with significant health problems. Early manifestations of zinc deficiency include decreased immunity resulting in increased susceptibility to infections such as diarrhea, common cold, acute lower respiratory infection and malaria. Zinc-deficient individuals also display dermatitis, delayed wound healing and alopecia. Prolonged deficiency leads to retardation of growth, genital development, hypogonadism and impaired neuropsychological functions (Prasad, 2008). Zinc deficiency in pregnancy retards fetal growth and postnatal development, causes neural tube defects and premature birth but the use of zinc supplementation in women still requires further studies (Osendarp et al., 2003; Uriu-Adams & Keen, 2010).

Zinc supplements are found in the forms of zinc gluconate, zinc sulfate, and zinc acetate, where the percentage of elemental zinc can varies (Haase et al., 2008). Studies have shown that supplementation with zinc corrects growth and gonadal development, improves immune functions and hastens recovery from diarrhea, common cold, acute lower respiratory infection and malaria (Black, 2003; Fischer Walker & Black, 2004). It is also used to treat genetic disorders such as acrodermatitis enteropathica (Maverakis et al., 2007) and Wilson's disease (Brewer, 2001). Zinc excess can induce copper deficiency and it is used in Wilson's disease to interfere with uptake of copper and subsequently reduce excessive copper accumulation. While zinc supplementation may be beneficial in certain conditions excessive zinc intake can pose serious health risks. Acute zinc toxicity causes gastrointestinal-related symptoms such as nausea, vomiting, tenesmus and diarrhea (Brown et al., 1964). Chronic zinc toxicity can lead to copper deficiency and its related hematological and neurological manifestations (Maret & Sandstead, 2006). Chronic high intake of zinc can also cause abnormalities of genitourinary functions (Johnson et al., 2007).

3. Zinc homeostasis and transport

Total zinc in human body is about 2-3 g for a 70 kg adult (Wastney et al., 1986). Ninety percent is incorporated in the muscle, most of which are poorly exchangeable and tightly bound to high molecular weight ligands such as metalloenzymes, metalloproteins, nucleoproteins and nucleic acids. The remaining 10% of zinc is readily exchangeable and loosely bound to amino acid and citrate (Frederickson, 1989; Outten & O'Halloran, 2001). This pool of zinc is found in plasma, liver and bone and is metabolically active, rapidly exchanged and sensitive to changes in the bioavailability of zinc in the diet. The prostate gland, pancreas, adrenal gland, certain areas of the brain, inner ear and eye, skin, nails, hair, red and white blood cells are known to accumulate high concentrations of zinc (Tapiero & Tew, 2003).

The concentrations of zinc are strictly regulated *in vivo* because dysregulation of zinc homeostasis can result in pathogenic consequences. Approximately 30-40% of intracellular zinc is localized in the nucleus, 50% in the cytosol and cytosolic organelles and the remainder are associated with cell membranes (Vallee & Falchuk, 1993). Zinc transporters play important roles in maintaining zinc homeostasis, as zinc ions are hydrophilic and do not cross cell membranes by passive diffusion (Cousins & McMahon, 2000). There are two known families of zinc transporters i.e. the ZIP (Zrt/Irt-like proteins (SLC39A)) family and the cation diffusion facilitator/Zinc transporter (CDF/ZnT (SLC30A)) family. At least 15 members of the ZIP family (Zn^{2+}-regulated metal transporter) (Cousins et al., 2006) and 10 members from the ZnT family (Eide, 2004) are found in mammalian cells. ZnT transporters regulate zinc efflux from cells or into intracellular vesicles, hence, reduce intracellular zinc availability, whereas ZIP members of the ZIP family participate in the transport of zinc, iron, and/or manganese. The human ZIP1, ZIP2, and ZIP4 proteins are involved in zinc uptake across the plasma membrane of various cell types (Eide, 2004).

4. Major functions of zinc

4.1 Structural and catalytic functions

Zinc has structural, catalytic and regulatory functions. It is a structural element found in many enzymes essential for DNA synthesis, transcription, aminoacyl-tRNA synthesis and ribosomal functions. It is found in zinc finger motifs of more than two thousands of transcription factors where these motifs provide a platform for interaction with DNA or other proteins (Vallee et al., 1991). Zincs are also found in LIM domains in proteins important for cytoskeletal organization, organ development and oncogenesis (Kadrmas & Beckerle, 2004). Zinc regulates cell proliferation and differentiation by modulating nucleic acid metabolisms and protein synthesis. It also controls cell growth by activating, transporting and modulating growth hormone, insulin-like growth factor-1, prolactin, testosterone and other steroid hormones (Costello et al., 1999; Ozturk et al., 2005; Prasad et al., 1996; Turgut et al., 2005). Zinc, unlike the highly reactive copper and iron, does not participate in redox reactions (Berg & Shi, 1996). The incorporation of zinc into proteins instead of these highly reactive elements helps prevent the generation of free radicals (Ho, 2004). Zinc, hence, has anti-oxidant activities. It maintains proper folding, stability and activity of zinc-dependent enzymes by protecting these enzymes from free radicals attacks (Coleman, 1992). Some of the zinc-dependent enzymes include superoxide dismutase, carbonic anhydrase, alkaline phosphatase, glutamic dehydrogenase, nucleotidase, carboxypeptidase A, retinal dehydrogenase and angiotensin-converting enzymes. Intracellular zinc also protects several compounds from oxidative damage and these include citrate in the prostate gland (Omu et al., 1998) and insulin in the secretory granules of the islet beta cells (Zalewski et al., 1994). In addition, zinc exerts its anti-oxidant abilities indirectly by maintaining an adequate level of the free radical scavengers such as metallothioneins (MTs) (Prasad, 1993; Tapiero & Tew, 2003). It also stabilizes cell membrane structure such as that of the red blood cells (Hennig et al., 1996) and sperm cells (Omu et al., 1998). Zinc-bound melanin granules of the skin, choroids, iris, retina, photoreceptors of the eye also provide protection against oxidative damage and apoptosis (Borovansky, 1994).

4.2 Zinc and immunity

Zinc is critical for immune function and is involved in many aspects of the immune system (Shankar & Prasad, 1998). Deficiency of zinc causes dysfunction of cells involved in innate immunity such as macrophages, neutrophils and natural killer (NK) cells and affects phagocytosis, intracellular killing, cytokine production, complement activity and delayed-type hypersensitivity. Zinc is also important for gene regulation in T lymphocytes. It activates pituitary growth hormone and thymulin, the thymic hormone that stimulates division, differentiation and maturation of T-cells, lymphocyte proliferation and cytotoxic activity of natural killer cells (Baum et al., 2000; Prasad, 1998). It also modulates the function of T-helper cells by regulating lymphokines, interleukin-2 (IL-2), interferon-gamma (IFN-γ) and tumour necrosis factor-alpha (TNF-α) in response to invasion of pathogens (Baum et al., 2000). It is also known that zinc helps in tissue repair and wound healing by stimulating keratinocyte proliferation and migration to the injured area (Tenaud et al., 2000) and scavenges proinflammatory cytokines-produced nitric oxide to prevent tissue damage (Yamaoka et al., 2000).

4.3 Zinc in cell signaling

Zinc is involved in many aspects of cell signaling, ranging from signal recognition, second messenger metabolisms to the regulation of gene expressions. It regulates signaling processes by directly modulating the activities of kinases, phosphatases, and transcription factors (Beyersmann & Haase, 2001) or acting on its own as an intracellular secondary messenger (Fukada et al., 2011; Yamasaki et al., 2007). Zinc initiates the signaling cascades by stimulating the activation of several receptors and ion channels and these include epidermal growth factor receptor (EGF-R) (Wu et al., 1999); insulin growth factor-1 receptor (IGF-1-R) (Haase & Maret, 2005); Gamma-AminoButyric Acid (GABA) receptor (Parviz & Gross, 2007); N-methyl-D-aspartate (NMDA) channels of the neuronal cells (Smart et al., 2004); voltage-gated Ca^{2+} (Magistretti et al., 2003), the calcium permeable α-amino-3-hydroxy-5-methyl-4-isoxazole-propionate (AMPA) channels (Blakemore & Trombley, 2004), transient receptor potential ankyrin (Hu et al., 2009) and ATP-sensitive K^+ channels (Prost et al., 2004). It also affects the activities of several second messengers. It is shown that zinc inhibits cyclic adenosine monophosphate (cAMP) signaling (Klein et al., 2002) and elevates cyclic guanosine monophosphate (cGMP) levels (Watjen et al., 2001).

Zinc regulates the transcription of genes important for cell proliferation and differentiation by modulating transcription factors such as metal response element-binding transcription factor-1, MTF-1 (Langmade et al., 2000); Egr-1 (Adamson et al., 2003); AP-1 and NF-κB (Herbein et al., 2006; Uzzo et al., 2006); Jun and ATF-2 (Samet et al., 1998). Among these, MTF-1 to date is the best-characterized zinc-activated transcription factors. MTF-1 responds acutely to changes in intracellular zinc concentrations by binding with zinc and translocates to nucleus. It then activates genes transcription by binding to promoters of other known zinc-responsive genes such as metallothioneins (MTs) and zinc transporter, ZnT-1 that regulate intracellular zinc concentrations (Langmade et al., 2000). Other zinc finger transcription factors such as Egr-1, AP-1 and NF-κB are important for the regulation of genes that control cells proliferation. Deregulation of these transcription factors contributes to cancer cells proliferation, metastasis and angiogenesis. How zinc affects the regulation of these transcription factors and their outcomes, however, varies. It is shown in a number of studies, that zinc at different concentrations activate or suppress the activities of NF-κB in different cell lines resulting in different cellular responses (Kim et al., 2007; Uzzo et al., 2006; Uzzo et al., 2002).

Zinc modulates kinases and phosphatases of major cells signaling pathways. A number of studies showed that zinc stimulates EGF receptor phosphorylation and activates members of the MAPKs family such as ERK (Hansson, 1996; Klein et al., 2006; Samet et al., 1998; Uzzo et al., 2006) and p38 kinase (Huang et al., 1999; Wu et al., 1999; Wu et al., 2005) activities in prostate cancer cells, murine fibroblasts, human bronchial epithelial cells, human airway epithelial cells and mouse cortical cells. Zinc also induces the phosphorylation of p70S6 kinase in murine fibroblasts, c-jun N-terminal kinase (JNK) in mouse cortical cells through phosphatidylinositol 3-kinase (P13K) signaling pathway (Eom et al., 2001; Kim et al., 2000), protein kinase C (PKC) activation (Csermely et al., 1988), protein kinase B (PKB) and glycogen synthase kinase (GSK)-3β activities in neuroblastoma cells (An et al., 2005). A number of studies also described the role of zinc in the modulation of phosphatases. Treatment of the human airway epithelial cells and C6 rat glioma cells with zinc increased protein tyrosine phosphorylation by inhibiting phosphatases such as PTP1B and SHP-1 (Haase & Maret, 2005) and zinc also inhibits the dual-specificity phosphatase VHR (Kim et al., 2000). These findings illustrate the extensive involvement of zinc on cellular signaling pathways and genes transcription. Balanced zinc homeostasis, therefore is vital for normal cell growth and differentiation; and deviations from optimal zinc levels may contribute to pathophysiologic consequences observed in many zinc-related diseases. Most of these zinc-affected pathways are also deregulated in many types of cancer and this further highlights the importance of zinc homeostasis in oncogenesis.

5. Zinc and the prostate gland

The human prostate gland is divided into three distinct morphological regions which include the peripheral, central and transition zones (McNeal, 1981). The peripheral zone contains the majority of the glandular tissues present in the normal prostate and accounts for 70% of the volume in the young adult prostate. The central zone consists of larger acini and has a more complex ductal branching while the transition zone comprises of glands lobules with shorter ducts in comparison to those in the peripheral zone. The central and transition zones account for 25% and 5% of the prostate volume, respectively.

The normal peripheral zone of the prostate gland accumulates the highest concentrations of zinc in comparison to other soft tissues of the body (Kar & Chowdhury, 1966; Lahtonen, 1985). The ability to accumulate zinc in the peripheral zone is due to the presence of highly specialized secretory epithelial cells that is not found in the central zone of the prostate. hZIP1 transporter is an important transporter for uptake from the circulation and accumulation in the prostate gland (Costello et al., 1999; Desouki et al., 2007) while hZIP-2 and hZIP-3 retain zinc in the cellular compartment (Desouki et al., 2007).

hZIP1 transporters are downregulated in adenocarcinoma cells and in prostate intra-epithelial neoplastic loci (PIN) (Rishi et al., 2003). This causes not only a decrease in zinc uptake (Franklin et al., 2005a; Franklin et al., 2003; Franklin et al., 2005b) but also reduces the capacity to accumulate zinc (Huang et al., 2006). The downregulation of hZIP1 is also associated with high prostate cancer risk in African American male population in comparison with Caucasians (Rishi et al., 2003). hZIP2, hZIP3 and ZnT4 are also found downregulated in malignant tissues in comparison to nonmalignant and Benign prostatic hyperplasia (BPH) tissues (Beck et al., 2004; Desouki et al., 2007). These findings collectively suggest that alterations of intracellular zinc due to changes in zinc transporters expression are associated to the development prostate cancer. It is suggested that human *ZIP1*, *ZIP2* and *ZIP3* genes may be tumor suppressor genes (Desouki et al., 2007) and zinc may be a tumor suppressor agent (Franklin & Costello, 2007).

5.1 Association of zinc with prostate cancer

It is still unclear of the role of zinc in malignant diseases but abnormal levels of zinc in serum of cancer patients and malignant tissues are widely reported. Serum zinc levels are increased in melanoma patients (Ros-Bullon et al., 1998) but more often, reduced serum zinc levels are reported in breast (Sharma et al., 1994; Yucel et al., 1994), gallbladder (Gupta et al., 2005), lung (Diez et al., 1989; Issell et al., 1981), Hodgkin's disease (Cunzhi et al., 2001), colorectal (Gupta et al., 1993), neck (Buntzel et al., 2007), leukemia (Zuo et al., 2006) and thyroid (Al-Sayer et al., 2004) cancer patients. Elevated zinc levels in malignant tissues are observed in breast (Margalioth et al., 1983), intestinal (Kucharzewski et al., 2003), metastatic nasopharyngeal (Bay et al., 1997) cancers but are decreased in kidney carcinoma tissues (Margalioth et al., 1983). It is also high in bone marrow of patients with non-Hodgkin lymphomas (Schmitt et al., 1993). In prostate cancer, decreased zinc levels are consistently observed in malignant tissue samples from different populations and at various stages of malignancy (Vartsky et al., 2003; Zaichick et al., 1997). Analysis of malignant prostate tissues showed a 60-70% reduction of zinc levels in comparison to those of the normal peripheral zone tissues (Zaichick et al., 1997). The plasma zinc level between patients with malignancy is also significantly lower than normal patients (Goel & Sankhwar, 2006).

5.1.1 Epidemiologic studies

It is reported that dietary zinc supplementation protects against oxidative damage, reduces cancer risk (Ho, 2004) and is beneficial against prostate tumorigenesis (Franklin & Costello, 2007). Findings from several epidemiologic studies, however, attain no consensus on the effectiveness of zinc against prostate cancer, partly because of differences in experimental design, amount of zinc administered and methods in determining plasma/serum zinc status (Haase et al., 2008). Several studies showed that there are either no beneficiary effects of zinc or there are no potential adverse effects of dietary zinc on prostate cancer risk (Andersson et al., 1996; Kolonel, 1996; Vlajinac et al., 1997; West et al., 1991). In contrast, there are reports which concluded that zinc reduces prostate cancer risk (Epstein et al., 2011; Key et al., 1997; Kristal et al., 1999). Gonzalez et al. (2009) reported that dietary zinc was not associated with prostate cancer and 10-year average intake of supplemental zinc does not reduce the overall risk of prostate cancer. However, they found that risk of advanced prostate cancer decreases with greater intake of supplemental zinc in their VITamins And Lifestyle (VITAL) cohort study (Gonzalez et al., 2009). There are also reports that showed high zinc intake increases the risk of advanced prostate cancer (Gallus et al., 2007; Lawson et al., 2007; Leitzmann et al., 2003) and higher intake of dietary zinc could also potentiate the development of BPH and progression towards cancer (Lagiou et al., 1999; Moyad, 2004). Although further studies are required in this area, these reports nevertheless, raised concern for potential detrimental outcomes of long-term use of high zinc-supplements in men.

5.1.2 *In vitro* studies

The beneficial effects of zinc in prostate cancer intervention and treatment were investigated *in vitro* and *in vivo* but yielded contradictory observations as well. Several *in vitro* zinc studies showed that zinc inhibits prostate cancer cells proliferation and invasion through the induction of necrotic cell death and caspase-mediated mitochondrial apoptogenesis (Feng et al., 2002; Feng et al., 2000; Iguchi et al., 1998; Liang et al., 1999). Other suggested inhibitory mechanisms include increased levels of Bax or decreased Bcl-2 and survivin expression-mediated apoptosis effect (Ku et al., 2010) and zinc-induced proteasomal degradation of HIF-1α, a protein often upregulated in tumors leading to more aggressive tumor growth and chemoresistance (Nardinocchi et al., 2010). In addition, zinc was reported to repress the metastatic potential of prostate cancer cells through various mechanisms. These include inhibition of NF-κB activities (Uzzo et al., 2006), suppression of the invasive potentials of human prostate aminopeptidase N and urokinase-type plasminogen activator (Ishii et al., 2001a; Ishii et al., 2001b) as well as inhibiting proteolytic activities of prostate specific antigen (PSA) (Ishii et al., 2004). In contrast, it is also reported that zinc promotes cancer cell growth by enhancing telomerase activity, an enzyme thought to be responsible for the continuous proliferation of tumor cells (Nemoto et al., 2000) and suppressing the inhibitory potential of bisphosphonates on tumor cell invasion (Boissier et al., 2000). Our studies also showed that restoration of high zinc for a prolonged period could only inhibit zinc proliferation transiently, after which the malignant cell growth was restored and acquired a more aggressive behaviour (Wong & Abubakar, 2008a; Wong & Abubakar, 2010).

5.1.3 *In vivo* studies

The association of zinc with prostate cancer and the therapeutic potentials of zinc in prostate cancer were also investigated *in vivo* (Table 1). Two early studies using xenograft mice inoculated with PC-3 cells (Feng et al., 2003) and PC-3-hZIP1 cells (Golovine et al., 2008) showed that zinc treatment resulted in inhibition of tumor growth. Feng et al. (2003) showed that inhibition of tumor growth was due to zinc-induced apoptosis. Golovine et al. (2008) showed that overexpression of hZIP1 transporter in PC3 cancer cells resulted in increased zinc uptake, decreased tumor volume and inhibition of NFκB activity which are usually high in PC3 cells at physiological zinc serum range (0.5–1.5 µg/ml). Direct intratumoral injection of zinc in mM range was also shown to halt prostate cancer cell growth in xenograft mice (Shah et al., 2009) but the practicality of using intratumoral administration in human remains in question. Prasad et al. (2010) used a more relevant mouse model i.e. transgenic adenocarcinoma of the mouse prostate (TRAMP) mice in their study to determine the role of zinc in the development of prostate cancer. TRAMP mice develop spontaneous autochtonous disease which enables studies on the transformation of normal prostatic cells, progression and metastasis of prostate cancer (Gingrich et al., 1996). These mice were given 0.85 ppm zinc (deficient), 30 ppm zinc (optimal) and 150 ppm zinc (high) for 14 weeks. Their results showed that prostate tumor weights were higher at both zinc-deficient and high zinc-supplemented mice which led them to suggest that zinc at optimal levels is preventive whereas at both deficient and higher levels it may enhance tumor growth (Prasad et al., 2010).

Animal models	Zinc concentrations given	Duration of treatment	Findings	References
Nude mice inoculated with PC3	0.25 μL/h	28 days (4 weeks)	Inhibition of tumor growth	Feng et al., 2003
C.B17/ICR-SCID mice inoculated with PC-3-hZIP1 in the flank region	2000 ppm	23 days (3.3 weeks)	Decreased tumor volume	Golovine et al., 2008
NOD/SCID inoculated with PC3 cells in the dorsum of animals	200 μL of 3 mM zinc acetate per injection	direct intratumoral injection every 48 hours for a period of two weeks	Halted prostate cancer cells growth	Shah et al., 2009
TRAMP mice	zinc deficient (0.85 ppm), optimal (normal) zinc (30 ppm) and high zinc (150 ppm)	14 weeks	Significantly higher tumor weights in zinc-deficient or high-zinc fed mice	Prasad et al., 2010
Sprague-Dawley rats using N-methyl-N-nitrosourea MNU+ testosterone (MNU + T)	100 ppm	3 times / week	Fewer incidences of hyperplasia, dysplasia, and prostatic intraepithelial neoplasia in the ventral prostate zinc-treated mice	Banudevi et al., 2011
Sprague-Dawley rats using MNU+ cyproterone acetate + testosterone propionate	227 mg/L (equivalent to 227 ppm)	20 weeks	Increased incidence of prostate intraepithelial neoplasm	Ko et al., 2010

Table 1. *In vivo* zinc studies using murine models

To investigate the chemopreventive potential of zinc, Banudevi et al. (2011) treated prostate cancer induced Sprague-Dawley rats using N-methyl-N-nitrosourea MNU+ testosterone (MNU + T) with zinc (100 ppm) thrice a week. The zinc-treated mice showed fewer incidences of hyperplasia, dysplasia, and prostatic intraepithelial neoplasia in the ventral prostate compared to the non-treated group (Banudevi et al., 2011). They concluded that zinc may act as a potential chemopreventive agent in targeting prostate cancer. However, in another study on prostate cancer induced Sprague-Dawley rats using MNU+ cyproterone acetate + testosterone propionate fed with zinc sulfate heptahydrate dissolved in drinking water (227 mg/L or 227 ppm) for 20 weeks, they found high dietary zinc increased intraprostatic zinc concentrations and promoted prostate intraepithelial neoplasm (Ko et al., 2010). A much higher zinc and longer duration of treatment may be responsible for the observations made by Ko et al. (2010), it nevertheless suggests that high zinc treatment for a prolonged period may have detrimental outcomes.

5.2 Mechanisms of zinc-induced prostate cancer pathogenesis

It is established that zinc deficiency is associated with prostate cancer development based on the observation of significantly low/absence of zinc in cancerous prostate tissues and indirect evidences from *in vitro* and animal studies. It remains to be unraveled whether the absence of zinc is a consequence of cells transformation or whether zinc deficiency directly contributes to transformation.

A number of studies showed that zinc exerts both growth and metabolic effects on prostate cells and contribute to the development of prostate malignancy by altering citrate metabolism (Costello et al., 2004; Singh et al., 2006). It is reported in these studies that zinc inhibits *in vitro* cultured human prostate cell lines (LNCaP, PC3 and BPH-1) and rat ventral prostate epithelium cells proliferation by inducing mitochondrial apoptogenesis by releasing cytochrome *c*, which then activates subsequent caspase mediated-apoptotic cascading events leading to apoptosis. It is also shown that zinc inhibits the gene expression and activity of m-aconitase in prostate cells (Costello et al., 1997; Tsui et al., 2006). These findings led to the proposal that the presence of high zinc in normal prostate limits citrate oxidation via the Krebs cycle resulting in accumulation of high citrate levels for the secretion of prostatic fluids (Costello et al., 1997). In the transformed prostate cells, where zinc concentration is very low or absent, citrate oxidation can proceed via the Krebs cycle to generate ATP, thus, providing unlimited energy for malignant cells growth (Costello et al., 2004; Costello & Franklin, 2006). Concurrently, as intracellular zinc decreases, the apoptogenic effects of zinc are also removed, hence encourages malignant cells proliferation (Costello et al., 2004). Based on these observations, these authors suggest that restoration of zinc to prostate may be an effective treatment for prostate cancer.

Although the proposed mechanisms are plausible, it is also discussed above that zinc has diverse effects on cellular processes and mediates various signaling transduction pathways including those that are implicated in the development and progression of prostate cancer. This point was exemplified in another study that showed the involvement of zinc in Akt pathway (Han et al., 2009). Akt/protein kinase B (PKB) gene is amplified in cancerous prostate tissues and increase in its kinase activities are associated with hormone-resistant prostate cancer (Edwards et al., 2003). Activation of Akt pathway promotes the survival and protection of cancer cells from apoptosis by inhibiting downstream death proteins such as Bad, caspase-9 and forkhead transcription factors (FHTF) (Cantley, 2002). Phosphatase and TENsin homolog (PTEN), a tumor suppressor, negatively regulate the phosphorylation of Akt and maintains it at basal level. Normal prostate cells accumulates high zinc and during zinc deficiency, Han et al. (2009) showed that Akt is hyperphosphorylated in prostate normal epithelial cells (PrEC) and led to Mdm2 phosphorylation and decreased nuclear accumulation of p53. This resulted in reduced tumor-suppressive effect of p53, hence, maintaining the progression of the cell cycle and promoting cell survival through an Akt-Mdm2-p53 signaling axis. In LNCaP prostate cancer cells where PTEN is deleted and mutated, Akt phosphorylation becomes uninhibited. In zinc-deficient LNCaP cells, it is suggested that Akt phosphorylates p21, inhibits its nuclear entry and promotes cytoplasmic degradation. Hence, zinc-deficient LNCaP cells could survive and progress through the G0/G1 phase of the cell cycle. This study showed that zinc is important in maintaining the survival of normal prostate cells and in its absence, the malignant cells uses alternative pathway to promote cell survival instead.

Difference in response to zinc between normal and malignant cells was also observed in our previous studies. We demonstrated an increasing percentage of senescent normal prostate PNT2 cells when treated with a high zinc concentration but this was not observed in LNCaP cells (Wong & Abubakar, 2008b). Hence, high zinc in the normal prostate regulates healthy prostate cell growth by maintaining senescence but this regulatory role is lost in zinc-deficient cancerous tissues. Han et al. (2009) also showed that cell growth was unchanged for LNCaP cells supplemented with high zinc although G2/M populations was depressed, which is similar to our observation (Wong & Abubakar, 2008a). Since there was no change in nuclear p21 level in high zinc-treated LNCaP cells in the study by Han et al., (2009), restoration of high zinc to LNCaP cells may have affected other pathways. We showed that restoration of high zinc to LNCaP for a longer period (5 weeks) resulted in upregulation of protein expression of Vaccinia H1-related (VHR) phosphatase, zeta chain-associated protein-70 (ZAP-70) kinase and phosphorylated extracellular signal-regulated protein kinase 1 and 2 (p-ERK 1 and 2) which declined after chelation of Zn^{2+}, highlighting the possible association of zinc with VHR/ZAP-70-associated pathways in the modulation of LNCaP prostate cancer cell growth.

To further determine the effects of prolonged high zinc treatment on global gene expressions in LNCaP prostate cancer cells, we continuously cultured LNCaP cells for at least five passages over a 5 week period in growth medium supplemented with supraphysiologic concentrations of Zn^{2+} (Wong & Abubakar, 2010). Various methods were employed to demonstrate the intracellular accumulation of zinc and these are correlated with the cancer cell growth and proliferation. Specific gene expression analysis using microarray was used to examine the different gene expression levels and validated using quantitative real time polymerase chain reaction amplification. Using this approach it was observed that high intracellular zinc initially inhibited prostate cell growth and colony formation on soft agar. The inhibition, however, is transient as the cancer cell growth rate recovers to the pre-zinc treatment cancerous cell growth rate. Results from microarray studies using these prolonged high zinc-treated cells suggest that the recovery is accompanied by high expression of genes known to promote prostate cancer cell proliferation, migration and aggressiveness. Genes such as *FASN, FAD, TACSTD1, FBL, ADRM1, E2F3, CD164* and *STEAP1* are highly expressed. In addition, *CD164, FBL* and *TACSTD1* were also found upregulated in increasing presence of high zinc in normal prostate PNT2 cells. Collectively, these findings suggest that zinc initially suppresses cell growth, perhaps by repressing the expressions of selected growth promoting genes but the ability of zinc to regulate these genes in the cancerous tissues are eventually lost, resulting in the superinduction of the expression of these genes which in turn promote the survival of the prostate cancer cells even when the intracellular zinc level is high. These observations, thus, support the epidemiologic findings that high zinc intake is associated with the progression to advanced aggressive prostate cancer. In another gene profiling study of normal human prostatic cell line HPR-1 and androgen-independent malignant prostate cancer PC3 cells treated with zinc (20 μM) for 1-6 hours, it was also observed that zinc affects many genes involved in oncogenesis pathways although genes associated with zinc accumulation and zinc-induced apoptosis are also found responsive (Lin et al., 2009). In their study, Fos, which codes for a transcription factor associated with AP-1, was dramatically up-regulated by short-term zinc treatment in PC-3 cells and up-regulation of c-Fos protein is known to occur in advanced human prostate cancer (Ouyang et al., 2008). They also showed that expression of the Akt1 and PIK3 genes, associated with the Akt pathway, was dramatically upregulated in normal cells but remained unaffected in the cancer cells. However, the long-term effect of zinc on the expression of these genes is not known since cells were only treated for 6 hours in this study. This observation nevertheless supports the role of zinc in regulating malignancy promoting genes in normal cells but its control is lost in the cancerous tissues. The consequences following the loss of zinc regulation of cancer-promoting genes warrant further research.

6. Conclusion

Despite the contrasting reports on the effects of zinc on prostate cancer cells, these studies collectively affirmed the importance of zinc in the regulation of prostate health under normal physiologic conditions. Adverse consequences are apparent with zinc deficiency as well as with high zinc supplementation. The diverse effects of zinc on prostate cells reflects the immensity of zinc interactions with various cellular kinases, phosphatases, signaling transduction molecules and transcription factors in the regulation of normal cellular processes and immune responses, thereby also affecting those of the tumor cells and tumor microenvironment (John et al., 2010) once the normal cells transformed. Because of the extensive involvement of zinc in cellular signaling networks which includes its potential role in regulating cancer-promoting genes, simple restoration of high intracellular zinc concentration to the cancerous tissues may not be corrective. Instead, it may further fuel aberrant signaling in cancer cells leading to deleterious consequences. The use of zinc therapy based on its ability to induce apoptosis is effective perhaps when given intratumorally but dietary supplementation of zinc faces with issues of bioavailability and difficulties in achieving therapeutically meaningful dose in diseased prostate. The effects of chronic use of zinc still require further research with standardized zinc preparations, methods of zinc measurement, patient selection and statistical analysis to achieve a final consensus of the effectiveness of zinc in prostate cancer prevention and treatment. On the other hand, research focus on developing methods of using endogenous zinc (Ghosh et al., 2010) for early detection and progression of prostate cancer in human as well as utilizing zinc-regulated genes for diagnosis or targeting them for treatment of prostate cancer may be more relevant in this regard.

7. Acknowledgement

The authors thank University of Malaya and Ministry of Science, Technology and Innovations, Malaysia for provision of research fundings received under Program of Research In Priority Area (IRPA) Grant No. 06-02-03-1025, VotF-382/2005C and VotF-0173/2003B.

8. References

Adamson, E., de Belle, I., Mittal, S., Wang, Y., Hayakawa, J., Korkmaz, K., O'Hagan, D., McClelland, M. & Mercola, D. (2003). Egr1 signaling in prostate cancer. *Cancer Biol Ther*, Vol. 2, No. 6. Nov-Dec, pp. 617-622, Issn 1538-4047 (Print) 1538-4047 (Linking)

Al-Sayer, H., Mathew, T. C., Asfar, S., Khourshed, M., Al-Bader, A., Behbehani, A. & Dashti, H. (2004). Serum changes in trace elements during thyroid cancers. *Mol Cell Biochem*, Vol. 260, No. 1-2. May, pp. 1-5, Issn 0300-8177 (Print) 0300-8177 (Linking)

An, W. L., Bjorkdahl, C., Liu, R., Cowburn, R. F., Winblad, B. & Pei, J. J. (2005). Mechanism of zinc-induced phosphorylation of p70 s6 kinase and glycogen synthase kinase 3beta in sh-sy5y neuroblastoma cells. *J Neurochem*, Vol. 92, No. 5. Mar, pp. 1104-1115, Issn 0022-3042 (Print) 0022-3042 (Linking)

Andersson, S. O., Wolk, A., Bergstrom, R., Giovannucci, E., Lindgren, C., Baron, J. & Adami, H. O. (1996). Energy, nutrient intake and prostate cancer risk: A population-based case-control study in Sweden. *Int J Cancer*, Vol. 68, No. 6. Dec 11, pp. 716-722, Issn 0020-7136 (Print)

Banudevi, S., Elumalai, P., Arunkumar, R., Senthilkumar, K., Gunadharini, D. N., Sharmila, G. & Arunakaran, J. (2011). Chemopreventive effects of zinc on prostate carcinogenesis induced by N-methyl-N-nitrosourea and testosterone in adult male sprague-dawley rats. *J Cancer Res Clin Oncol*, Vol. 137, No. 4. Apr, pp. 677-686, Issn 1432-1335 (Electronic) 0171-5216 (Linking)

Baum, M. K., Shor-Posner, G. & Campa, A. (2000). Zinc status in human immunodeficiency virus infection. *J Nutr*, Vol. 130, No. 5S Suppl. May, pp. 1421S-1423S, Issn 0022-3166 (Print) 0022-3166 (Linking)

Bay, B., Chan, Y., Fong, C. & Leong, H. (1997). Differential cellular zinc levels in metastatic and primary nasopharyngeal carcinoma. *Int J Oncol*, Vol. 11, No. 4. Oct, pp. 745-748, Issn 1019-6439 (Print) 1019-6439 (Linking)

Beck, F. W., Prasad, A. S., Butler, C. E., Sakr, W. A., Kucuk, O. & Sarkar, F. H. (2004). Differential expression of hZnT-4 in human prostate tissues. *Prostate*, Vol. 58, No. 4. Mar 1, pp. 374-381, Issn 0270-4137 (Print)

Berg, J. M. & Shi, Y. (1996). The galvanization of biology: A growing appreciation for the roles of zinc. *Science*, Vol. 271, No. 5252. Feb 23, pp. 1081-1085, Issn 0036-8075 (Print) 0036-8075 (Linking)

Beyersmann, D. & Haase, H. (2001). Functions of zinc in signaling, proliferation and differentiation of mammalian cells. *Biometals*, Vol. 14, No. 3-4. Sep-Dec, pp. 331-341, Issn 0966-0844 (Print) 0966-0844 (Linking)

Black, R. E. (2003). Zinc deficiency, infectious disease and mortality in the developing world. *J Nutr*, Vol. 133, No. 5 Suppl 1. May, pp. 1485S-1489S, Issn 0022-3166 (Print) 0022-3166 (Linking)

Blakemore, L. J. & Trombley, P. Q. (2004). Diverse modulation of olfactory bulb AMPA receptors by zinc. *Neuroreport*, Vol. 15, No. 5. Apr 9, pp. 919-923, Issn 0959-4965 (Print)

Boissier, S., Ferreras, M., Peyruchaud, O., Magnetto, S., Ebetino, F. H., Colombel, M., Delmas, P., Delaisse, J. M. & Clezardin, P. (2000). Bisphosphonates inhibit breast and prostate carcinoma cell invasion, an early event in the formation of bone metastases. *Cancer Res*, Vol. 60, No. 11. Jun 1, pp. 2949-2954, Issn 0008-5472 (Print) 0008-5472 (Linking)

Borovansky, J. (1994). Zinc in pigmented cells and structures, interactions and possible roles. *Sb Lek*, Vol. 95, No. 4. pp. 309-320, Issn 0036-5327 (Print) 0036-5327 (Linking)

Brewer, G. J. (2001). Zinc acetate for the treatment of Wilson's disease. *Expert Opin Pharmacother*, Vol. 2, No. 9. Sep, pp. 1473-1477, Issn 1465-6566 (Print)

Brown, M. A., Thom, J. V., Orth, G. L., Cova, P. & Juarez, J. (1964). Food poisoning involving zinc contamination. *Arch Environ Health*, Vol. 8, May, pp. 657-660, Issn 0003-9896 (Print)

Buntzel, J., Bruns, F., Glatzel, M., Garayev, A., Mucke, R., Kisters, K., Schafer, U., Schonekaes, K. & Micke, O. (2007). Zinc concentrations in serum during head and neck cancer progression. *Anticancer Res*, Vol. 27, No. 4A. Jul-Aug, pp. 1941-1943, Issn 0250-7005 (Print) 0250-7005 (Linking)

Cantley, L. C. (2002). The phosphoinositide 3-kinase pathway. *Science*, Vol. 296, No. 5573. May 31, pp. 1655-1657, Issn 1095-9203 (Electronic) 0036-8075 (Linking)

Coleman, J. E. (1992). Zinc proteins: Enzymes, storage proteins, transcription factors, and replication proteins. *Annu Rev Biochem*, Vol. 61, pp. 897-946, Issn 0066-4154 (Print)

Costello, L. C., Feng, P., Milon, B., Tan, M. & Franklin, R. B. (2004). Role of zinc in the pathogenesis and treatment of prostate cancer: Critical issues to resolve. *Prostate Cancer Prostatic Dis*, Vol. 7, No. 2. pp. 111-117, Issn 1365-7852 (Print)

Costello, L. C. & Franklin, R. B. (1998). Novel role of zinc in the regulation of prostate citrate metabolism and its implications in prostate cancer. *Prostate*, Vol. 35, No. 4. Jun 1, pp. 285-296, Issn 0270-4137 (Print) 0270-4137 (Linking)

Costello, L. C. & Franklin, R. B. (2006). The clinical relevance of the metabolism of prostate cancer; zinc and tumor suppression: Connecting the dots. *Mol Cancer*, Vol. 5, No., pp. 17, Issn 1476-4598 (Electronic)

Costello, L. C., Liu, Y., Franklin, R. B. & Kennedy, M. C. (1997). Zinc inhibition of mitochondrial aconitase and its importance in citrate metabolism of prostate epithelial cells. *J Biol Chem*, Vol. 272, No. 46. Nov 14, pp. 28875-28881, Issn 0021-9258 (Print) 0021-9258 (Linking)

Costello, L. C., Liu, Y., Zou, J. & Franklin, R. B. (1999). Evidence for a zinc uptake transporter in human prostate cancer cells which is regulated by prolactin and testosterone. *J Biol Chem*, Vol. 274, No. 25. Jun 18, pp. 17499-17504, Issn 0021-9258 (Print)

Cousins, R. J., Liuzzi, J. P. & Lichten, L. A. (2006). Mammalian zinc transport, trafficking, and signals. *J Biol Chem*, Vol. 281, No. 34. Aug 25, pp. 24085-24089, Issn 0021-9258 (Print) 0021-9258 (Linking)

Cousins, R. J. & McMahon, R. J. (2000). Integrative aspects of zinc transporters. *J Nutr*, Vol. 130, No. 5S Suppl. May, pp. 1384S-1387S, Issn 0022-3166 (Print) 0022-3166 (Linking)

Csermely, P., Szamel, M., Resch, K. & Somogyi, J. (1988). Zinc can increase the activity of protein kinase C and contributes to its binding to plasma membranes in T lymphocytes. *J Biol Chem*, Vol. 263, No. 14. May 15, pp. 6487-6490, Issn 0021-9258 (Print)

Cunzhi, H., Jiexian, J., Xianwen, Z., Jingang, G. & Suling, H. (2001). Classification and prognostic value of serum copper/zinc ratio in Hodgkin's disease. *Biol Trace Elem Res*, Vol. 83, No. 2. Nov, pp. 133-138, Issn 0163-4984 (Print)

Desouki, M. M., Geradts, J., Milon, B., Franklin, R. B. & Costello, L. C. (2007). hZip2 and hZip3 zinc transporters are down regulated in human prostate adenocarcinomatous glands. *Mol Cancer*, Vol. 6, pp. 37, Issn 1476-4598 (Electronic)

Deutsch, E., Maggiorella, L., Eschwege, P., Bourhis, J., Soria, J. C. & Abdulkarim, B. (2004). Environmental, genetic, and molecular features of prostate cancer. *Lancet Oncol*, Vol. 5, No. 5. May, pp. 303-313, Issn 1470-2045 (Print) 1470-2045 (Linking)

Diez, M., Arroyo, M., Cerdan, F. J., Munoz, M., Martin, M. A. & Balibrea, J. L. (1989). Serum and tissue trace metal levels in lung cancer. *Oncology*, Vol. 46, No. 4. pp. 230-234, Issn 0030-2414 (Print) 0030-2414 (Linking)

Edwards, J., Krishna, N. S., Witton, C. J. & Bartlett, J. M. (2003). Gene amplifications associated with the development of hormone-resistant prostate cancer. *Clin Cancer Res*, Vol. 9, No. 14. Nov 1, pp. 5271-5281, Issn 1078-0432 (Print) 1078-0432 (Linking)

Eide, D. J. (2004). The slc39 family of metal ion transporters. *Pflugers Arch*, Vol. 447, No. 5. Feb, pp. 796-800, Issn 0031-6768 (Print) 0031-6768 (Linking)

Eom, S. J., Kim, E. Y., Lee, J. E., Kang, H. J., Shim, J., Kim, S. U., Gwag, B. J. & Choi, E. J. (2001). Zn(2+) induces stimulation of the c-jun n-terminal kinase signaling pathway through phosphoinositide 3-kinase. *Mol Pharmacol*, Vol. 59, No. 5. May, pp. 981-986, Issn 0026-895X (Print) 0026-895X (Linking)

Epstein, M. M., Kasperzyk, J. L., Andren, O., Giovannucci, E. L., Wolk, A., Hakansson, N., Andersson, S. O., Johansson, J. E., Fall, K. & Mucci, L. A. (2011). Dietary zinc and prostate cancer survival in a swedish cohort. *Am J Clin Nutr*, Vol. 93, No. 3. Mar, pp. 586-593, Issn 1938-3207 (Electronic) 0002-9165 (Linking)

Feng, P., Li, T. L., Guan, Z. X., Franklin, R. B. & Costello, L. C. (2002). Direct effect of zinc on mitochondrial apoptogenesis in prostate cells. *Prostate*, Vol. 52, No. 4. Sep 1, pp. 311-318, Issn 0270-4137 (Print)

Feng, P., Li, T. L., Guan, Z. X., Franklin, R. B. & Costello, L. C. (2003). Effect of zinc on prostatic tumorigenicity in nude mice. *Ann N Y Acad Sci*, Vol. 1010, No., Dec, pp. 316-320, Issn 0077-8923 (Print) 0077-8923 (Linking)

Feng, P., Liang, J. Y., Li, T. L., Guan, Z. X., Zou, J., Franklin, R. & Costello, L. C. (2000). Zinc induces mitochondria apoptogenesis in prostate cells. *Mol Urol*, Vol. 4, No. 1. Spring, pp. 31-36, Issn 1091-5362 (Print)

Feustel, A. & Wennrich, R. (1984). Determination of the distribution of zinc and cadmium in cellular fractions of BPH, normal prostate and prostatic cancers of different histologies by atomic and laser absorption spectrometry in tissue slices. *Urol Res*, Vol. 12, No. 5. pp. 253-256, Issn 0300-5623 (Print)

Fischer Walker, C. & Black, R. E. (2004). Zinc and the risk for infectious disease. *Annu Rev Nutr*, Vol. 24, pp. 255-275, Issn 0199-9885 (Print)

Food and Nutrition Board, Institute of Medicine, National Academies. (2010a). Dietary Reference Intakes (DRIs): Recommended Dietary Allowances and Adequate Intakes and Vitamins, In: *United States Department of Agriculture, National Agriculture Library*, 24.06.2011, Available from: http://fnic.nal.usda.gov

Food and Nutrition Board, Institute of Medicine, National Academies. (2010b). Dietary Reference Intakes (DRIs): Tolerable Upper Intake Levels, Elements, In: *United States Department of Agriculture, National Agriculture Library*, 24.06.2011, Available from: http://fnic.nal.usda.gov

Franklin, R. B. & Costello, L. C. (2007). Zinc as an anti-tumor agent in prostate cancer and in other cancers. *Arch Biochem Biophys*, Vol. 463, No. 2. Jul 15, pp. 211-217, Issn 0003-9861 (Print)

Franklin, R. B., Feng, P., Milon, B., Desouki, M. M., Singh, K. K., Kajdacsy-Balla, A., Bagasra, O. & Costello, L. C. (2005a). Hzip1 zinc uptake transporter down regulation and zinc depletion in prostate cancer. *Mol Cancer*, Vol. 4, pp. 32, Issn 1476-4598 (Electronic)

Franklin, R. B., Ma, J., Zou, J., Guan, Z., Kukoyi, B. I., Feng, P. & Costello, L. C. (2003). Human Zip1 is a major zinc uptake transporter for the accumulation of zinc in prostate cells. *J Inorg Biochem*, Vol. 96, No. 2-3. Aug 1, pp. 435-442, Issn 0162-0134 (Print)

Franklin, R. B., Milon, B., Feng, P. & Costello, L. C. (2005b). Zinc and zinc transporters in normal prostate and the pathogenesis of prostate cancer. *Front Biosci*, Vol. 10, pp. 2230-2239, Issn 1093-4715 (Electronic)

Frederickson, C. J. (1989). Neurobiology of zinc and zinc-containing neurons. *Int Rev Neurobiol*, Vol. 31, pp. 145-238, Issn 0074-7742 (Print)

Fukada, T., Yamasaki, S., Nishida, K., Murakami, M. & Hirano, T. (2011). Zinc homeostasis and signaling in health and diseases: Zinc signaling. *J Biol Inorg Chem*, Vol., Jun 10, pp., Issn 1432-1327 (Electronic) 0949-8257 (Linking)

Gallus, S., Foschi, R., Negri, E., Talamini, R., Franceschi, S., Montella, M., Ramazzotti, V., Tavani, A., Dal Maso, L. & La Vecchia, C. (2007). Dietary zinc and prostate cancer risk: A case-control study from Italy. *Eur Urol*, Vol. 52, No. 4. Oct, pp. 1052-1056, Issn 0302-2838 (Print)

Ghosh, S. K., Kim, P., Zhang, X. A., Yun, S. H., Moore, A., Lippard, S. J. & Medarova, Z. (2010). A novel imaging approach for early detection of prostate cancer based on endogenous zinc sensing. *Cancer Res*, Vol. 70, No. 15. Aug 1, pp. 6119-6127, Issn 1538-7445 (Electronic) 0008-5472 (Linking)

Gingrich, J. R., Barrios, R. J., Morton, R. A., Boyce, B. F., DeMayo, F. J., Finegold, M. J., Angelopoulou, R., Rosen, J. M. & Greenberg, N. M. (1996). Metastatic prostate cancer in a transgenic mouse. *Cancer Res*, Vol. 56, No. 18. Sep 15, pp. 4096-4102, Issn 0008-5472 (Print) 0008-5472 (Linking)

Giovannucci, E. (2001). Medical history and etiology of prostate cancer. *Epidemiol Rev*, Vol. 23, No. 1. pp. 159-162, Issn 0193-936X (Print) 0193-936X (Linking)

Goel, T. & Sankhwar, S. N. (2006). Comparative study of zinc levels in benign and malignant lesions of the prostate. *Scand J Urol Nephrol*, Vol. 40, No. 2. pp. 108-112, Issn 0036-5599 (Print) 0036-5599 (Linking)

Golovine, K., Makhov, P., Uzzo, R. G., Shaw, T., Kunkle, D. & Kolenko, V. M. (2008). Overexpression of the zinc uptake transporter hZip1 inhibits Nuclear Factor-kappaB and reduces the malignant potential of prostate cancer cells in vitro and in vivo. *Clin Cancer Res*, Vol. 14, No. 17. Sep 1, pp. 5376-5384, Issn 1078-0432 (Print)

Gonzalez, A., Peters, U., Lampe, J. W. & White, E. (2009). Zinc intake from supplements and diet and prostate cancer. *Nutr Cancer*, Vol. 61, No. 2. pp. 206-215, Issn 1532-7914 (Electronic) 0163-5581 (Linking)

Gupta, S. K., Shukla, V. K., Vaidya, M. P., Roy, S. K. & Gupta, S. (1993). Serum and tissue trace elements in colorectal cancer. *J Surg Oncol*, Vol. 52, No. 3. Mar, pp. 172-175, Issn 0022-4790 (Print) 0022-4790 (Linking)

Gupta, S. K., Singh, S. P. & Shukla, V. K. (2005). Copper, zinc, and cu/zn ratio in carcinoma of the gallbladder. *J Surg Oncol*, Vol. 91, No. 3. Sep 1, pp. 204-208, Issn 0022-4790 (Print) 0022-4790 (Linking)

Haase, H. & Maret, W. (2005). Protein tyrosine phosphatases as targets of the combined insulinomimetic effects of zinc and oxidants. *Biometals*, Vol. 18, No. 4. Aug, pp. 333-338, Issn 0966-0844 (Print) 0966-0844 (Linking)

Haase, H., Overbeck, S. & Rink, L. (2008). Zinc supplementation for the treatment or prevention of disease: Current status and future perspectives. *Exp Gerontol*, Vol. 43, No. 5. May, pp. 394-408, Issn 0531-5565 (Print) 0531-5565 (Linking)

Han, C. T., Schoene, N. W. & Lei, K. Y. (2009). Influence of zinc deficiency on Akt-Mdm2-p53 and Akt-p21 signaling axes in normal and malignant human prostate cells. *Am J Physiol Cell Physiol*, Vol. 297, No. 5. Nov, pp. C1188-1199, Issn 1522-1563 (Electronic) 0363-6143 (Linking)

Hansson, A. (1996). Extracellular zinc ions induces mitogen-activated protein kinase activity and protein tyrosine phosphorylation in bombesin-sensitive swiss 3T3 fibroblasts. *Arch Biochem Biophys*, Vol. 328, No. 2. Apr 15, pp. 233-238, Issn 0003-9861 (Print)

Hennig, B., Toborek, M. & McClain, C. J. (1996). Antiatherogenic properties of zinc: Implications in endothelial cell metabolism. *Nutrition*, Vol. 12, No. 10. Oct, pp. 711-717, Issn 0899-9007 (Print) 0899-9007 (Linking)

Herbein, G., Varin, A. & Fulop, T. (2006). NF-kappaB, AP-1, zinc-deficiency and aging. *Biogerontology*, Vol. 7, No. 5-6. Oct-Dec, pp. 409-419, Issn 1389-5729 (Print)

Ho, E. (2004). Zinc deficiency, DNA damage and cancer risk. *J Nutr Biochem*, Vol. 15, No. 10. Oct, pp. 572-578, Issn 0955-2863 (Print)

Hu, H., Bandell, M., Petrus, M. J., Zhu, M. X. & Patapoutian, A. (2009). Zinc activates damage-sensing TRPA1 ion channels. *Nat Chem Biol*, Vol. 5, No. 3. Mar, pp. 183-190, Issn 1552-4469 (Electronic) 1552-4450 (Linking)

Huang, L., Kirschke, C. P. & Zhang, Y. (2006). Decreased intracellular zinc in human tumorigenic prostate epithelial cells: A possible role in prostate cancer progression. *Cancer Cell Int*, Vol. 6, No., pp. 10, Issn 1475-2867 (Electronic) 1475-2867 (Linking)

Huang, S., Maher, V. M. & McCormick, J. (1999). Involvement of intermediary metabolites in the pathway of extracellular Ca2+-induced mitogen-activated protein kinase activation in human fibroblasts. *Cell Signal*, Vol. 11, No. 4. Apr, pp. 263-274, Issn 0898-6568 (Print)

Iguchi, K., Hamatake, M., Ishida, R., Usami, Y., Adachi, T., Yamamoto, H., Koshida, K., Uchibayashi, T. & Hirano, K. (1998). Induction of necrosis by zinc in prostate carcinoma cells and identification of proteins increased in association with this induction. *Eur J Biochem*, Vol. 253, No. 3. May 1, pp. 766-770, Issn 0014-2956 (Print) 0014-2956 (Linking)

Ishii, K., Otsuka, T., Iguchi, K., Usui, S., Yamamoto, H., Sugimura, Y., Yoshikawa, K., Hayward, S. W. & Hirano, K. (2004). Evidence that the prostate-specific antigen (PSA)/Zn2+ axis may play a role in human prostate cancer cell invasion. *Cancer Lett*, Vol. 207, No. 1. Apr 15, pp. 79-87, Issn 0304-3835 (Print)

Ishii, K., Usui, S., Sugimura, Y., Yamamoto, H., Yoshikawa, K. & Hirano, K. (2001a). Inhibition of Aminopeptidase N (AP-N) and Urokinase-type Plasminogen Activator (UPA) by zinc suppresses the invasion activity in human urological cancer cells. *Biol Pharm Bull*, Vol. 24, No. 3. Mar, pp. 226-230, Issn 0918-6158 (Print)

Ishii, K., Usui, S., Sugimura, Y., Yoshida, S., Hioki, T., Tatematsu, M., Yamamoto, H. & Hirano, K. (2001b). Aminopeptidase N regulated by zinc in human prostate participates in tumor cell invasion. *Int J Cancer*, Vol. 92, No. 1. Apr 1, pp. 49-54, Issn 0020-7136 (Print)

Issell, B. F., MacFadyen, B. V., Gum, E. T., Valdivieso, M., Dudrick, S. J. & Bodey, G. P. (1981). Serum zinc levels in lung cancer patients. *Cancer*, Vol. 47, No. 7. Apr 1, pp. 1845-1848, Issn 0008-543X (Print) 0008-543X (Linking)

Jemal, A., Siegel, R., Xu, J. & Ward, E. (2010). Cancer statistics, 2010. *CA Cancer J Clin*, Vol. 60, No. 5. Sep-Oct, pp. 277-300, Issn 1542-4863 (Electronic) 0007-9235 (Linking)

John, E., Laskow, T. C., Buchser, W. J., Pitt, B. R., Basse, P. H., Butterfield, L. H., Kalinski, P. & Lotze, M. T. (2010). Zinc in innate and adaptive tumor immunity. *J Transl Med*, Vol. 8, pp. 118, Issn 1479-5876 (Electronic)

Johnson, A. R., Munoz, A., Gottlieb, J. L. & Jarrard, D. F. (2007). High Dose Zinc Increases Hospital Admissions Due To Genitourinary Complications. J Urol, Vol. 177, No. 2, Feb 2007, pp. 639-643, ISSN 0022-5347 (Print)

Kadrmas, J. L. & Beckerle, M. C. (2004). The LIM domain: From the cytoskeleton to the nucleus. *Nat Rev Mol Cell Biol*, Vol. 5, No. 11. Nov, pp. 920-931, Issn 1471-0072 (Print)

Kar, A. B. & Chowdhury, A. R. (1966). The distribution of zinc in the subcellular fractions of the rhesus monkey and rat prostate. *J Urol*, Vol. 96, No. 3. Sep, pp. 370-371, Issn 0022-5347 (Print) 0022-5347 (Linking)

Key, T. J., Silcocks, P. B., Davey, G. K., Appleby, P. N. & Bishop, D. T. (1997). A case-control study of diet and prostate cancer. *Br J Cancer*, Vol. 76, No. 5. pp. 678-687, Issn 0007-0920 (Print) 0007-0920 (Linking)

Kim, J. H., Cho, H., Ryu, S. E. & Choi, M. U. (2000). Effects of metal ions on the activity of protein tyrosine phosphatase VHR: Highly potent and reversible oxidative inactivation by Cu2+ ion. *Arch Biochem Biophys*, Vol. 382, No. 1. Oct 1, pp. 72-80, Issn 0003-9861 (Print)

Kim, Y. M., Cao, D., Reed, W., Wu, W., Jaspers, I., Tal, T., Bromberg, P. A. & Samet, J. M. (2007). Zn2+-induced NF-kappaB-dependent transcriptional activity involves site-specific p65/RelA phosphorylation. *Cell Signal*, Vol. 19, No. 3. Mar, pp. 538-546, Issn 0898-6568 (Print)

Klein, C., Creach, K., Irintcheva, V., Hughes, K. J., Blackwell, P. L., Corbett, J. A. & Baldassare, J. J. (2006). Zinc induces ERK-dependent cell death through a specific ras isoform. *Apoptosis*, Vol. 11, No. 11. Nov, pp. 1933-1944, Issn 1360-8185 (Print)

Klein, C., Sunahara, R. K., Hudson, T. Y., Heyduk, T. & Howlett, A. C. (2002). Zinc inhibition of CAMP signaling. *J Biol Chem*, Vol. 277, No. 14. Apr 5, pp. 11859-11865, Issn 0021-9258 (Print)

Ko, Y. H., Woo, Y. J., Kim, J. W., Choi, H., Kang, S. H., Lee, J. G., Kim, J. J., Park, H. S. & Cheon, J. (2010). High-dose dietary zinc promotes prostate intraepithelial neoplasia in a murine tumor induction model. *Asian J Androl*, Vol. 12, No. 2. Mar, pp. 164-170, Issn 1745-7262 (Electronic) 1008-682X (Linking)

Kolonel, L. N. (1996). Nutrition and prostate cancer. *Cancer Causes Control*, Vol. 7, No. 1. Jan, pp. 83-44, Issn 0957-5243 (Print) 0957-5243 (Linking)

Kristal, A. R., Stanford, J. L., Cohen, J. H., Wicklund, K. & Patterson, R. E. (1999). Vitamin and mineral supplement use is associated with reduced risk of prostate cancer. *Cancer Epidemiol Biomarkers Prev*, Vol. 8, No. 10. Oct, pp. 887-892, Issn 1055-9965 (Print) 1055-9965 (Linking)

Ku, J. H., Seo, S. Y., Kwak, C. & Kim, H. H. (2010). The role of survivin and bcl-2 in zinc-induced apoptosis in prostate cancer cells. *Urol Oncol*, Vol., Sep 3, pp., Issn 1873-2496 (Electronic) 1078-1439 (Linking)

Kucharzewski, M., Braziewicz, J., Majewska, U. & Gozdz, S. (2003). Selenium, copper, and zinc concentrations in intestinal cancer tissue and in colon and rectum polyps. *Biol Trace Elem Res*, Vol. 92, No. 1. Apr, pp. 1-10, Issn 0163-4984 (Print) 0163-4984 (Linking)

Lagiou, P., Wuu, J., Trichopoulou, A., Hsieh, C. C., Adami, H. O. & Trichopoulos, D. (1999). Diet and benign prostatic hyperplasia: A study in greece. *Urology*, Vol. 54, No. 2. Aug, pp. 284-290, Issn 1527-9995 (Electronic)

Lahtonen, R. (1985). Zinc and cadmium concentrations in whole tissue and in separated epithelium and stroma from human benign prostatic hypertrophic glands. *Prostate*, Vol. 6, No. 2. pp. 177-183, Issn 0270-4137 (Print) 0270-4137 (Linking)

Langmade, S. J., Ravindra, R., Daniels, P. J. & Andrews, G. K. (2000). The transcription factor MTF-1 mediates metal regulation of the mouse Znt1 gene. *J Biol Chem*, Vol. 275, No. 44. Nov 3, pp. 34803-34809, Issn 0021-9258 (Print)

Lawson, K. A., Wright, M. E., Subar, A., Mouw, T., Hollenbeck, A., Schatzkin, A. & Leitzmann, M. F. (2007). Multivitamin use and risk of prostate cancer in the National Institutes of Health-AARP diet and health study. *J Natl Cancer Inst*, Vol. 99, No. 10. May 16, pp. 754-764, Issn 1460-2105 (Electronic) 0027-8874 (Linking)

Leitzmann, M. F., Stampfer, M. J., Wu, K., Colditz, G. A., Willett, W. C. & Giovannucci, E. L. (2003). Zinc supplement use and risk of prostate cancer. *J Natl Cancer Inst*, Vol. 95, No. 13. Jul 2, pp. 1004-1007, Issn 1460-2105 (Electronic)

Liang, J. Y., Liu, Y. Y., Zou, J., Franklin, R. B., Costello, L. C. & Feng, P. (1999). Inhibitory effect of zinc on human prostatic carcinoma cell growth. *Prostate*, Vol. 40, No. 3. Aug 1, pp. 200-207, Issn 0270-4137 (Print)

Lin, S. F., Wei, H., Maeder, D., Franklin, R. B. & Feng, P. (2009). Profiling of zinc-altered gene expression in human prostate normal vs. cancer cells: A time course study. *J Nutr Biochem*, Vol. 20, No. 12. Dec, pp. 1000-1012, Issn 1873-4847 (Electronic) 0955-2863 (Linking)

Magistretti, J., Castelli, L., Taglietti, V. & Tanzi, F. (2003). Dual effect of Zn2+ on multiple types of voltage-dependent ca2+ currents in rat palaeocortical neurons. *Neuroscience*, Vol. 117, No. 2. pp. 249-264, Issn 0306-4522 (Print)

Maret, W. & Sandstead, H. H. (2006). Zinc requirements and the risks and benefits of zinc supplementation. *J Trace Elem Med Biol*, Vol. 20, No. 1. pp. 3-18, Issn 0946-672X (Print) 0946-672X (Linking)

Margalioth, E. J., Schenker, J. G. & Chevion, M. (1983). Copper and zinc levels in normal and malignant tissues. *Cancer*, Vol. 52, No. 5. Sep 1, pp. 868-872, Issn 0008-543X (Print) 0008-543X (Linking)

Maverakis, E., Fung, M. A., Lynch, P. J., Draznin, M., Michael, D. J., Ruben, B. & Fazel, N. (2007). Acrodermatitis enteropathica and an overview of zinc metabolism. *J Am Acad Dermatol*, Vol. 56, No. 1. Jan, pp. 116-124, Issn 1097-6787 (Electronic) 0190-9622 (Linking)

McNeal, J. E. (1981). The zonal anatomy of the prostate. *Prostate*, Vol. 2, No. 1. pp. 35-49, Issn 0270-4137 (Print) 0270-4137 (Linking)

Moyad, M. A. (2004). Zinc for prostate disease and other conditions: A little evidence, a lot of hype, and a significant potential problem. *Urol Nurs*, Vol. 24, No. 1. Feb, pp. 49-52, Issn 1053-816X (Print)

Nardinocchi, L., Pantisano, V., Puca, R., Porru, M., Aiello, A., Grasselli, A., Leonetti, C., Safran, M., Rechavi, G., Givol, D., Farsetti, A. & D'Orazi, G. (2010). Zinc downregulates HIF-1alpha and inhibits its activity in tumor cells in vitro and in vivo. *PLoS ONE*, Vol. 5, No. 12. pp. e15048, Issn 1932-6203 (Electronic)

Nemoto, K., Kondo, Y., Himeno, S., Suzuki, Y., Hara, S., Akimoto, M. & Imura, N. (2000). Modulation of telomerase activity by zinc in human prostatic and renal cancer cells. *Biochem Pharmacol*, Vol. 59, No. 4. Feb 15, pp. 401-405, Issn 0006-2952 (Print)

Omu, A. E., Dashti, H. & Al-Othman, S. (1998). Treatment of asthenozoospermia with zinc sulphate: Andrological, immunological and obstetric outcome. *Eur J Obstet Gynecol Reprod Biol*, Vol. 79, No. 2. Aug, pp. 179-184, Issn 0301-2115 (Print) 0301-2115 (Linking)

Osendarp, S. J., West, C. E. & Black, R. E. (2003). The need for maternal zinc supplementation in developing countries: An unresolved issue. *J Nutr*, Vol. 133, No. 3. Mar, pp. 817S-827S, Issn 0022-3166 (Print) 0022-3166 (Linking)

Outten, C. E. & O'Halloran, T. V. (2001). Femtomolar sensitivity of metalloregulatory proteins controlling zinc homeostasis. *Science*, Vol. 292, No. 5526. Jun 29, pp. 2488-2492, Issn 0036-8075 (Print) 0036-8075 (Linking)

Ouyang, X., Jessen, W. J., Al-Ahmadie, H., Serio, A. M., Lin, Y., Shih, W. J., Reuter, V. E., Scardino, P. T., Shen, M. M., Aronow, B. J., Vickers, A. J., Gerald, W. L. & Abate-Shen, C. (2008). Activator Protein-1 transcription factors are associated with progression and recurrence of prostate cancer. *Cancer Res*, Vol. 68, No. 7. Apr 1, pp. 2132-2144, Issn 1538-7445 (Electronic) 0008-5472 (Linking)

Ozturk, A., Baltaci, A. K., Mogulkoc, R., Oztekin, E. & Kul, A. (2005). The effects of zinc deficiency and testosterone supplementation on leptin levels in castrated rats and their relation with LH, FSH and testosterone. *Neuro Endocrinol Lett*, Vol. 26, No. 5. Oct, pp. 548-554, Issn 0172-780X (Print)

Parviz, M. & Gross, G. W. (2007). Quantification of zinc toxicity using neuronal networks on microelectrode arrays. *Neurotoxicology*, Vol. 28, No. 3. May, pp. 520-531, Issn 0161-813X (Print) 0161-813X (Linking)

Prasad, A. S. (1993). Zinc in human health and disease. *J Assoc Physicians India*, Vol. 41, No. 8. Aug, pp. 519-521, Issn 0004-5772 (Print) 0004-5772 (Linking)

Prasad, A. S. (1998). Zinc and immunity. *Mol Cell Biochem*, Vol. 188, No. 1-2. Nov, pp. 63-69, Issn 0300-8177 (Print) 0300-8177 (Linking)

Prasad, A. S. (2008). Clinical, immunological, anti-inflammatory and antioxidant roles of zinc. *Exp Gerontol*, Vol. 43, No. 5. May, pp. 370-377, Issn 0531-5565 (Print) 0531-5565 (Linking)

Prasad, A. S., Halsted, J. A. & Nadimi, M. (1961). Syndrome of iron deficiency anemia, hepatosplenomegaly, hypogonadism, dwarfism and geophagia. *Am J Med*, Vol. 31, Oct, pp. 532-546, Issn 0002-9343 (Print)

Prasad, A. S., Mantzoros, C. S., Beck, F. W., Hess, J. W. & Brewer, G. J. (1996). Zinc status and serum testosterone levels of healthy adults. *Nutrition*, Vol. 12, No. 5. May, pp. 344-348, Issn 0899-9007 (Print) 0899-9007 (Linking)

Prasad, A. S., Mukhtar, H., Beck, F. W., Adhami, V. M., Siddiqui, I. A., Din, M., Hafeez, B. B. & Kucuk, O. (2010). Dietary zinc and prostate cancer in the TRAMP mouse model. *J Med Food*, Vol. 13, No. 1. Feb, pp. 70-76, Issn 1557-7600 (Electronic) 1096-620X (Linking)

Prasad, A. S., Schulert, A. R., Miale, A., Jr., Farid, Z. & Sandstead, H. H. (1963). Zinc and iron deficiencies in male subjects with dwarfism and hypogonadism but without ancylostomiasis, schistosomiasis or severe anemia. *Am J Clin Nutr*, Vol. 12, Jun, pp. 437-444, Issn 0002-9165 (Print)

Prost, A. L., Bloc, A., Hussy, N., Derand, R. & Vivaudou, M. (2004). Zinc is both an intracellular and extracellular regulator of KATP channel function. *J Physiol*, Vol. 559, No. Pt 1. Aug 15, pp. 157-167, Issn 0022-3751 (Print) 0022-3751 (Linking)

Rishi, I., Baidouri, H., Abbasi, J. A., Bullard-Dillard, R., Kajdacsy-Balla, A., Pestaner, J. P., Skacel, M., Tubbs, R. & Bagasra, O. (2003). Prostate cancer in African american men is associated with downregulation of zinc transporters. *Appl Immunohistochem Mol Morphol*, Vol. 11, No. 3. Sep, pp. 253-260, Issn 1541-2016 (Print) 1533-4058 (Linking)

Ros-Bullon, M. R., Sanchez-Pedreno, P. & Martinez-Liarte, J. H. (1998). Serum zinc levels are increased in melanoma patients. *Melanoma Res*, Vol. 8, No. 3. Jun, pp. 273-277, Issn 0960-8931 (Print) 0960-8931 (Linking)

Samet, J. M., Graves, L. M., Quay, J., Dailey, L. A., Devlin, R. B., Ghio, A. J., Wu, W., Bromberg, P. A. & Reed, W. (1998). Activation of mapks in human bronchial epithelial cells exposed to metals. *Am J Physiol*, Vol. 275, No. 3 Pt 1. Sep, pp. L551-558, Issn 0002-9513 (Print) 0002-9513 (Linking)

Sandstrom, B. (1997). Bioavailability of zinc. *Eur J Clin Nutr*, Vol. 51 Suppl 1, Jan, pp. S17-19, Issn 0954-3007 (Print)

Schmitt, Y., Haug, M. & Kruse-Jarres, J. D. (1993). Determination of the trace elements zinc, copper, nickel and chromium in bone marrow and plasma of patients with non-hodgkin lymphomas. *J Trace Elem Electrolytes Health Dis*, Vol. 7, No. 4. Dec, pp. 223-228, Issn 0931-2838 (Print) 0931-2838 (Linking)

Shah, M.R., Kriedt, C.L., Lents, N.H., Hoyer, M.K., Jamaluddin, N., Klein, C. & Baldassare, J. (2009). Direct intra-tumoral injection of zinc-acetate halts tumor growth in a xenograft model of prostate cancer. *J Exp Clin Cancer Res*, Vol. 28, Jun 17, pp. 84, Issn 1756-9966 (Electronic) 0392-9078 (Linking)

Shankar, A. H. & Prasad, A. S. (1998). Zinc and immune function: The biological basis of altered resistance to infection. *Am J Clin Nutr*, Vol. 68, No. 2 Suppl. Aug, pp. 447S-463S, Issn 0002-9165 (Print) 0002-9165 (Linking)

Sharma, K., Mittal, D. K., Kesarwani, R. C., Kamboj, V. P. & Chowdhery. (1994). Diagnostic and prognostic significance of serum and tissue trace elements in breast malignancy. *Indian J Med Sci*, Vol. 48, No. 10. Oct, pp. 227-232, Issn 0019-5359 (Print) 0019-5359 (Linking)

Singh, K. K., Desouki, M. M., Franklin, R. B. & Costello, L. C. (2006). Mitochondrial aconitase and citrate metabolism in malignant and nonmalignant human prostate tissues. *Mol Cancer*, Vol. 5, No., pp. 14, Issn 1476-4598 (Electronic) 1476-4598 (Linking)

Smart, T. G., Hosie, A. M. & Miller, P. S. (2004). Zn2+ ions: Modulators of excitatory and inhibitory synaptic activity. *Neuroscientist*, Vol. 10, No. 5. Oct, pp. 432-442, Issn 1073-8584 (Print) 1073-8584 (Linking)

Tapiero, H. & Tew, K. D. (2003). Trace elements in human physiology and pathology: Zinc and metallothioneins. *Biomed Pharmacother*, Vol. 57, No. 9. Nov, pp. 399-411, Issn 0753-3322 (Print) 0753-3322 (Linking)

Tenaud, I., Leroy, S., Chebassier, N. & Dreno, B. (2000). Zinc, copper and manganese enhanced keratinocyte migration through a functional modulation of keratinocyte integrins. *Exp Dermatol*, Vol. 9, No. 6. Dec, pp. 407-416, Issn 0906-6705 (Print) 0906-6705 (Linking)

Tsui, K. H., Chang, P. L. & Juang, H. H. (2006). Zinc blocks gene expression of mitochondrial aconitase in human prostatic carcinoma cells. *Int J Cancer*, Vol. 118, No. 3. Feb 1, pp. 609-615, Issn 0020-7136 (Print) 0020-7136 (Linking)

Turgut, S., Kaptanoglu, B., Turgut, G., Emmungil, G. & Genc, O. (2005). Effects of cadmium and zinc on plasma levels of growth hormone, insulin-like growth factor-1, and insulin-like growth factor-binding protein 3. *Biol Trace Elem Res*, Vol. 108, No. 1-3. Winter, pp. 197-204, Issn 0163-4984 (Print)

Uriu-Adams, J. Y. & Keen, C. L. (2010). Zinc and Reproduction: Effects of Zinc Deficiency on Prenatal and Early Postnatal Development. *Birth Defects Res B Dev Reprod Toxicol*, Vol. 89, No. 4, Aug 2010, pp. 313-325, ISSN 1542-9741 (Electronic)

Uzzo, R. G., Crispen, P. L., Golovine, K., Makhov, P., Horwitz, E. M. & Kolenko, V. M. (2006). Diverse effects of zinc on NF-kappaB and AP-1 transcription factors: Implications for prostate cancer progression. *Carcinogenesis*, Vol. 27, No. 10. Oct, pp. 1980-1990, Issn 0143-3334 (Print)

Uzzo, R. G., Leavis, P., Hatch, W., Gabai, V. L., Dulin, N., Zvartau, N. & Kolenko, V. M. (2002). Zinc inhibits Nuclear Factor-kappa B activation and sensitizes prostate cancer cells to cytotoxic agents. Clin Cancer Res, Vol. 8, No. 11. Nov, pp. 3579-3583, Issn 1078-0432 (Print)

Vallee, B. L., Coleman, J. E. & Auld, D. S. (1991). Zinc fingers, zinc clusters, and zinc twists in DNA-binding protein domains. *Proc Natl Acad Sci U S A*, Vol. 88, No. 3. Feb 1, pp. 999-1003, Issn 0027-8424 (Print) 0027-8424 (Linking)

Vallee, B. L. & Falchuk, K. H. (1993). The biochemical basis of zinc physiology. *Physiol Rev*, Vol. 73, No. 1. Jan, pp. 79-118, Issn 0031-9333 (Print) 0031-9333 (Linking)

Vartsky, D., Shilstein, S., Bercovich, A., Huszar, M., Breskin, A., Chechik, R., Korotinsky, S., Malnick, S. D. & Moriel, E. (2003). Prostatic zinc and prostate specific antigen: An experimental evaluation of their combined diagnostic value. *J Urol*, Vol. 170, No. 6 Pt 1. Dec, pp. 2258-2262, Issn 0022-5347 (Print) 0022-5347 (Linking)

Vlajinac, H. D., Marinkovic, J. M., Ilic, M. D. & Kocev, N. I. (1997). Diet and prostate cancer: A case-control study. *Eur J Cancer*, Vol. 33, No. 1. Jan, pp. 101-107, Issn 0959-8049 (Print) 0959-8049 (Linking)

Wastney, M. E., Aamodt, R. L., Rumble, W. F. & Henkin, R. I. (1986). Kinetic analysis of zinc metabolism and its regulation in normal humans. *Am J Physiol*, Vol. 251, No. 2 Pt 2. Aug, pp. R398-408, Issn 0002-9513 (Print) 0002-9513 (Linking)

Watjen, W., Benters, J., Haase, H., Schwede, F., Jastorff, B. & Beyersmann, D. (2001). Zn2+ and Cd2+ increase the cyclic GMP level in PC12 cells by inhibition of the cyclic nucleotide phosphodiesterase. *Toxicology*, Vol. 157, No. 3. Jan 26, pp. 167-175, Issn 0300-483X (Print)

West, D. W., Slattery, M. L., Robison, L. M., French, T. K. & Mahoney, A. W. (1991). Adult dietary intake and prostate cancer risk in Utah: A case-control study with special emphasis on aggressive tumors. *Cancer Causes Control*, Vol. 2, No. 2. Mar, pp. 85-94, Issn 0957-5243 (Print)

Wise, A. (1995). Phytate and zinc bioavailability. *Int J Food Sci Nutr*, Vol. 46, No. 1. Feb, pp. 53-63, Issn 0963-7486 (Print) 0963-7486 (Linking)

Wong, P. F. & Abubakar, S. (2008a). High intracellular Zn2+ ions modulate the VHR, ZAP-70 and ERK activities of lncap prostate cancer cells. *Cell Mol Biol Lett*, Vol. 13, No. 3. pp. 375-390, Issn 1689-1392 (Electronic)

Wong, P. F. & Abubakar, S. (2008b). LNCaP prostate cancer cells are insensitive to zinc-induced senescence. *J Trace Elem Med Biol*, Vol. 22, No. 3. pp. 242-247, Issn 0946-672X (Print)

Wong, P. F. & Abubakar, S. (2010). Comparative transcriptional study of the effects of high intracellular zinc on prostate carcinoma cells. *Oncol Rep*, Vol. 23, No. 6. Jun, pp. 1501-1516, Issn 1791-2431 (Electronic) 1021-335X (Linking)

Wu, W., Graves, L. M., Jaspers, I., Devlin, R. B., Reed, W. & Samet, J. M. (1999). Activation of the EGF receptor signaling pathway in human airway epithelial cells exposed to metals. *Am J Physiol*, Vol. 277, No. 5 Pt 1. Nov, pp. L924-931, Issn 0002-9513 (Print)

Wu, W., Silbajoris, R. A., Whang, Y. E., Graves, L. M., Bromberg, P. A. & Samet, J. M. (2005). p38 and EGF receptor kinase-mediated activation of the phosphatidylinositol 3-kinase/Akt pathway is required for Zn2+-induced cyclooxygenase-2 expression. *Am J Physiol Lung Cell Mol Physiol*, Vol. 289, No. 5. Nov, pp. L883-889, Issn 1040-0605 (Print)

Yamaoka, J., Kume, T., Akaike, A. & Miyachi, Y. (2000). Suppressive effect of zinc ion on inos expression induced by interferon-gamma or tumor necrosis factor-alpha in murine keratinocytes. *J Dermatol Sci*, Vol. 23, No. 1. May, pp. 27-35, Issn 0923-1811 (Print) 0923-1811 (Linking)

Yamasaki, S., Sakata-Sogawa, K., Hasegawa, A., Suzuki, T., Kabu, K., Sato, E., Kurosaki, T., Yamashita, S., Tokunaga, M., Nishida, K. & Hirano, T. (2007). Zinc is a novel intracellular second messenger. *J Cell Biol*, Vol. 177, No. 4. May 21, pp. 637-645, Issn 0021-9525 (Print) 0021-9525 (Linking)

Yucel, I., Arpaci, F., Ozet, A., Doner, B., Karayilanoglu, T., Sayar, A. & Berk, O. (1994). Serum copper and zinc levels and copper/zinc ratio in patients with breast cancer. *Biol Trace Elem Res*, Vol. 40, No. 1. Jan, pp. 31-38, Issn 0163-4984 (Print) 0163-4984 (Linking)

Zaichick, V., Sviridova, T. V. & Zaichick, S. V. (1997). Zinc in the human prostate gland: Normal, hyperplastic and cancerous. *Int Urol Nephrol*, Vol. 29, No. 5. pp. 565-574, Issn 0301-1623 (Print)

Zalewski, P. D., Millard, S. H., Forbes, I. J., Kapaniris, O., Slavotinek, A., Betts, W. H., Ward, A. D., Lincoln, S. F. & Mahadevan, I. (1994). Video image analysis of labile zinc in viable pancreatic islet cells using a specific fluorescent probe for zinc. *J Histochem Cytochem*, Vol. 42, No. 7. Jul, pp. 877-884, Issn 0022-1554 (Print) 0022-1554 (Linking)

Zuo, X. L., Chen, J. M., Zhou, X., Li, X. Z. & Mei, G. Y. (2006). Levels of selenium, zinc, copper, and antioxidant enzyme activity in patients with leukemia. *Biol Trace Elem Res*, Vol. 114, No. 1-3. Winter, pp. 41-53, Issn 0163-4984 (Print) 0163-4984 (Linking)

9

The Potential Target Therapy
of Prostate Cancer Stem Cells

Luis A. Espinoza[1], Christopher Albanese[2,3] and Olga C. Rodriguez[2]
[1]Department of Biochemistry and Molecular & Cell Biology
[2]Department of Oncology
[3]Department of Pathology Georgetown University, NW Washington, DC
USA

1. Introduction

Prostate cancer is the most commonly diagnosed cancer in men and the second leading cause of cancer related mortality (Byers et al., 2006; McDavid et al., 2004; Sedjo et al., 2007). Localized prostate cancer is treated by either radical prostatectomy or radiotherapy. For aggressive prostate cancer, hormonal therapy is the standard treatment however; approximately 30% of these tumors become hormone–independent (hormone-refractory) (HRPC). Furthermore, prostate cancer cells that survive chemotherapy or radiation treatment may be able to repair most of the radiation-induced DNA breaks (Kimura et al., 1999; Kimura & Gelmann, 2000). Therefore, a primary goal in the diagnosis and management of prostate cancer is the identification of biomarkers that can reliably predict the degree of malignancy of the tumor and can also be used as potential molecular targets to improve the response to therapy. This necessity has arisen from the fact that for American males, prostate cancer is the most diagnosed neoplasia and the second leading cause of cancer-related deaths (Kendal & Mai, 2010; Sajid et al., 2011).

Risk factors associated with increased prostate cancer incidences include both age and a sub-Saharan African ancestry, with African-American men having the highest reported incidence rates of all ethnic groups in the United States (239.8 cases/100,000) (Chu et al., 2003; Odedina et al., 2009). Furthermore, deaths from prostate cancer following surgery are more than 2-fold higher in African-American men (56.3/100,000) succumbing to the disease compared to white men (23.9/100,000) (Abbott et al., 1998; Chornokur et al., 2011; Talcott et al., 2007). Death from prostate cancer is generally due to metastatic disease that results from resistance to treatment such as anti-hormonal therapy. Since African American men are two-times more likely to die of prostate cancer, identifying the mechanisms that support indolent against aggressive disease is an important area of research.

Increasing evidence suggests that primary and metastatic tumors may be initiated and sustained by a subpopulation of low abundance cancer cells with stem-like properties (Clarke et al., 2006; Clevers, 2005). These cells, known as cancer stem cells (CSC) or tumor-initiating cells (TIC), share some characteristics with normal stem cells, such as the potential of self-renewal, the capacity to clonally expand, and the ability of multi-lineage differentiation (Dalerba et al., 2007; Lang et al., 2009; Weissman et al., 2001). In addition, through acquired genetic and epigenetic changes, these cells can exhibit abnormal behavior like increased resistance to apoptosis, decreased senescence, and capacity to escape from immune surveillance. All these features can contribute to tumor dissemination, resistance to therapy, and disease recurrence.

There is little doubt that identification and characterization of CSCs is of enormous interest because they may provide important information related to the aggressiveness of the disease as well as be relevant for the development of targeted drugs to treat metastatic tumors and reduce recurrence (Park et al., 2009; Wang, 2007). It is important to note that several anticancer therapies are frequently used to eliminate prostate cancer cells; however; a number of these cells with malignant phenotypes can survive and may eventually lead to tumor regrowth (Dean et al., 2005; Dingli & Michor, 2006). Therefore, the recognition of markers for CSC and cell proliferation during the processes of prostate tumor initiation and progression is of vital importance to track CSCs for the development and improvement of therapies. It is also important to remark that subpopulations of prostate tumor cells with cancer progenitor properties are thought to support refractory response to a given treatment, leading to prostate tumor recurrence; therefore, new approaches to identifying and targeting these cancer subpopulations might provide an avenue to managing metastatic and recurrent disease refractive to treatment (Chaffer & Weinberg, 2011; Lang et al., 2009; Polyak & Hahn, 2006). This chapter will discuss the potential applications of CSC markers that may predict risk of clinical outcome and provide a guide for appropriate therapy of prostate neoplasias.

2. Stem cells in the prostate

One of the best-accepted models to explain the origin of the different cell types that make up a given tissue is the stem cell model (Reya et al., 2001; Weissman et al., 2001). In this model, most of the differentiated cell subtypes that give raise to the tissues can trace their origin to a few low-abundance progenitor cells and no longer term tissue maintenance is supported through normal adult stem cells that have the capacity for self-renewal and multi-lineage differentiation. These stem cells or progenitor cells are characterized by the high expression of specific embryonic markers and by a marked degree of plasticity that allows them to differentiate into the specific cell types required at a given point in time. According to the prostate stem cell model (Isaacs & Coffey, 1989), the progenitor cells reside primarily within the basal layer of the prostatic epithelium and have the capacity to give rise to all basal, luminal and neuroendocrine epithelial cells (Figure 1).

Prostate progenitor stem cells are androgen-independent and express high levels of stem cell markers (Table 1) such as prominin-1 (CD133), stem cell antigen (Sca1), cluster of differentiation 44 (CD44), integrin alpha2beta1 ($\alpha2\beta1$) and nestin (Collins et al., 2005; Li et al., 2008). As these progenitor cells differentiate into luminal secretory cells, they acquire the capacity to express androgen receptor (AR), prostatic specific antigen (PSA), prostatic acid phosphatase (PAP), cluster of differentiation 57 (CD57), 15-lipoxygenase 2 (15-LOX2), and cytokeratins 8 (CK8) and 18 (CK18). When the adult stem cells commit instead to the generation of non-secretory basal cells, they primarily express CD44, tumor protein 63 (p63), cytokeratin 5 (CK5) and 14 (CK14) but not AR, PSA, and PAP (Liu et al., 1997; Signoretti et al., 2000). There is a cell subtype intermediate between basal and luminal that shows expression of the CK5, CK8 and CK18 but not CK14 (Schalken, 2005). Neuroendocrine (NE) cells are found dispersed throughout the epithelium and can be identified by their expression of chromogranin A, synaptophysin, and neuron-specific enolase (NSE) (Bonkhoff et al., 1995; di Sant' Agnese, 1996). NE cells also express some peptide hormones such as somatostatin, calcitonin and serotonin. However, they do not express AR or PSA. The prostate also contains several types of stromal cell including fibroblasts, myofibroblasts, and smooth muscle cells that guide the growth and differentiation of the epithelium.

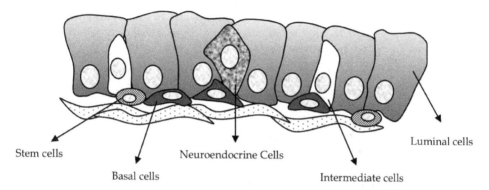

Fig. 1. The prostate epithelium niche contains a low percentage of prostate stem cells that express embryonic markers and are capable of generating the different cellular types, which compose this microenvironment. Cell types that are believed to arise from the differentiation of prostate stem cells are the basal, NE cells, and luminal secretory cells. Intermediate cells are believed to be a transitional type between basal and luminal cells.

The debate regarding the location, phenotype, number, nature, and presence of stem cells in the adult prostate still persist. However, consistent evidence supporting the existence of SC in the prostate has been reported in adult rodent prostate (English et al., 1987; Hudson, 2003; Miki, 2010). After several rounds of castration-induced regression and testosterone-induced regeneration in this animal model, a small proportion of cells (CSCs), were able to proliferate and also gave rise to differentiated and non-proliferative glandular epithelial cells. Although, the majority of luminal cells undergo apoptosis after androgen deprivation, the remaining androgen-independent epithelial cells contain a high proportion of basal cells (Montpetit et al., 1988; Webber et al., 1997a, 1997b). After regression, the remaining epithelial population appears to regenerate the prostate following androgen replacement.

The cycle of prostatic involution and regeneration can be repeated many times, indicating that the androgen-independent stem cells survive androgen deprivation and have an extensive proliferative and regenerative capacity, as well as multipotency. The identification and utilization of different types of biological markers in different in vivo models has led to the hypothesis that prostate stem cells reside within the basal cell layer of the gland. Indeed, mice null for p63, the progenitor gene for the tumor suppressor p53 family, are born without prostate or mammary glands (Mills et al., 2002; Signoretti et al., 2000). Both progenitors and basal cells of the prostate express p63, however this protein is lost during prostate differentiation and is not expressed in malignant prostatic lesions (Signoretti et al., 2000).

In humans prostate basal cells express B-cell lymphoma 2 (BCL2), an anti-apoptotic protein that is frequently expressed by stem cells and is inversely related to androgen stimulation (Lu et al., 1996). While administration of a pulse of bromodeoxyuridine (BrDU) identifies rapid proliferating transit-amplifying cells in the luminal compartment, a region that is close to the urethra, and also contains stem cells (Tsujimura et al., 2002). Because stem cells are maintained in a quiescent state, the high expression of transforming growth factor beta (TGF-β) by smooth muscle cells that form the proximal region of the prostatic ducts was proposed as a mechanism that modulates proliferation of prostatic epithelial stem cells. Indeed, blocking of TGF-β expression in the prostate induced an excessive proliferation of prostatic epithelial cells in the proximal region of the prostate (Kundu et al., 2000). Additional observations have shown that stem cells are also located in different regions of the prostate, which have the ability to survive androgen ablation and can regenerate prostatic tissue after androgen is replaced (Goto et al., 2006).

Markers expressed by prostate epithelial cells				
Stem Cells	Basal Cells	Neuroendocrine Cells	Intermediate Cells	Luminal Cells
CD133+	p63+	AR-	CD133+	AR+
CD117+	CD44+	CK18+	α2β1+	CK8+
CD49f+	CD117+	chromogranin A+	CK5+	CK18+
nestin+	CK5+	synaptophysin +	CK8+	CD57+
α2β1+	CK14+	serotonin+	CK14-	PSA+
ALDH+	AR-	somastostatin+	CK18+	PAP-
Trop-2+	PSA-			p27+
CK5+	PAP-			Sca1
CK8+				
CK14+				
CK18+				
CK19+				
AR-				
p63-				
PSA-				
PAP-				

Table 1. Complex expression of markers associated with different prostatic epithelial cells

The prolonged regenerative capacity of prostate progenitor stem cells may increase their susceptibility to accumulate genetic or epigenetic alterations during their life cycle, events that may help to promote increased proliferative rates, decreased cell death, and overall survival advantages over prostate progenitor stem cells, contributing thus to transformation (Al-Hajj & Clarke, 2004; Bapat et al., 2005; Beachy et al., 2004; Miller et al., 2005; Mimeault & Batra, 2006b, 2007a; Odedina et al., 2009). The tumor associated stem cell compartment may therefore, represent a self-replicating reservoir of malignant cells, which may accumulate further genetic and epigenetic aberrations that can thus result in therapy-resistant, tumor recurrence and/or metastasis (Hsieh et al., 2007; Rajan et al., 2009; Witte, 2009). It is believed that tumor stem cells maintain many of the features and capabilities of their normal counterpart, including long-term self-renewal and multipotency. Stem-like functions of CSCs inherited from their normal stem cells counterparts may be critical for survival during long periods of time in tissues (Hsieh et al., 2007; O'Brien et al., 2010; Rajan et al., 2009; Rosen & Jordan, 2009; Vermeulen et al., 2008; Witte, 2009). In this regard, the generation of cancer cells and their success in tumor growth are probably dependent on dysregulations affecting cells with stem-like characteristics and have the ability to promote tumor and support tumor development (Dalerba et al., 2007; Lang et al., 2009; Weissman et al., 2001). In fact, malignant tumors, like normal tissue, frequently contain cells at various stages of differentiation, a mechanism that mimics dedifferentiation of mature cell types and presumes a hierarchical organization (Clarke et al., 2006; Clevers, 2005). Because there is the possibility that CSCs share various signaling characteristics with normal stem cells, several methods are frequently utilized to identify putative CSCs in human prostate cancer tissues, human and animal cell lines, and *in vivo* cancer animal models.

3. Assaying prostate cancer stem cells

The determination of cancer stem cells in primary tumors is a difficult task, with many variables and potential for confounding results. CSCs constitute a minority proportion of the constituent cells of tumors, and therefore their analysis can only be undertaken after isolation and propagation in tissue culture or *in vivo* systems. Several methods are being used to identify, enrich, and propagate these tumor cells and to study their biology as crucial players in tumorigenesis (Table 2).

3.1 Enrichment of CSCs from cancer cell lines and primary tumors

Human immortalized prostate cancer cell lines have been accessible and frequently utilized as biological models to investigate cancer biology and to test the efficacy of potential anticancer drugs. Most of cancer cell lines available have been continuously cultured under different conditions, and only a minor percentage of cells preserve their clonal growth, clonogenic potential, and the ability to form tumors when transplanted in animal hosts. Criticisms to cancer cell lines arise due to the high potential for culture contamination by other cell lines (Borrell, 2010; Li et al., 2009). These cells represent highly selected subgroup of cells that may have accumulated additional genetic abnormalities as they adapt to an artificial environment. Nevertheless, the utilization of cancer cell lines is an important tool used by researchers to study CSCs and carry out mechanistic studies.

Following isolation, analysis of CSCs is performed by culturing primary tumor cells *in vitro*, either as monolayers or as spheres, both of which are particularly difficult in the case of prostate cancer cells derived from primary tissues (Miki et al., 2007; Tokar et al., 2005). Indeed, most human prostate cancer cell lines utilized to dissect the events associated to cancer progression and metastasis has been established from metastatic lesions or from xenograft tumors (Sobel & Sadar, 2005a, 2005b). An efficient cell immortalization culture based on the inhibition of the serine/threonine kinase ROCK have been shown to reversibly immortalize primary human keratinocytes and to increase the cloning efficiency of murine prostate cells (Chapman et al., 2010). Since immortalized keratinocytes are genetically and functionally similar to the primary tissues they were derived from, this method is an advance over the traditional procedures that promote genetic changes. Strict parameters defining CSCs require that upon isolation these cells exhibit certain biological characteristics such as self-renewal and proliferative potential, as well the capacity, under the proper conditions, to differentiate into other cell types. These capabilities can be determined *in vitro* through the use of colony formation assays. However, the stem-like features of these cells is confirmed through experimental approaches in which these cancer cells in a very low number have the capacity to generate tumors in *in vivo* systems.

The most commonly used *in vivo* system used to propagate these tumorigenic cells are xenograft models, either subcutaneous in the renal capsule or orthotopic. For these isolated putative CSCs to be established as such, certain conditions must be met. Isolation of CSCs should be capable of generating a tumor *in vivo*, and successful serial transplantation of these tumors must be possible for several generations. Importantly, a number of variables that can affect the outcome of these *in vivo* assays includes: the manner in which cells are isolated; whether these cells are initially propagated *in vitro* before transplantation, which can cause them to become more aggressive as a result of new acquired mutations; the procedure employed to inoculate the mice; the strain of mice employed, etc, that is often taken, in particular during the experimental planning phase and analysis process.

Assaying Prostate Cancer Stem Cells
Isolation through stem cell markers expression
CD44+
Integrin $\alpha1\beta2+$
CD133+
CD44+/$\alpha1\beta2+$
CD44+/CD24-
$\alpha1\beta2+$/CD133+
CD44+/$\alpha1\beta2+$/CD133+
Isolation of cancer stem cells
Established human cancer cell lines
Fresh human surgical samples
Culture in ultra-low attachment surface
Isolation of holoclones
Limiting dilution assay
Hoechst 33342 dye and exclusion
Rhodamine 123
Methods to measure proliferation, growth rate, invasion
Fluorescent activated cell sorting
Matrigel invasion
Matrigel 3-D culture
Sphere formation anchorage independent growth protasphere
Methods to identify gene signatures and/or protein expression
Microarray
Quantitative RT-PCR
Sequencing
Tissue microarray
Flow cytometry
Immunohistochemistry
Immunofluorescent analysis
Immunoblotting
Animals models (into immunocompromised mice)
Transplantation
Xenografts

Table 2. Methods utilized for the enrichment of prostatic cancer stem cells.

3.2 Determining the frequency of CSCs based on limiting dilution assay and spherogenecity

The rarity of cancer stem cells within the tumor bulk in many cases makes the utilization of the limiting dilution assay (LDA) necessary. This type of analysis has the ability to estimate the frequency of CSCs among a population of cancer cells (Hope & Bhatia, 2011; Schroeder, 2011). LDA can also be utilized to estimate the ability of a single tumor cell to form spheroids in serum-free cultures. Importantly, to reduce possible variations and calculate the frequency of CSCs, LDA needs to be tested in both bulk and fractionated cancer cells for each individual tumor (O'Brien et al., 2010). Since CSCs are a rare population with low numbers of cells, the injection of unsorted tumor cells into mice has been used to expand these cancer cells before applying LDA. It is important to consider that even if serial dilutions of tumor cells are injected into groups of animals, the development of a tumor in a recipient animal implies that the inoculum contained at least one reproductively intact cell (Porter & Berry, 1963). The LDA can also provide important information regarding the existence of cooperation among tumor cells that may be critical for the surviving and proliferation of cells that generate a tumor, therefore validating the existence of a single CSC (Hu & Smyth, 2009).

Several experimental approaches are being utilized to study the properties of cancer stem cells *in vitro*. For example, utilizing low adherence cultures, growth in soft agar, suspension cultures, and the use of ultra low adherence plates. In general, a serum-free media containing epidermal growth factor (EGF) and fibroblast growth factor (FGF), specifically formulated for the culture of pure populations of stem cells, is utilized to enrich and grow putative CSCs (Tropepe et al., 1999). The success of these methodologies is quite relative. Because the cells grow in these stringent conditions cannot be kept in culture for long periods of time. Recent evidence has demonstrated that sphere cells with stem-like properties from prostate cancer cells can be generated and propagated without the addition of growth factors (Rybak et al., 2011). This new culturing condition also supported a long-term culture of prostate stem-like cells, adding an important tool to investigate the biology and the expression of specific cell surface markers in CSCs. Similarly, inhibition of ROCK activity in culture (Chapman et al., 2010) enabled an 8-fold increase in *in vitro* prostate colony assay, and also significantly increased the cloning efficiency of prostate stem cells from mice (Zhang et al., 2011).

3.3 Protaspheres

The utilization of spheres assay is an important tool for the in serial in vivo transplantation to verify self-renewal potential. Although, sphere cells are generated, serially passaged, and maintained in undifferentiated phenotype under appropriate cell culture conditions, they need to be inoculated into animal models to confirm their ability to generate tumor growth. In this regard, it is necessary to ensure the best animal model available in order to reproduce tumor CSCs biology as it occurs in humans. It is important to note that variation on experimental conditions would certainly influence frequency estimates. In fact, it was suggested that limiting dilution data might be dramatically affected by the duration of data analysis (Yamazaki et al., 2009) or by modification of xenotransplantation assay in non-obese diabetic severe combined immunodeficient (NOD/SCID) mice (Quintana et al., 2008). Therefore, a main concern for the application of this methodology is that sometimes, the animal models overstate the biology of cancer formation in humans.

Prostate cancer cell lines are frequently used to investigate the mechanisms that modulate protaspheres in non-adherent cultures. Several reports have shown that most of these cells have the ability to form spheres; however, the frequency of cells that form spheres is very heterogeneous across all cell lines. It is possible that adaptation of these cells to non-adherent culture conditions may be a determinant in forming spheres (Bisson & Prowse, 2009). It has also been shown that holoclone-forming cells, cells whose progeny forms almost exclusively growing colonies, in prostate cancer specimens with the highest clonogenic potential were associated with stem cell phenotypes (Patrawala et al., 2007). More, the presence of large holoclones was also consistently observed in prostate cancer cell protaspheres (Li et al., 2008; Zhang & Waxman, 2010), suggesting that spheres with stem cell-like features have a higher proliferative potential. Indeed, protaspheres were capable of forming new generations of protaspheres and retained proliferative capacity as well as clonogenic potential after serial passages (Guzman-Ramirez et al., 2009).

3.4 Identification of cancer stem cell signatures using microarray technology

The utilization of microarray analysis has allowed for screening the expression profile of numerous genes in prostate tumors (Glinsky, 2007; Mendes et al., 2008; Witte, 2009). By using gene expression microarray technology, the expression levels of thousands of genes are analyzed in a single experiment and evidences of certain degree of relevance to cancer progression may be also obtained (Borst & Wessels, 2010; Witte, 2009; Zieger, 2008). Because cancer cells and somatic stem cells share the biological characteristics of self-renewal and proliferation, the principles of stem cell biology can be applied to improve our understanding of cancer biology (Liang et al., 2009). Although several cell surface markers have been utilized for the isolation of putative cancer stem cells, the identification of key molecules and pathways that play pivotal roles in prostate cancer progression towards an aggressive stage is crucial for a more precise prognosis in patients with prostate cancer (Ladanyi, 2008; Rubin, 2008). As a matter of fact, the identification of molecular signatures has allowed the identification of androgen subtypes of cancers that have not been distinguished by pathological criteria (Alizadeh et al., 2009; Goodison et al., 2010; Perou et al., 2010; Wegiel et al., 2010; Yang et al., 2010) and in prostate tumors, the microarray technology has identified androgen-regulated genes in prostate tumor models (Elek et al., 2000).

Laboratory animals have been used to mimic natural aspects of human prostate cancer development. The evaluation of gene expression in samples derived from these animal models has provided for the identification of gene signatures, which are represented in the altered expression in a large group of genes (Ladanyi, 2008; Mendes et al., 2008; Witte, 2009). These data can be useful to compare *in vitro* results with intact animal expression changes and the different signatures that may eventually be predictors of cancer progression. More recently, a major effort towards this end addresses global analyses of gene expression profiles. However, the large body of data sometimes does not provide clear information about the specific genes that may be associated with the aggressive growth of prostate tumors. In this regard, the identification of poor prognosis using an interspecies comparison of prostate cancer gene-expression profiles has been a valuable tool to predict the association of potential oncogenic events to an aggressive phenotype of prostate cancer (Kela et al., 2009).

Because gene expression is a complex process characterized by a high degree of regulation, studying which genes are active and which are inactive during tumor progression helps to understand both how these cells may function normally and how they are affected when several genes do not perform properly. In addition, gene expression profiles can provide key information in the identification of a signature that can be used to assess corresponding biological responses in other potential candidate(s), which may be indicative of cancer progression effects and pathological endpoints (Goodison et al., 2010; Hsieh et al., 2007; Mendes et al., 2008). Therefore, there is no doubt that microarray technology is a new tool for the clinical lab and also can improve the accuracy of classical diagnostic techniques by identifying potential novel tumor specific markers. Therefore, it is important that microarray data be publicly available. The establishment of specific criteria is important to identify genes associated to diseases. This may facilitate the classification by the identification of only relevant genes, improving the tumor classification accuracy and reducing the dimensionality of the data set (Wang et al., 2005).

3.5 The side population dilemma to isolate CSCs

An innovative approach frequently utilized to isolate stem cells is the side population (SP) assay (Goodell et al., 1996). This controversial technique had generated excitement because of its enormous potential to isolate putative CSCs. Cells with and SP phenotype, which is associated with primitive and undifferentiated stem cells characteristic are enriched based on their highest efflux activity to dyes such as Hoechst 33342 or Rhodamine 123. This approach had allowed the identification of a small subset of quiescent and replicating Hoechst-staining CD34-negative in murine cells that efflux the dye, allowing defined separation of this subset from the rest of the bone marrow (Goodell et al., 1996). This subset presented a very homogeneous pattern compared to cell surface markers. Using this approach, a subset of cells with similar phenotype to mouse was also identified in human bone marrow. This conserved SP phenotype was proposed as a common molecular feature for stem cells possessing multi-organ plasticity. The assessment of the molecular basis for SP phenotype found that the ATP-binding cassette (ABC) protein breast cancer resistant protein (Bcrp1) transporter expression is highly conserved in primitive stem cells from murine bone marrow, skeletal muscle, and cultured ES cells. While Bcrp1 expression is exclusive of the primitive subset CD34+ and was developmentally regulated, enforced expression of Bcrp-1 expanded the SP phenotype in bone-marrow cells (Zhou et al., 2001).

Other ABC transporters, including the multidrug resistance 1 (Mdr1a/1b, mouse; MDR1, human) and the multidrug resistant protein (MRP) are also able to efflux Hoechst 33342, which have been indicated as contributors for multidrug resistance of tumor cells (Schinkel et al., 1997). However, in the Mdr1a/b/Bcrp1 triple knockout mice model, some bone marrow cells still retained the SP phenotype. This redundancy suggested that the influence of transporters in the SP phenotype is probably not exclusive on the expression of ABC transporter proteins. Latter experiments using knock down of the Bcrp1 gene expression animal model proved that the Bcrp1 gene, and not Mdr1a/1b, drastically reduced the number of SP cells in the bone marrow and in skeletal muscle. This study also evidenced that Bcrp1 expression is crucial in protecting early hematopoietic cells against chemotherapeutic drugs such as topotecan, mitoxantrone, or 5-fluorouracil (5-FU) (Zhou et al., 2002).

It has been proposed that the lower affinity of MDR-1-encoded transporter rather than the ATP-binding cassette, sub-family G (WHITE), member 2 (ABCG2) transporter for the Hoechst dye may explain its reduced effect in the SP phenotype. Indeed, enforced expression of a MDR1 retroviral vector in murine bone marrow cells *in vitro* increased SP cells only to 3.6% of the total population (Bunting et al., 2000), a very low percentage compared with the impressive levels provided when the ABCG2 vector (62.5% SP cells) was utilized (Zhou et al., 2001). In fact, SP cells isolated from normal prostate tissues isolated from radical prostatectomy were enriched in ABCG2 expression. The gene expression signature of the ABCG2 subpopulation showed a consistent number of markers associated with stem-like phenotype (Pascal et al., 2007), suggesting the feasibility of the SP assay to identify and isolate cells with stem-like phenotype in the prostate.

Reports associating SP cells with tumorigenicity and/or aggressiveness have also been established in many tissues including breast, colorectal, glioma, medulloblastoma, ovarian, and thyroid (Chiba et al., 2006; Hirschmann-Jax et al., 2004; Kondo et al., 2004; Mitsutake et al., 2007; Szotek et al., 2006). In prostate tumor cell lines and human tissues, the utilization of the SP assay has also allowed the enrichment of cells with stem-like characteristics, which expressed high levels of different types of transporters such as ABCG2, ATP-binding cassette, sub-family A (ABC1), member 2 (ABCA2), MDR-1 and MRP-1 (Mathew et al., 2009; Oates et al., 2009; Patrawala et al., 2005). The prostate cancer SP phenotype possessed self-renewal capacities *in vitro* and *in vivo* intrinsic properties of stem cells as evidence by the activity of Wnt and Hedgehog signaling pathways, high proliferation rate, and tumorigenic potential ((Bhatt et al., 2003; Brown et al., 2007; Patrawala et al., 2005). These findings implied that the SP subpopulation is enriched with tumorigenic stem-like cancer cells that may be resistant against therapies.

Cells with stem-like characteristics have also been enriched in SP subsets but were not exclusive for breast, thyroid, and breast cancer cell lines in which some of the non-SP cells had the ability to generate cells with SP phenotypes (Mitsutake et al., 2007; Patrawala et al., 2005). Interestingly, non-SP cells also preserved their tumorigenic potential. Although contamination might be responsible for these unexpected results, a critical concern in this endeavor is that SP assay does not isolate cells by a definitive cell surface profile; because of that, the population being isolated is very heterogeneous (Challen & Little, 2006). It was also reported that both SP and non-SP fractions from malignant mesothelioma and lung adenocarcinomas cell lines were also equally able to form spheres, have a high tumorigenic potential, and are resistant to chemotherapeutic agents (Pan et al., 2010). More intriguing was the fact that no evidence of stem-like characteristics was found in gastrointestinal cancer cell lines in which lifespan in tissue culture and tumorigenesis potential are not exclusively associated with the SP phenotype (Haraguchi et al., 2006). This leads to the next question: are other types of cells also involved in key events during cancer evolution? These results also indicate that the SP assay is not appropriate for the identification and enrichment of putative CSCs in lung tumors (Kai et al., 2010).

Together, these results raise the inevitable question: is it correct to affirm that SP enriches a subpopulation with potential stem-like characteristics? One potential explanation for these conflicting results was provided by the kinetic analysis of Hoechst 33342 on bone marrow over a dye incubation period (Ibrahim et al., 2007). This approach demonstrated that bone marrow nuclear cells evidenced an identical staining pattern at varying rates, even under conditions where SP fraction was depleted, suggesting that the SP phenotype is not unique to stem cells. These data may be indicative of a transient feature of marrow cells when exposed to Hoechst 33342 for varying amounts of time. It is also possible that cells not exhibiting SP phenotype may have their membrane pumps overwhelmed or perhaps the dye efflux mechanism is inactivated.

All the biological assays discussed above may have important clinical implications. Indeed, proliferation assays could be included in the routine assays of pathologists to provide the most accurate diagnosis to patients with prostate cancer. As a matter of fact, the grading of prostate tumors (low versus high) is analyzed based on tubule formation, nuclear grade, and mitotic count. The mitosis cell evaluation is carried out basically by scoring the number of mitotic cells present within a giving sample. Considering that the worst histologic grade dictates the biologic behavior of prostate cancer (Chan et al., 2000; Harnden et al., 2007; Hattab et al., 2006; Pan et al., 2000; Sim et al., 2008), the inclusion of appropriate assays to identify proliferative signatures may improve the clinical diagnosis/prognosis of prostate cancer that may help to reduce misdiagnosis, missed diagnosis, or decrease the rates of overdiagnosis.

4. Prostatic cancer stem cells

A challenge in studying solid neoplasias is the heterogeneity observed in the tumor bulk where multiple cell types coexist, each exhibiting unique proliferation rates, invasion, and metastatic potential. This is the result of diverse combinations of genetic and epigenetic aberrations that arise from stressors such as inflammation, oxidative stress, aging and environmental influence.

Although several commonly mutated genes involved in the tumorigenesis process have been identified, there is no clear evidence that the transformed cells specifically responsible for tumor initiation and maintenance of solid malignant neoplasias have been clearly identified or isolated thus far. Therefore, it is crucial for the understanding of cancer evolution to provide new insights into the molecular mechanisms by which CSCs modulate cancer development. In this respect, efforts are being made toward the identification of reliable biomarkers (Keysar & Jimeno, 2010; Marhaba et al., 2008; Zoller, 2011) for the accurate identification of malignant progenitor tumor cells and also to use them as possible molecular targets to improve response to therapy. These potential markers of stem cells or CSC markers obviously preserve specific biological functions, but these have yet to be discovered as only limited research has been conducted to explore the process of their roles in tumor initiation and progression. Moreover, the limited number of cancer stem cells within the tumor, the heterogeneity of androgen receptors, the phenotypic characteristics of the tumor bulk and different genetic signatures are also important aspects that restrict the identification of this unique subset of cancer cells in prostatic cancer.

Numerous reports have described several types of tumors including prostate cancers, biological markers that can recognize a small population of cancer cells in the tumor bulk with stem-like characteristics (Miki et al., 2007; Patrawala et al., 2006; Patrawala et al., 2007; Vander Griend et al., 2008). Many of these markers associated with stem cells are cell surface proteins (i.e., CD44, CD133, CD166, etc), which is facilitating the identification of tumor subpopulations with stem-like phenotypes. In addition, signaling pathways activated by the core pluripotent transcription factors Nanog, Oct4, and Sox2, which are very important components of the machinery that modulates cell-renewal and maintains pluripotency in both embryos and stem cells, are also frequently overexpressed in poorly differentiated tumor cells (Jeter et al., 2009; Jeter et al., 2011). However, the nuclear localization of these transcription factors precludes their utilization for the enrichment of CSC.

Cancer stem cells have been enriched from human cancer prostate based on the expression of α2β1 integrin or CD133 (Collins et al., 2005). In addition, holoclones from the prostatic cell line PC3 that were tumorigenic in xenograft assays showed increased expression of α2β1, β-catenin, and CD44 (Li et al., 2008). Although CD44 expression was also associated with enrichment of cancer stem cells in other prostatic epithelial cell lines, this subset of cells displayed low efficiency in formation of xenograft tumors (Hurt et al., 2008; Patrawala et al., 2007). Prostate tumor cells expressing the CD133 isolated from $\alpha2\beta1^{hi}$ cells were capable of expanding in culture. These prostatic putative stem cells were able to drive the reconstitution of prostatic-like acini in immunocompromised male nude mice (Richardson et al., 2004). Even when controversial reports have challenged the role of CD133 as a cancer stem cell marker, several evidences have supported that CD133 expression is generally detected in prostate cancers (Guzman-Ramirez et al., 2009). In fact, this subset of cells had the ability to form protaspheres from single cells. However, protaspheres generated from freshly isolated cancer prostate cells that were either CD133+ or CD133-, suggested that neoplastic transformation can confer self-renewal potential also to CD133- progenitor cells (Tang et al., 2007).

A comparison of clonogenic cells isolated from primary prostate cancer populations identified only tumor-derived $\alpha2\beta1^{high}$/CD133+/CD44+. This cellular subpopulation also presented a phenotype similar to normal prostate stem cells and was also capable of self-renewal and extensive proliferation compared to more differentiated cells did not form *in vitro* secondary colonies (Collins et al., 2005). The differentiation of this subpopulation with serum and dihydrotestosterone to an androgen receptor-positive phenotype promoted in these cells the expression of AR+/PAP+/CK18+, which suggests that they were derived from a more primitive multipotent population of CSCs. In support for these findings, Patrawala et al., (Patrawala et al., 2006) reported that a highly purified CD44+ prostate cancer subset from xenografts of a human tumor, as well as from multiple cultured cell lines are enriched in tumorigenic and metastatic progenitor cells. The CD44+ subpopulation was more invasive than CD44- cells and also expressed high levels of several stem-like genes such as Oct3/4, Bmi, and β-catenin.

In addition, clonally derived human prostate cancer specimens from epithelial cell lines expressing the embryonic stem markers Nanog, Oct4, and Sox2 as well as other early progenitor cell markers such as CD44, CD133, c-kit, and Nestin were able to recapitulate human prostate tumors in SCID mice and were also categorized according to Gleason score (Gu et al., 2007). In fact, these cell lines formed tumors that contained basal, luminal, and NE epithelial cell lineage of the prostate, and retained their capacity of proliferation through serial transplantations. This is consistent with studies showing that high levels of Nanog is expressed in human primary prostate cancers cells and it also have a functional role for tumor growth (Jeter et al., 2009; Jeter et al., 2011). Interestingly, the putative prostate cancer stem cells do not express AR and p63, similar to that reported for prostate stem cells (Barbieri & Pietenpol, 2006; Rizzo et al., 2005). In support of these findings, increased expression of CD133 and the stromal cell-derived factor-1 receptor (CXCR4) were detected in a subpopulation of clinical prostate specimens that do not express AR (Miki et al., 2007). It is therefore conceivable to predict that the heterogeneous nature of prostate cancer, a common characteristics of this disease may have a stem cell compartment. Therefore, it is unlikely that a single marker can be used for the identification of cancer stem cells' subpopulations within the tumor mass.

5. Therapy targeting prostate cancer stem cells

The dysregulation of the cell cycle regulatory machinery that impact tumor cell proliferation also participates in the accelerated growth observed in most malignant tumors. Although the exact genes that comprise the proliferation status may differ in different type of tumors, evidence has demonstrated that the cell cycle regulation is frequently altered in prostate cancers, in part, by the interplay of activation of oncogenic cascades with diverse hormones, growth factors, and cytokines. These events may eventually lead to a more poorly differentiated and aggressive tumor behavior, leading to overall higher rates of progression and worse prognosis, irrespective of the size of the lesion (Flavin et al., 2010, 2011; Niu et al., 2010; Saeki et al., 2010). Therefore, inhibitors of cell cycle regulatory proteins has become an area of increased interest in targeting both cancer cells per se and CSCs (Malumbres & Barbacid, 2009). For example, we have recently demonstrated the efficacy of a novel dansylated VMY-1-103, a CDK1, CDK2 inhibitor, based on purvalanol B (Ringer et al., 2010), at very low concentrations in inhibiting Erb-2/Erb-3/heregulin-induced cell proliferation in LNCaP prostate cancer cells. It was also observed that VMY-1-103 induced apoptosis via decreased mitochondrial membrane polarity, induced p53 phosphorylation, caspase-3 activation, and PARP cleavage in these prostatic tumor cells, which express p53 wild type. More, VMY-1-103 was also effective inducing cell cycle arrest in prostate cancer cell lines compromised for p53 function, however, VMY-1-103 failed to induce apoptosis in p53-null prostate cell lines PC3 (Ringer et al., 2010). These results, strongly suggest that VMY-1-103 may be an effective therapeutic, either alone or in combinations with other drugs, in treating prostate cancer. Importantly, we have also found that VMY-1-103 is also effective in inducing apoptosis in spheroid cultures (Ringer et al., unpublished data). Given the critical role of CDK1 in proper timing of mitosis in all cells, VMY-1-103 may also be able to efficiently target CSC's, and this exciting possibility is being addressed both *in vitro* and *in vivo*.

Cancer usually treated using chemotherapy, radiotherapy, or surgery had limited effect on most primary tumors, which have already spread to other organs, leading to recurrent disease in the majority of patients. The reduced number of individuals that benefit of standard therapies may be improved with targeted clinical trials (Simon & Maitournam, 2004). In this respect, the identification of potential biological markers by microarray or sequencing technologies would help to restrict the number of patients that might response to a specific drug. However, the limited knowledge in tumor cell biology, in which multiples abnormalities need to be targeted simultaneously make difficult to predict which patients are most likely to respond to a given regimen (Sparreboom & Verweij, 2009; Woodward & Sulman, 2008). For instance, the significant therapeutic advances in patients with diverse types of localized cancers have been limited by relapse due to the persistence of cancer cells in primary tumors and micrometastases that may have intrinsic or acquisition of a resistant phenotype to current therapies available (Gray-Schopfer et al., 2007; Mimeault & Batra, 2006a, 2007b; Mimeault et al., 2007; van Leenders et al., 2001; Yang et al., 2010).

Despite recent therapeutic approaches that have significantly increased survival, most prostate aggressive tumors become resistant to current treatment protocols and the proportion of cancers that progress is significantly higher in the African American population (Chornokur et al., 2011; Gurel et al., 2008). Prostate cancers that initially respond to standard chemotherapy often recur with selective outgrowth of tumor cell subpopulations that are resistant not only to the original chemotherapeutic agents but also to other therapeutics. Thus, for example, most patients that relapses with castration-resistant cancer metastatic tumors for which there are no curative treatment. In this regard, it has been suggested that the cancer stem cell model may be responsible for the degree of sensitivity to anti-androgen therapy (Schalken, 2005). Although different cellular events involving pathways may effectively activate a different path to androgen independence probably through a paracrine androgen-independent pathway, the multifocality and heterogeneity of prostate cancer may also account for hormone therapy resistance. In a human prostate cancer progression xenograft model, most of androgen-responsive genes that were initially downregulated under conditions of androgen deprivation were later re-expressed in recurrence tumors, indicating failure of androgen-derivation therapy as well as acceleration of tumor progression (Mousses et al., 2001). Another microarray-based profiling found that increase in AR transcript, as well as protein levels are essential for accruing resistance to anti-androgen therapy (Chen et al., 2004). Indeed, multiple cellular signaling pathways including AR, Akt, mitogen-activated protein kinase (MAPK), the nuclear factor kappa B (NF-κB), TGF-β, vascular endothelial growth factor (VEGF), and Wnt have been shown to enhance AR signaling and confer development of hormone-independent/castration-resistance in preclinical models (Mellado et al., 2009; Wegiel et al., 2010). More recently, it has been reported that Nanog induction promoted castration-resistant tumor phenotype and tumor regeneration in the human tumor cell line LNCaP. These findings support the notion that AR expression in prostate tumors is modulated by CSCs (Maitland & Collins, 2008).

The most challenging problem in prostate cancer is the identification of which cell or cells are transformed and initiate carcinogenesis. In addition, tumor heterogeneity appears to mask a minor tumor population (CSCs) that have the ability to self-renew and form a tumor but are typically in a quiescent state. This has been suggested as a critical mechanism by which CSCs are resistant to conventional chemotherapy or radiation treatments. Thus, prostate CSCs are likely to modulate resistant to androgen deprivation therapy and promote recurrence as hormone-refractory tumors and metastatic lesions. Even though prostatic CSCs do not express AR or PSA (Lawson & Witte, 2007; Tang et al., 2007), it appears contradictive to propose that these cells are the modulators of tumor progression in castrate resistance. Nevertheless, three potential mechanisms have been proposed to explain poor outcome in prostate cancer patients (Sharifi et al., 2006): 1) Clonal selection to anti-androgen therapy may occur in transit-amplifying cells, which arise from the stem cells and divide a finite number of times until they become differentiated. Because of the limited growth of transit-amplifying cells, it is possible that CSCs may produce them in response to castration therapy; 2) Growth factor released by surrounding AR responsive cells may provide the resistance response to this type of therapy; and 3) CSCs produce cells that have a more differentiated morphology and express AR.

The diagnosis and treatment of prostate cancer are currently based on clinical stage, biopsy Gleason grade, and serum PSA levels, which do not provide accurate information about the status of the tumor. Several studies have identified by microarray, genetic signatures of prostate cancer that appear to provide a more accurate pathological distinction based on different degrees of severity (Lapointe et al., 2004; Singh et al., 2002). The identification of relevant cell signaling pathways signatures that are overexpressed in subpopulation with stem-like characteristics may also provide mechanistic information regarding their roles in tumor progression and metastasis (Birnie et al., 2008; Sharad et al., 2011). Therefore, it has been suggested that sophisticated therapy approaches involving specific DNA damaging agents in combination with DNA repair inhibitors may also improve available therapies against prostate cancer (Berry et al., 2008; Cano et al., 2007). In addition, the combination of targeting cancer stem cells and androgen ablation may kill tumor cells and disrupt those cells that support tumor growth and survival (Berry et al., 2008).

6. Conclusions

CSCs are believed to be a subpopulation of cancer cells that modulate malignancy and resistance to current anticancer treatments and, therefore, indicators of inferior prognosis. Although some of the mutated target genes have been identified, there is no clear evidence regarding the identification and isolation of cells that initiate tumor formation in solid malignant neoplasias. Therefore, even the role of CSC in tumorigenesis has been very well accepted, thought it remains controversial whether cancer mass arises specifically from stem cells. It is believed that in tumor bulk, there are particular subsets of cells (CSC) that may have the potential to promote tumor progression and resistance to conventional therapies. After completion of a treatment, the surviving tumor cells may have acquired even more mutations during the drug treatment. The additional genetic changes in this particular tumor subpopulation may explain why the conventional therapies fail in eradicating the cancer, a frequent concern in the diagnosis of prostate cancer and the rapid regrowth of the tumor but this time with a more aggressive phenotype. Since standard therapies applied to cancer are usually based on radiologic documentation of tumor shrinkage, the presence of CSCs may explain failure of tumor eradication. Thus, there is still an immediate priority for the identification of robust prognostic biomarkers to optimize cancer therapies to effectively target CSCs and their environment to improve prostate cancer treatment.

7. References

Abbott, R. R., Taylor, D. K., and Barber, K. (1998). A comparison of prostate knowledge of African-American and Caucasian men: changes from prescreening baseline to postintervention. *Cancer J Sci Am, 4*, 175-177.

Al-Hajj, M., and Clarke, M. F. (2004). Self-renewal and solid tumor stem cells. *Oncogene, 23*, 7274-7282.

Alizadeh, A. A., Gentles, A. J., Lossos, I. S., and Levy, R. (2009). Molecular outcome prediction in diffuse large-B-cell lymphoma. *N Engl J Med, 360*, 2794-2795.

Bapat, S. A., Mali, A. M., Koppikar, C. B., and Kurrey, N. K. (2005). Stem and progenitor-like cells contribute to the aggressive behavior of human epithelial ovarian cancer. *Cancer Res, 65*, 3025-3029.

Barbieri, C. E., and Pietenpol, J. A. (2006). p63 and epithelial biology. *Exp Cell Res, 312*, 695-706.

Beachy, P. A., Karhadkar, S. S., and Berman, D. M. (2004). Tissue repair and stem cell renewal in carcinogenesis. *Nature, 432*, 324-331.

Berry, P. A., Maitland, N. J., and Collins, A. T. (2008). Androgen receptor signalling in prostate: effects of stromal factors on normal and cancer stem cells. *Mol Cell Endocrinol, 288*, 30-37.

Bhatt, R. I., Brown, M. D., Hart, C. A., Gilmore, P., Ramani, V. A., George, N. J., and Clarke, N. W. (2003). Novel method for the isolation and characterisation of the putative prostatic stem cell. *Cytometry A, 54*, 89-99.

Birnie, R., Bryce, S. D., Roome, C., Dussupt, V., Droop, A., Lang, S. H., Berry, P. A., Hyde, C. F., Lewis, J. L., Stower, M. J., Maitland, N. J., and Collins, A. T. (2008). Gene expression profiling of human prostate cancer stem cells reveals a pro-inflammatory phenotype and the importance of extracellular matrix interactions. *Genome Biol, 9*, R83.

Bisson, I., and Prowse, D. M. (2009). WNT signaling regulates self-renewal and differentiation of prostate cancer cells with stem cell characteristics. *Cell Res, 19*, 683-697.

Bonkhoff, H., Stein, U., and Remberger, K. (1995). Endocrine-paracrine cell types in the prostate and prostatic adenocarcinoma are postmitotic cells. *Hum Pathol, 26*, 167-170.

Borrell, B. (2010). How accurate are cancer cell lines? *Nature, 463*, 858.

Borst, P., and Wessels, L. (2010). Do predictive signatures really predict response to cancer chemotherapy? *Cell Cycle, 9*, 4836-4840.

Brown, M. D., Gilmore, P. E., Hart, C. A., Samuel, J. D., Ramani, V. A., George, N. J., and Clarke, N. W. (2007). Characterization of benign and malignant prostate epithelial Hoechst 33342 side populations. *Prostate, 67*, 1384-1396.

Bunting, K. D., Zhou, S., Lu, T., and Sorrentino, B. P. (2000). Enforced P-glycoprotein pump function in murine bone marrow cells results in expansion of side population stem cells in vitro and repopulating cells in vivo. *Blood, 96*, 902-909.

Byers, T., Barrera, E., Fontham, E. T., Newman, L. A., Runowicz, C. D., Sener, S. F., Thun, M. J., Winborn, S., and Wender, R. C. (2006). A midpoint assessment of the American Cancer Society challenge goal to halve the U.S. cancer mortality rates between the years 1990 and 2015. *Cancer, 107*, 396-405.

Cano, P., Godoy, A., Escamilla, R., Dhir, R., and Onate, S. A. (2007). Stromal-epithelial cell interactions and androgen receptor-coregulator recruitment is altered in the tissue microenvironment of prostate cancer. *Cancer Res, 67*, 511-519.

Chaffer, C. L., and Weinberg, R. A. (2011). A perspective on cancer cell metastasis. *Science, 331*, 1559-1564.

Challen, G. A., and Little, M. H. (2006). A side order of stem cells: the SP phenotype. *Stem Cells, 24*, 3-12.

Chan, T. Y., Partin, A. W., Walsh, P. C., and Epstein, J. I. (2000). Prognostic significance of Gleason score 3+4 versus Gleason score 4+3 tumor at radical prostatectomy. *Urology, 56*, 823-827.

Chapman, S., Liu, X., Meyers, C., Schlegel, R., and McBride, A. A. (2010). Human keratinocytes are efficiently immortalized by a Rho kinase inhibitor. *J Clin Invest, 120*, 2619-2626.

Chen, C. D., Welsbie, D. S., Tran, C., Baek, S. H., Chen, R., Vessella, R., Rosenfeld, M. G., and Sawyers, C. L. (2004). Molecular determinants of resistance to antiandrogen therapy. *Nat Med, 10*, 33-39.

Chiba, T., Kita, K., Zheng, Y. W., Yokosuka, O., Saisho, H., Iwama, A., Nakauchi, H., and Taniguchi, H. (2006). Side population purified from hepatocellular carcinoma cells harbors cancer stem cell-like properties. *Hepatology, 44*, 240-251.

Chornokur, G., Dalton, K., Borysova, M. E., and Kumar, N. B. (2011). Disparities at presentation, diagnosis, treatment, and survival in African American men, affected by prostate cancer. *Prostate, 71*, 985-997.

Chu, K. C., Tarone, R. E., and Freeman, H. P. (2003). Trends in prostate cancer mortality among black men and white men in the United States. *Cancer, 97*, 1507-1516.

Clarke, M. F., Dick, J. E., Dirks, P. B., Eaves, C. J., Jamieson, C. H., Jones, D. L., Visvader, J., Weissman, I. L., and Wahl, G. M. (2006). Cancer stem cells--perspectives on current status and future directions: AACR Workshop on cancer stem cells. *Cancer Res, 66*, 9339-9344.

Clevers, H. (2005). Stem cells, asymmetric division and cancer. *Nat Genet, 37*, 1027-1028.

Collins, A. T., Berry, P. A., Hyde, C., Stower, M. J., and Maitland, N. J. (2005). Prospective identification of tumorigenic prostate cancer stem cells. *Cancer Res, 65*, 10946-10951.

Dalerba, P., Cho, R. W., and Clarke, M. F. (2007). Cancer stem cells: models and concepts. *Annu Rev Med, 58*, 267-284.

Dean, M., Fojo, T., and Bates, S. (2005). Tumour stem cells and drug resistance. *Nat Rev Cancer, 5*, 275-284.

di Sant' Agnese, P. A. (1996). Neuroendocrine differentiation in the precursors of prostate cancer. *Eur Urol, 30*, 185-190.

Dingli, D., and Michor, F. (2006). Successful therapy must eradicate cancer stem cells. *Stem Cells, 24*, 2603-2610.

Elek, J., Park, K. H., and Narayanan, R. (2000). Microarray-based expression profiling in prostate tumors. *In Vivo, 14*, 173-182.

English, H. F., Santen, R. J., and Isaacs, J. T. (1987). Response of glandular versus basal rat ventral prostatic epithelial cells to androgen withdrawal and replacement. *Prostate, 11*, 229-242.

Flavin, R., Zadra, G., and Loda, M. (2010). Metabolic alterations and targeted therapies in prostate cancer. *J Pathol*.

Flavin, R., Zadra, G., and Loda, M. (2011). Metabolic alterations and targeted therapies in prostate cancer. *J Pathol, 223*, 283-294.

Glinsky, G. V. (2007). Stem cell origin of death-from-cancer phenotypes of human prostate and breast cancers. *Stem Cell Rev, 3*, 79-93.

Goodell, M. A., Brose, K., Paradis, G., Conner, A. S., and Mulligan, R. C. (1996). Isolation and functional properties of murine hematopoietic stem cells that are replicating in vivo. *J Exp Med, 183*, 1797-1806.

Goodison, S., Sun, Y., and Urquidi, V. (2010). Derivation of cancer diagnostic and prognostic signatures from gene expression data. *Bioanalysis, 2*, 855-862.

Goto, K., Salm, S. N., Coetzee, S., Xiong, X., Burger, P. E., Shapiro, E., Lepor, H., Moscatelli, D., and Wilson, E. L. (2006). Proximal prostatic stem cells are programmed to regenerate a proximal-distal ductal axis. *Stem Cells, 24*, 1859-1868.

Gray-Schopfer, V., Wellbrock, C., and Marais, R. (2007). Melanoma biology and new targeted therapy. *Nature, 445*, 851-857.

Gu, G., Yuan, J., Wills, M., and Kasper, S. (2007). Prostate cancer cells with stem cell characteristics reconstitute the original human tumor in vivo. *Cancer Res, 67*, 4807-4815.

Gurel, B., Iwata, T., Koh, C. M., Yegnasubramanian, S., Nelson, W. G., and De Marzo, A. M. (2008). Molecular alterations in prostate cancer as diagnostic, prognostic, and therapeutic targets. *Adv Anat Pathol, 15*, 319-331.

Guzman-Ramirez, N., Voller, M., Wetterwald, A., Germann, M., Cross, N. A., Rentsch, C. A., Schalken, J., Thalmann, G. N., and Cecchini, M. G. (2009). In vitro propagation and characterization of neoplastic stem/progenitor-like cells from human prostate cancer tissue. *Prostate, 69*, 1683-1693.

Haraguchi, N., Utsunomiya, T., Inoue, H., Tanaka, F., Mimori, K., Barnard, G. F., and Mori, M. (2006). Characterization of a side population of cancer cells from human gastrointestinal system. *Stem Cells, 24*, 506-513.

Harnden, P., Shelley, M. D., Coles, B., Staffurth, J., and Mason, M. D. (2007). Should the Gleason grading system for prostate cancer be modified to account for high-grade tertiary components? A systematic review and meta-analysis. *Lancet Oncol, 8,* 411-419.

Hattab, E. M., Koch, M. O., Eble, J. N., Lin, H., and Cheng, L. (2006). Tertiary Gleason pattern 5 is a powerful predictor of biochemical relapse in patients with Gleason score 7 prostatic adenocarcinoma. *J Urol, 175,* 1695-1699; discussion 1699.

Hirschmann-Jax, C., Foster, A. E., Wulf, G. G., Nuchtern, J. G., Jax, T. W., Gobel, U., Goodell, M. A., and Brenner, M. K. (2004). A distinct "side population" of cells with high drug efflux capacity in human tumor cells. *Proc Natl Acad Sci U S A, 101,* 14228-14233.

Hope, K., and Bhatia, M. (2011). Clonal interrogation of stem cells. *Nat Methods, 8,* S36-40.

Hsieh, A. C., Small, E. J., and Ryan, C. J. (2007). Androgen-response elements in hormone-refractory prostate cancer: implications for treatment development. *Lancet Oncol, 8,* 933-939.

Hu, Y., and Smyth, G. K. (2009). ELDA: extreme limiting dilution analysis for comparing depleted and enriched populations in stem cell and other assays. *J Immunol Methods, 347,* 70-78.

Hudson, D. L. (2003). Prostate epithelial stem cell culture. *Cytotechnology, 41,* 189-196.

Hurt, E. M., Kawasaki, B. T., Klarmann, G. J., Thomas, S. B., and Farrar, W. L. (2008). CD44+ CD24(-) prostate cells are early cancer progenitor/stem cells that provide a model for patients with poor prognosis. *Br J Cancer, 98,* 756-765.

Ibrahim, S. F., Diercks, A. H., Petersen, T. W., and van den Engh, G. (2007). Kinetic analyses as a critical parameter in defining the side population (SP) phenotype. *Exp Cell Res, 313,* 1921-1926.

Isaacs, J. T., and Coffey, D. S. (1989). Etiology and disease process of benign prostatic hyperplasia. *Prostate Suppl, 2,* 33-50.

Jeter, C. R., Badeaux, M., Choy, G., Chandra, D., Patrawala, L., Liu, C., Calhoun-Davis, T., Zaehres, H., Daley, G. Q., and Tang, D. G. (2009). Functional evidence that the self-renewal gene NANOG regulates human tumor development. *Stem Cells, 27,* 993-1005.

Jeter, C. R., Liu, B., Liu, X., Chen, X., Liu, C., Calhoun-Davis, T., Repass, J., Zaehres, H., Shen, J. J., and Tang, D. G. (2011). NANOG promotes cancer stem cell characteristics and prostate cancer resistance to androgen deprivation. *Oncogene.*

Kai, K., D'Costa, S., Yoon, B. I., Brody, A. R., Sills, R. C., and Kim, Y. (2010). Characterization of side population cells in human malignant mesothelioma cell lines. *Lung Cancer, 70,* 146-151.

Kela, I., Harmelin, A., Waks, T., Orr-Urtreger, A., Domany, E., and Eshhar, Z. (2009). Interspecies comparison of prostate cancer gene-expression profiles reveals genes associated with aggressive tumors. *Prostate, 69,* 1034-1044.

Kendal, W. S., and Mai, K. T. (2010). Histological subtypes of prostatic cancer: a comparative survival study. *Can J Urol, 17,* 5355-5359.

Keysar, S. B., and Jimeno, A. (2010). More than markers: biological significance of cancer stem cell-defining molecules. *Mol Cancer Ther, 9,* 2450-2457.

Kimura, K., Bowen, C., Spiegel, S., and Gelmann, E. P. (1999). Tumor necrosis factor-alpha sensitizes prostate cancer cells to gamma-irradiation-induced apoptosis. *Cancer Res, 59,* 1606-1614.

Kimura, K., and Gelmann, E. P. (2000). Tumor necrosis factor-alpha and Fas activate complementary Fas-associated death domain-dependent pathways that enhance apoptosis induced by gamma-irradiation. *J Biol Chem, 275*, 8610-8617.

Kondo, T., Setoguchi, T., and Taga, T. (2004). Persistence of a small subpopulation of cancer stem-like cells in the C6 glioma cell line. *Proc Natl Acad Sci U S A, 101*, 781-786.

Kundu, S. D., Kim, I. Y., Yang, T., Doglio, L., Lang, S., Zhang, X., Buttyan, R., Kim, S. J., Chang, J., Cai, X., Wang, Z., and Lee, C. (2000). Absence of proximal duct apoptosis in the ventral prostate of transgenic mice carrying the C3(1)-TGF-beta type II dominant negative receptor. *Prostate, 43*, 118-124.

Ladanyi, M. (2008). Targeted therapy of cancer: new roles for pathologists. *Mod Pathol, 21 Suppl 2*, S1.

Lang, S. H., Frame, F. M., and Collins, A. T. (2009). Prostate cancer stem cells. *J Pathol, 217*, 299-306.

Lapointe, J., Li, C., Higgins, J. P., van de Rijn, M., Bair, E., Montgomery, K., Ferrari, M., Egevad, L., Rayford, W., Bergerheim, U., Ekman, P., DeMarzo, A. M., Tibshirani, R., Botstein, D., Brown, P. O., Brooks, J. D., and Pollack, J. R. (2004). Gene expression profiling identifies clinically relevant subtypes of prostate cancer. *Proc Natl Acad Sci U S A, 101*, 811-816.

Lawson, D. A., and Witte, O. N. (2007). Stem cells in prostate cancer initiation and progression. *J Clin Invest, 117*, 2044-2050.

Li, H., Chen, X., Calhoun-Davis, T., Claypool, K., and Tang, D. G. (2008). PC3 human prostate carcinoma cell holoclones contain self-renewing tumor-initiating cells. *Cancer Res, 68*, 1820-1825.

Li, H., Jiang, M., Honorio, S., Patrawala, L., Jeter, C. R., Calhoun-Davis, T., Hayward, S. W., and Tang, D. G. (2009). Methodologies in assaying prostate cancer stem cells. *Methods Mol Biol, 568*, 85-138.

Liang, Y., Russell, I., Walworth, C., and Chen, C. (2009). Gene expression in stem cells. *Crit Rev Eukaryot Gene Expr, 19*, 289-300.

Liu, A. Y., True, L. D., LaTray, L., Nelson, P. S., Ellis, W. J., Vessella, R. L., Lange, P. H., Hood, L., and van den Engh, G. (1997). Cell-cell interaction in prostate gene regulation and cytodifferentiation. *Proc Natl Acad Sci U S A, 94*, 10705-10710.

Lu, Q. L., Abel, P., Foster, C. S., and Lalani, E. N. (1996). bcl-2: role in epithelial differentiation and oncogenesis. *Hum Pathol, 27*, 102-110.

Maitland, N. J., and Collins, A. T. (2008). Prostate cancer stem cells: a new target for therapy. *J Clin Oncol, 26*, 2862-2870.

Malumbres, M., and Barbacid, M. (2009). Cell cycle, CDKs and cancer: a changing paradigm. *Nat Rev Cancer, 9*, 153-166.

Marhaba, R., Klingbeil, P., Nuebel, T., Nazarenko, I., Buechler, M. W., and Zoeller, M. (2008). CD44 and EpCAM: cancer-initiating cell markers. *Curr Mol Med, 8*, 784-804.

Mathew, G., Timm, E. A., Jr., Sotomayor, P., Godoy, A., Montecinos, V. P., Smith, G. J., and Huss, W. J. (2009). ABCG2-mediated DyeCycle Violet efflux defined side population in benign and malignant prostate. *Cell Cycle, 8*, 1053-1061.

McDavid, K., Lee, J., Fulton, J. P., Tonita, J., and Thompson, T. D. (2004). Prostate cancer incidence and mortality rates and trends in the United States and Canada. *Public Health Rep, 119*, 174-186.

Mellado, B., Codony, J., Ribal, M. J., Visa, L., and Gascon, P. (2009). Molecular biology of androgen-independent prostate cancer: the role of the androgen receptor pathway. *Clin Transl Oncol, 11,* 5-10.

Mendes, A., Scott, R. J., and Moscato, P. (2008). Microarrays--identifying molecular portraits for prostate tumors with different Gleason patterns. *Methods Mol Med, 141,* 131-151.

Miki, J. (2010). Investigations of prostate epithelial stem cells and prostate cancer stem cells. *Int J Urol, 17,* 139-147.

Miki, J., Furusato, B., Li, H., Gu, Y., Takahashi, H., Egawa, S., Sesterhenn, I. A., McLeod, D. G., Srivastava, S., and Rhim, J. S. (2007). Identification of putative stem cell markers, CD133 and CXCR4, in hTERT-immortalized primary nonmalignant and malignant tumor-derived human prostate epithelial cell lines and in prostate cancer specimens. *Cancer Res, 67,* 3153-3161.

Miller, S. J., Lavker, R. M., and Sun, T. T. (2005). Interpreting epithelial cancer biology in the context of stem cells: tumor properties and therapeutic implications. *Biochim Biophys Acta, 1756,* 25-52.

Mills, A. A., Qi, Y., and Bradley, A. (2002). Conditional inactivation of p63 by Cre-mediated excision. *Genesis, 32,* 138-141.

Mimeault, M., and Batra, S. K. (2006a). Concise review: recent advances on the significance of stem cells in tissue regeneration and cancer therapies. *Stem Cells, 24,* 2319-2345.

Mimeault, M., and Batra, S. K. (2006b). Recent advances on multiple tumorigenic cascades involved in prostatic cancer progression and targeting therapies. *Carcinogenesis, 27,* 1-22.

Mimeault, M., and Batra, S. K. (2007a). Functions of tumorigenic and migrating cancer progenitor cells in cancer progression and metastasis and their therapeutic implications. *Cancer Metastasis Rev, 26,* 203-214.

Mimeault, M., and Batra, S. K. (2007b). Interplay of distinct growth factors during epithelial mesenchymal transition of cancer progenitor cells and molecular targeting as novel cancer therapies. *Ann Oncol, 18,* 1605-1619.

Mimeault, M., Hauke, R., Mehta, P. P., and Batra, S. K. (2007). Recent advances in cancer stem/progenitor cell research: therapeutic implications for overcoming resistance to the most aggressive cancers. *J Cell Mol Med, 11,* 981-1011.

Mitsutake, N., Iwao, A., Nagai, K., Namba, H., Ohtsuru, A., Saenko, V., and Yamashita, S. (2007). Characterization of side population in thyroid cancer cell lines: cancer stem-like cells are enriched partly but not exclusively. *Endocrinology, 148,* 1797-1803.

Montpetit, M., Abrahams, P., Clark, A. F., and Tenniswood, M. (1988). Androgen-independent epithelial cells of the rat ventral prostate. *Prostate, 12,* 13-28.

Mousses, S., Wagner, U., Chen, Y., Kim, J. W., Bubendorf, L., Bittner, M., Pretlow, T., Elkahloun, A. G., Trepel, J. B., and Kallioniemi, O. P. (2001). Failure of hormone therapy in prostate cancer involves systematic restoration of androgen responsive genes and activation of rapamycin sensitive signaling. *Oncogene, 20,* 6718-6723.

Niu, Y., Chang, T. M., Yeh, S., Ma, W. L., Wang, Y. Z., and Chang, C. (2010). Differential androgen receptor signals in different cells explain why androgen-deprivation therapy of prostate cancer fails. *Oncogene, 29,* 3593-3604.

O'Brien, C. A., Kreso, A., and Jamieson, C. H. (2010). Cancer stem cells and self-renewal. *Clin Cancer Res, 16,* 3113-3120.

Oates, J. E., Grey, B. R., Addla, S. K., Samuel, J. D., Hart, C. A., Ramani, V. A., Brown, M. D., and Clarke, N. W. (2009). Hoechst 33342 side population identification is a conserved and unified mechanism in urological cancers. *Stem Cells Dev, 18*, 1515-1522.

Odedina, F. T., Akinremi, T. O., Chinegwundoh, F., Roberts, R., Yu, D., Reams, R. R., Freedman, M. L., Rivers, B., Green, B. L., and Kumar, N. (2009). Prostate cancer disparities in Black men of African descent: a comparative literature review of prostate cancer burden among Black men in the United States, Caribbean, United Kingdom, and West Africa. *Infect Agent Cancer, 4 Suppl 1*, S2.

Pan, C. C., Potter, S. R., Partin, A. W., and Epstein, J. I. (2000). The prognostic significance of tertiary Gleason patterns of higher grade in radical prostatectomy specimens: a proposal to modify the Gleason grading system. *Am J Surg Pathol, 24*, 563-569.

Pan, J., Zhang, Q., Wang, Y., and You, M. (2010). 26S proteasome activity is down-regulated in lung cancer stem-like cells propagated in vitro. *PLoS One, 5*, e13298.

Park, C. Y., Tseng, D., and Weissman, I. L. (2009). Cancer stem cell-directed therapies: recent data from the laboratory and clinic. *Mol Ther, 17*, 219-230.

Pascal, L. E., Oudes, A. J., Petersen, T. W., Goo, Y. A., Walashek, L. S., True, L. D., and Liu, A. Y. (2007). Molecular and cellular characterization of ABCG2 in the prostate. *BMC Urol, 7*, 6.

Patrawala, L., Calhoun, T., Schneider-Broussard, R., Li, H., Bhatia, B., Tang, S., Reilly, J. G., Chandra, D., Zhou, J., Claypool, K., Coghlan, L., and Tang, D. G. (2006). Highly purified CD44+ prostate cancer cells from xenograft human tumors are enriched in tumorigenic and metastatic progenitor cells. *Oncogene, 25*, 1696-1708.

Patrawala, L., Calhoun, T., Schneider-Broussard, R., Zhou, J., Claypool, K., and Tang, D. G. (2005). Side population is enriched in tumorigenic, stem-like cancer cells, whereas ABCG2+ and ABCG2- cancer cells are similarly tumorigenic. *Cancer Res, 65*, 6207-6219.

Patrawala, L., Calhoun-Davis, T., Schneider-Broussard, R., and Tang, D. G. (2007). Hierarchical organization of prostate cancer cells in xenograft tumors: the CD44+alpha2beta1+ cell population is enriched in tumor-initiating cells. *Cancer Res, 67*, 6796-6805.

Perou, C. M., Parker, J. S., Prat, A., Ellis, M. J., and Bernard, P. S. (2010). Clinical implementation of the intrinsic subtypes of breast cancer. *Lancet Oncol, 11*, 718-719; author reply 720-711.

Polyak, K., and Hahn, W. C. (2006). Roots and stems: stem cells in cancer. *Nat Med, 12*, 296-300.

Porter, E. H., and Berry, R. J. (1963). The Efficient Design of Transplantable Tumour Assays. *Br J Cancer, 17*, 583-595.

Quintana, E., Shackleton, M., Sabel, M. S., Fullen, D. R., Johnson, T. M., and Morrison, S. J. (2008). Efficient tumour formation by single human melanoma cells. *Nature, 456*, 593-598.

Rajan, P., Elliott, D. J., Robson, C. N., and Leung, H. Y. (2009). Alternative splicing and biological heterogeneity in prostate cancer. *Nat Rev Urol, 6*, 454-460.

Reya, T., Morrison, S. J., Clarke, M. F., and Weissman, I. L. (2001). Stem cells, cancer, and cancer stem cells. *Nature, 414*, 105-111.

Richardson, G. D., Robson, C. N., Lang, S. H., Neal, D. E., Maitland, N. J., and Collins, A. T. (2004). CD133, a novel marker for human prostatic epithelial stem cells. *J Cell Sci, 117*, 3539-3545.

Ringer, L., Sirajuddin, P., Yenugonda, V. M., Ghosh, A., Divito, K., Trabosh, V., Patel, Y., Brophy, A., Grindrod, S., Lisanti, M. P., Rosenthal, D., Brown, M. L., Avantaggiati, M. L., Rodriguez, O., and Albanese, C. (2010). VMY-1-103, a dansylated analog of purvalanol B, induces caspase-3-dependent apoptosis in LNCaP prostate cancer cells. *Cancer Biol Ther, 10,* 320-325.

Rizzo, S., Attard, G., and Hudson, D. L. (2005). Prostate epithelial stem cells. *Cell Prolif, 38,* 363-374.

Rosen, J. M., and Jordan, C. T. (2009). The increasing complexity of the cancer stem cell paradigm. *Science, 324,* 1670-1673.

Rubin, M. A. (2008). Targeted therapy of cancer: new roles for pathologists--prostate cancer. *Mod Pathol, 21 Suppl 2,* S44-55.

Rybak, A. P., He, L., Kapoor, A., Cutz, J. C., and Tang, D. (2011). Characterization of sphere-propagating cells with stem-like properties from DU145 prostate cancer cells. *Biochim Biophys Acta, 1813,* 683-694.

Saeki, N., Gu, J., Yoshida, T., and Wu, X. (2010). Prostate stem cell antigen: a Jekyll and Hyde molecule? *Clin Cancer Res, 16,* 3533-3538.

Sajid, S., Mohile, S. G., Szmulewitz, R., Posadas, E., and Dale, W. (2011). Individualized decision-making for older men with prostate cancer: balancing cancer control with treatment consequences across the clinical spectrum. *Semin Oncol, 38,* 309-325.

Schalken, J. A. (2005). Validation of molecular targets in prostate cancer. *BJU Int, 96 Suppl 2,* 23-29.

Schinkel, A. H., Mayer, U., Wagenaar, E., Mol, C. A., van Deemter, L., Smit, J. J., van der Valk, M. A., Voordouw, A. C., Spits, H., van Tellingen, O., Zijlmans, J. M., Fibbe, W. E., and Borst, P. (1997). Normal viability and altered pharmacokinetics in mice lacking mdr1-type (drug-transporting) P-glycoproteins. *Proc Natl Acad Sci U S A, 94,* 4028-4033.

Schroeder, T. (2011). Long-term single-cell imaging of mammalian stem cells. *Nat Methods, 8,* S30-35.

Sedjo, R. L., Byers, T., Barrera, E., Jr., Cohen, C., Fontham, E. T., Newman, L. A., Runowicz, C. D., Thorson, A. G., Thun, M. J., Ward, E., Wender, R. C., and Eyre, H. J. (2007). A midpoint assessment of the American Cancer Society challenge goal to decrease cancer incidence by 25% between 1992 and 2015. *CA Cancer J Clin, 57,* 326-340.

Sharad, S., Srivastava, A., Ravulapalli, S., Parker, P., Chen, Y., Li, H., Petrovics, G., and Dobi, A. (2011). Prostate cancer gene expression signature of patients with high body mass index. *Prostate Cancer Prostatic Dis, 14,* 22-29.

Sharifi, N., Kawasaki, B. T., Hurt, E. M., and Farrar, W. L. (2006). Stem cells in prostate cancer: resolving the castrate-resistant conundrum and implications for hormonal therapy. *Cancer Biol Ther, 5,* 901-906.

Signoretti, S., Waltregny, D., Dilks, J., Isaac, B., Lin, D., Garraway, L., Yang, A., Montironi, R., McKeon, F., and Loda, M. (2000). p63 is a prostate basal cell marker and is required for prostate development. *Am J Pathol, 157,* 1769-1775.

Sim, H. G., Telesca, D., Culp, S. H., Ellis, W. J., Lange, P. H., True, L. D., and Lin, D. W. (2008). Tertiary Gleason pattern 5 in Gleason 7 prostate cancer predicts pathological stage and biochemical recurrence. *J Urol, 179,* 1775-1779.

Simon, R., and Maitournam, A. (2004). Evaluating the efficiency of targeted designs for randomized clinical trials. *Clin Cancer Res, 10,* 6759-6763.

Singh, D., Febbo, P. G., Ross, K., Jackson, D. G., Manola, J., Ladd, C., Tamayo, P., Renshaw, A. A., D'Amico, A. V., Richie, J. P., Lander, E. S., Loda, M., Kantoff, P. W., Golub, T. R., and Sellers, W. R. (2002). Gene expression correlates of clinical prostate cancer behavior. *Cancer Cell, 1*, 203-209.

Sobel, R. E., and Sadar, M. D. (2005a). Cell lines used in prostate cancer research: a compendium of old and new lines--part 1. *J Urol, 173*, 342-359.

Sobel, R. E., and Sadar, M. D. (2005b). Cell lines used in prostate cancer research: a compendium of old and new lines--part 2. *J Urol, 173*, 360-372.

Sparreboom, A., and Verweij, J. (2009). Advances in cancer therapeutics. *Clin Pharmacol Ther, 85*, 113-117.

Szotek, P. P., Pieretti-Vanmarcke, R., Masiakos, P. T., Dinulescu, D. M., Connolly, D., Foster, R., Dombkowski, D., Preffer, F., Maclaughlin, D. T., and Donahoe, P. K. (2006). Ovarian cancer side population defines cells with stem cell-like characteristics and Mullerian Inhibiting Substance responsiveness. *Proc Natl Acad Sci U S A, 103*, 11154-11159.

Talcott, J. A., Spain, P., Clark, J. A., Carpenter, W. R., Do, Y. K., Hamilton, R. J., Galanko, J. A., Jackman, A., and Godley, P. A. (2007). Hidden barriers between knowledge and behavior: the North Carolina prostate cancer screening and treatment experience. *Cancer, 109*, 1599-1606.

Tang, D. G., Patrawala, L., Calhoun, T., Bhatia, B., Choy, G., Schneider-Broussard, R., and Jeter, C. (2007). Prostate cancer stem/progenitor cells: identification, characterization, and implications. *Mol Carcinog, 46*, 1-14.

Tokar, E. J., Ancrile, B. B., Cunha, G. R., and Webber, M. M. (2005). Stem/progenitor and intermediate cell types and the origin of human prostate cancer. *Differentiation, 73*, 463-473.

Tropepe, V., Sibilia, M., Ciruna, B. G., Rossant, J., Wagner, E. F., and van der Kooy, D. (1999). Distinct neural stem cells proliferate in response to EGF and FGF in the developing mouse telencephalon. *Dev Biol, 208*, 166-188.

Tsujimura, A., Koikawa, Y., Salm, S., Takao, T., Coetzee, S., Moscatelli, D., Shapiro, E., Lepor, H., Sun, T. T., and Wilson, E. L. (2002). Proximal location of mouse prostate epithelial stem cells: a model of prostatic homeostasis. *J Cell Biol, 157*, 1257-1265.

van Leenders, G. J., Aalders, T. W., Hulsbergen-van de Kaa, C. A., Ruiter, D. J., and Schalken, J. A. (2001). Expression of basal cell keratins in human prostate cancer metastases and cell lines. *J Pathol, 195*, 563-570.

Vander Griend, D. J., Karthaus, W. L., Dalrymple, S., Meeker, A., DeMarzo, A. M., and Isaacs, J. T. (2008). The role of CD133 in normal human prostate stem cells and malignant cancer-initiating cells. *Cancer Res, 68*, 9703-9711.

Vermeulen, L., Sprick, M. R., Kemper, K., Stassi, G., and Medema, J. P. (2008). Cancer stem cells--old concepts, new insights. *Cell Death Differ, 15*, 947-958.

Wang, J. C. (2007). Evaluating therapeutic efficacy against cancer stem cells: new challenges posed by a new paradigm. *Cell Stem Cell, 1*, 497-501.

Wang, Y., Tetko, I. V., Hall, M. A., Frank, E., Facius, A., Mayer, K. F., and Mewes, H. W. (2005). Gene selection from microarray data for cancer classification--a machine learning approach. *Comput Biol Chem, 29*, 37-46.

Webber, M. M., Bello, D., and Quader, S. (1997a). Immortalized and tumorigenic adult human prostatic epithelial cell lines: characteristics and applications Part 2. Tumorigenic cell lines. *Prostate, 30*, 58-64.

Webber, M. M., Bello, D., and Quader, S. (1997b). Immortalized and tumorigenic adult human prostatic epithelial cell lines: characteristics and applications. Part 3. Oncogenes, suppressor genes, and applications. *Prostate, 30,* 136-142.

Wegiel, B., Evans, S., Hellsten, R., Otterbein, L. E., Bjartell, A., and Persson, J. L. (2010). Molecular pathways in the progression of hormone-independent and metastatic prostate cancer. *Curr Cancer Drug Targets, 10,* 392-401.

Weissman, I. L., Anderson, D. J., and Gage, F. (2001). Stem and progenitor cells: origins, phenotypes, lineage commitments, and transdifferentiations. *Annu Rev Cell Dev Biol, 17,* 387-403.

Witte, J. S. (2009). Prostate cancer genomics: towards a new understanding. *Nat Rev Genet, 10,* 77-82.

Woodward, W. A., and Sulman, E. P. (2008). Cancer stem cells: markers or biomarkers? *Cancer Metastasis Rev, 27,* 459-470.

Yamazaki, J., Mizukami, T., Takizawa, K., Kuramitsu, M., Momose, H., Masumi, A., Ami, Y., Hasegawa, H., Hall, W. W., Tsujimoto, H., Hamaguchi, I., and Yamaguchi, K. (2009). Identification of cancer stem cells in a Tax-transgenic (Tax-Tg) mouse model of adult T-cell leukemia/lymphoma. *Blood, 114,* 2709-2720.

Yang, S. Y., Adelstein, J., and Kassis, A. I. (2010). Putative molecular signatures for the imaging of prostate cancer. *Expert Rev Mol Diagn, 10,* 65-74.

Zhang, K., and Waxman, D. J. (2010). PC3 prostate tumor-initiating cells with molecular profile FAM65Bhigh/MFI2low/LEF1low increase tumor angiogenesis. *Mol Cancer, 9,* 319.

Zhang, L., Valdez, J. M., Zhang, B., Wei, L., Chang, J., and Xin, L. (2011). ROCK inhibitor Y-27632 suppresses dissociation-induced apoptosis of murine prostate stem/progenitor cells and increases their cloning efficiency. *PLoS One, 6,* e18271.

Zhou, S., Morris, J. J., Barnes, Y., Lan, L., Schuetz, J. D., and Sorrentino, B. P. (2002). Bcrp1 gene expression is required for normal numbers of side population stem cells in mice, and confers relative protection to mitoxantrone in hematopoietic cells in vivo. *Proc Natl Acad Sci U S A, 99,* 12339-12344.

Zhou, S., Schuetz, J. D., Bunting, K. D., Colapietro, A. M., Sampath, J., Morris, J. J., Lagutina, I., Grosveld, G. C., Osawa, M., Nakauchi, H., and Sorrentino, B. P. (2001). The ABC transporter Bcrp1/ABCG2 is expressed in a wide variety of stem cells and is a molecular determinant of the side-population phenotype. *Nat Med, 7,* 1028-1034.

Zieger, K. (2008). High throughput molecular diagnostics in bladder cancer - on the brink of clinical utility. *Mol Oncol, 1,* 384-394.

Zoller, M. (2011). CD44: can a cancer-initiating cell profit from an abundantly expressed molecule? *Nat Rev Cancer, 11,* 254-267.

Permissions

The contributors of this book come from diverse backgrounds, making this book a truly international effort. This book will bring forth new frontiers with its revolutionizing research information and detailed analysis of the nascent developments around the world.

We would like to thank Philippe E. Spiess, for lending his expertise to make the book truly unique. He has played a crucial role in the development of this book. Without his invaluable contribution this book wouldn't have been possible. He has made vital efforts to compile up to date information on the varied aspects of this subject to make this book a valuable addition to the collection of many professionals and students.

This book was conceptualized with the vision of imparting up-to-date information and advanced data in this field. To ensure the same, a matchless editorial board was set up. Every individual on the board went through rigorous rounds of assessment to prove their worth. After which they invested a large part of their time researching and compiling the most relevant data for our readers. Conferences and sessions were held from time to time between the editorial board and the contributing authors to present the data in the most comprehensible form. The editorial team has worked tirelessly to provide valuable and valid information to help people across the globe.

Every chapter published in this book has been scrutinized by our experts. Their significance has been extensively debated. The topics covered herein carry significant findings which will fuel the growth of the discipline. They may even be implemented as practical applications or may be referred to as a beginning point for another development. Chapters in this book were first published by InTech; hereby published with permission under the Creative Commons Attribution License or equivalent.

The editorial board has been involved in producing this book since its inception. They have spent rigorous hours researching and exploring the diverse topics which have resulted in the successful publishing of this book. They have passed on their knowledge of decades through this book. To expedite this challenging task, the publisher supported the team at every step. A small team of assistant editors was also appointed to further simplify the editing procedure and attain best results for the readers.

Our editorial team has been hand-picked from every corner of the world. Their multi-ethnicity adds dynamic inputs to the discussions which result in innovative outcomes. These outcomes are then further discussed with the researchers and contributors who give their valuable feedback and opinion regarding the same. The feedback is then collaborated with the researches and they are edited in a comprehensive manner to aid the understanding of the subject.

Apart from the editorial board, the designing team has also invested a significant amount of their time in understanding the subject and creating the most relevant covers. They scrutinized every image to scout for the most suitable representation of the subject and create an appropriate cover for the book.

The publishing team has been involved in this book since its early stages. They were actively engaged in every process, be it collecting the data, connecting with the contributors or procuring relevant information. The team has been an ardent support to the editorial, designing and production team. Their endless efforts to recruit the best for this project, has resulted in the accomplishment of this book. They are a veteran in the field of academics and their pool of knowledge is as vast as their experience in printing. Their expertise and guidance has proved useful at every step. Their uncompromising quality standards have made this book an exceptional effort. Their encouragement from time to time has been an inspiration for everyone.

The publisher and the editorial board hope that this book will prove to be a valuable piece of knowledge for researchers, students, practitioners and scholars across the globe.

List of Contributors

Jacqueline R. Ha, Yu Hao D. Huang and Sujata Persad
University of Alberta, Department of Pediatrics, Canada

Santiago Vilar-González and Alberto Pérez-Rozos
Instituto de Medicina Oncológica y Molecular de Asturias.IMOMA, Spain

Yin-Quan Tang and Shamala Devi Sekaran
University of Malaya, Malaysia

Tsutomu Nishiyama
Division of Urology, Department of Regenerative and Transplant Medicine, Niigata University Graduate School of Medical and Dental Sciences, Niigata, Japan

Mustafa Ozen
Department of Medical Genetics Istanbul University Cerrahpasa Medical School, Istanbul, Turkey
Bezmialem Vakif University, Istanbul, Turkey
Department of Pathology & Immunology Baylor College of Medicine, Houston, TX, USA

Serhat Sevli
Department of Medical Genetics Istanbul University Cerrahpasa Medical School, Istanbul, Turkey

Sophia L. Maund and Scott D. Cramer
Wake Forest University School of Medicine, University of Colorado, DenverAnschutz Medical Campus, USA

Jorge A. R. Salvador
Laboratório de Química Farmacêutica, Faculdade de Farmácia da, Universidade de Coimbra Pólo das Ciências da Saúde Azinhaga de Santa Comba, Coimbra, Portugal
Centro de Neurociências e Biologia Celular, Universidade de Coimbra, Coimbra, Portugal

Vânia M. Moreira
Laboratório de Química Farmacêutica, Faculdade de Farmácia da Universidade de Coimbra Pólo das Ciências da Saúde Azinhaga de Santa Comba, Coimbra, Portugal
Centro de Química de Coimbra, Faculdade de Ciências e Tecnologia da Universidade de Coimbra Rua Larga, Coimbra, Portugal

Wong Pooi-Fong
Department of Pharmacology, Faculty of Medicine, University of Malaya, Malaysia

AbuBakar Sazaly
Department of Medical Microbiology, Faculty of Medicine, University of Malaya, Malaysia

Luis A. Espinoza
Department of Biochemistry and Molecular & Cell Biology, USA

Christopher Albanese
Department of Oncology, USA
Department of Pathology Georgetown University, NW Washington, DC, USA

Olga C. Rodriguez
Department of Oncology, USA